AF902265

# CONTEMPORARY TOPICS OF PNEUMONIA

Edited by **Zissis C. Chroneos**

**Contemporary Topics of Pneumonia**
http://dx.doi.org/10.5772/66055
Edited by Zissis C. Chroneos

**Contributors**

Valério Monteiro-Neto, Lídio Lima-Neto, Afonso Abreu, Cinara Regina Monteiro, Salim Surani, Mauricio Rodriguez, Patricia Silveyra, Nathalie Fuentes, Lidys Rivera, Mihaela Ileana Ionescu, Akira Takeda, Anurag Payasi, Gazalla Ayub, Manu Chaudhary, Sameera M. Al Johani, Javed Akhter, Jean-Marie Ntumba Kayembe, Harry César Kayembe Ntumba

**Published by InTech**
Janeza Trdine 9, 51000 Rijeka, Croatia

**© The Editor(s) and the Author(s) 2017**
The moral rights of the editor(s) and the author(s) have been asserted.
All rights to the book as a whole are reserved by InTech. The book as a whole (compilation) cannot be reproduced, distributed or used for commercial or non-commercial purposes without InTech's written permission. Enquiries concerning the use of the book should be directed to InTech's rights and permissions department (permissions@intechopen.com).
Violations are liable to prosecution under the governing Copyright Law.

Individual chapters of this publication are distributed under the terms of the Creative Commons Attribution 3.0 Unported License which permits commercial use, distribution and reproduction of the individual chapters, provided the original author(s) and source publication are appropriately acknowledged. More details and guidelines concerning content reuse and adaptation can be found at http://www.intechopen.com/copyright-policy.html.

**Notice**

Statements and opinions expressed in the chapters are these of the individual contributors and not necessarily those of the editors or publisher. No responsibility is accepted for the accuracy of information contained in the published chapters. The publisher assumes no responsibility for any damage or injury to persons or property arising out of the use of any materials, instructions, methods or ideas contained in the book.

**Publishing Process Manager** Romina Rovan
**Technical Editor** SPi Global
**Cover** InTech Design team

First published December, 2017
Printed in Croatia
Legal deposit, Croatia: National and University Library in Zagreb

Additional hard copies can be obtained from orders@intechopen.com

Contemporary Topics of Pneumonia, Edited by Zissis C. Chroneos
p. cm.
Print ISBN 978-953-51-3707-8
Online ISBN 978-953-51-3708-5

# We are IntechOpen, the world's leading publisher of Open Access books

# Built by scientists, for scientists

**4,200+**
Open access books available

**116,000+**
International authors and editors

**125M+**
Downloads

**151**
Countries delivered to

Our authors are among the

**Top 1%**
most cited scientists

**12.2%**
Contributors from top 500 universities

CLARIVATE ANALYTICS BOOK CITATION INDEX INDEXED

WEB OF SCIENCE™

Selection of our books indexed in the Book Citation Index in Web of Science™ Core Collection (BKCI)

Interested in publishing with us?
Contact book.department@intechopen.com

Numbers displayed above are based on latest data collected.
For more information visit www.intechopen.com

For EU product safety concerns:
IN TECH d.o.o., Prolaz Marije Krucifikse Kozulić 3, 51000 Rijeka, Croatia,
info@intechopen.com or visit our website at intechopen.com.

# Meet the editor

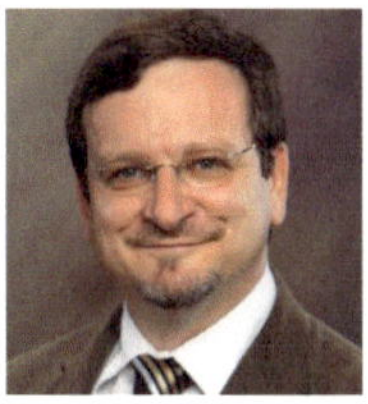

After completing doctoral studies in Chemistry at the University of South Carolina, Zissis C. Chroneos pursued postdoctoral studies at Vanderbilt University College of Medicine and Cincinnati Children's Medical Center to elucidate the mechanisms by which surfactant proteins modulate host defense and inflammation in the lung. These studies led to his discovery of the surfactant protein A receptor SP-R210 and its identification as cell-surface isoforms of Myosin 18A that modulate innate receptor dynamics and polarization in macrophages. He is currently an associate professor of Pediatrics, Microbiology and Immunology at Pennsylvania State University College of Medicine investigating host factors and SP-R210–mediated mechanisms that modulate surfactant metabolism, macrophage differentiation, and pathogenesis of viral and bacterial infections in the lung.

# Contents

**Preface IX**

**Section 1 Intersection of Environment and Pneumonia 1**

Chapter 1 **Understanding the Intersection of Environmental Pollution, Pneumonia, and Inflammation: Does Gender Play a Role? 3**
Patricia Silveyra, Nathalie Fuentes and Lidys Rivera

Chapter 2 **Pneumonia: A Challenging Health Concern with the Climate Change 35**
Jean-Marie Ntumba Kayembe and Harry-César Ntumba Kayembe

**Section 2 Drug-Resistant Pneumonia 51**

Chapter 3 **The Emerging Problems of Carbapenem-Resistant Gram-Negative Bacillary Pneumonia 53**
Mihaela Ileana Ionescu

Chapter 4 **Multidrug-Resistant Gram-Negative Pneumonia and Infection in Intensive Care Unit 77**
Mauricio Rodriguez and Salim R. Surani

Chapter 5 **Microbiology of Ventilator-Associated Pneumonia 105**
Valério Monteiro-Neto, Lídio G. Lima-Neto, Afonso G. Abreu and Cinara Regina A. V. Monteiro

Chapter 6 **Advancing in the Direction of Right Solutions: Treating Multidrug-Resistant Pneumonia 125**
Manu Chaudhary, Gazalla Ayub and Anurag Payasi

**Section 3 Idiopathic and Viral Etiologies of Pneumonia 143**

Chapter 7 **Interstitial Pneumonia Associated with Connective Tissue Disease: An Overview and an Insight 145**
Akira Takeda and Yoshiki Ishii

Chapter 8 **Pneumonia of Viral Etiologies 191**
Al Johani Sameera and Akhter Javed

# Preface

Pneumonia is a life-threatening inflammation of the air sacs, small airways, and surrounding connective tissue. Pneumonia is caused by bacterial and viral organisms or by immune system–related interstitial disease of idiopathic origin. Infectious pneumonia afflicts millions of people worldwide across age groups. The highest mortality rates occur in children under 5 years of age, the elderly, and critically ill patients in hospitals. Environmental and socioeconomic factors and access to health care underlie differences in morbidity and mortality rates from pneumonia in different parts of the world. The increasing incidence of antibiotic resistance and limitations in existing therapies are major public health concerns in the clinical management of pneumonias.

The book *Contemporary Topics of Pneumonia* consists of eight chapters that combine systematic reviews and investigations; global and clinical perspectives on bacterial, viral, and interstitial pneumonias; drug resistance; and natural remedies to eradicate carbapenem-resistant Enterobacteriaceae. In Section I, chapters examine the influence of environmental pollution, gender and hormonal influences, and the prospect of climate change on epidemiology and susceptibility to infectious and inflammatory lung disease. In Section II, chapters cover clinical, epidemiologic, diagnostic, bacteriological, multidrug resistance, and ecological aspects of community and health care–associated bacterial infections that devastate the efforts of medical practitioners in critical care facilities. Two chapters in Section II appraise the increasing prevalence, acquisition, and ecological aspects of carbapenem resistance in the microbiome and evaluate the use of essential oils and nonantibiotic adjuvant chemotherapy as complementary approaches for the treatment of drug-resistant infection. Section III includes a comprehensive chapter on interstitial pneumonia as an autoimmune connective tissue disease and a chapter that reviews viral etiologies of pneumonia.

Written by clinical and research scientists who are directly involved in patient care and research on pneumonia, the compilation of topics in this book brings together reference, educational, and research materials that meet the investigational interests of specialists, researchers, and students and informational needs of patients and general public. I would like to thank the authors for their contributions and diligent efforts in preparing the chapters and Romina Rovan at InTechOpen for facilitating the editorial process.

**Zissis C. Chroneos, PhD**
Associate Professor of Pediatrics, Microbiology and Immunology,
Pennsylvania State University College of Medicine, USA

Section 1

# Intersection of Environment and Pneumonia

Chapter 1

# Understanding the Intersection of Environmental Pollution, Pneumonia, and Inflammation: Does Gender Play a Role?

Patricia Silveyra, Nathalie Fuentes and Lidys Rivera

Additional information is available at the end of the chapter

http://dx.doi.org/10.5772/intechopen.69627

**Abstract**

Accumulating evidence indicates that exposure to air pollution is associated with increased mortality from respiratory disease. Exposure to ambient pollutants, such as ozone, particulate matter, sulfur dioxide, nitrogen dioxide, and other agents has been associated with decrease in lung function and immunity, and with increased rates of hospitalization for lung disease, including pneumonia. Furthermore, sex differences in frequency and severity of pulmonary disease and infection have been reported, suggesting a role of sex hormones in mediating these differences. Pneumonia, which is commonly caused by bacterial infection and subsequent lung inflammation leading to hospitalization and death, occurs at different rates in men and women. In this context, male and female hormones can have direct effects on the immunity system by binding to receptors in immune cells, and these responses can be modulated by environmental exposures. This chapter summarizes clinical, animal, and epidemiological studies linking exposure to air pollution and pneumonia in both males and females. Understanding sex-specific mechanisms in pneumonia pathogenesis and environmental responses can help in the development of more effective therapeutics and treatment options to reduce negative health outcomes in men and women.

**Keywords:** sex differences, ozone, particulate matter, air pollution, sex hormones, community-acquired pneumonia, environmental exposures

## 1. Introduction

Regulation of the lung inflammatory response is critical to the successful resolution of pneumonia. Exposure to air pollutants has been linked to negative lung health outcomes, and both male

INTECH
open science | open minds

© 2017 The Author(s). Licensee InTech. This chapter is distributed under the terms of the Creative Commons Attribution License (http://creativecommons.org/licenses/by/3.0), which permits unrestricted use, distribution, and reproduction in any medium, provided the original work is properly cited.

and female sex hormones have been shown to control the lung immune response [1, 2]. This chapter combines evidence of three areas: pneumonia infection, air pollution, and hormonal control of sex-specific immune responses. We will discuss common pathogens responsible for pneumonia and associations with environmental exposures, and lessons learned from animal models of infection and exposure to various air pollutants. Together, this information could help better explain the differences observed in susceptibility to pneumonia between men and women, and help in the development of better treatment options for male and female patients.

## 2. Pneumonia in the clinic: classification, comorbidities, and pathogenesis

### 2.1. Classification

Pneumonia is classified according to the patient population affected as: (a) community-acquired pneumonia (CAP), (b) hospital-acquired pneumonia (HAP), (c) ventilator-associated pneumonia (VAP), and (d) nursing home-associated pneumonia (NHAP) [3]. Of these classifications, CAP is the most frequently found, predominantly affecting young children because of the immaturity of their immune system, and older adults due to their immunosenescence and comorbidities of aging [4].

Community-acquired pneumonia is a common infection that affects the lower respiratory tract and it is acquired outside of the hospital or within 48 h of admission, and it is primarily associated with the presence of a new infiltrate on the chest radiograph [2, 3]. Community-acquired pneumonia is often caused by pathogens of the not multidrug-resistant type (MDR), which is an important distinction from the other types of pneumonia. However, some patients with recent antibiotic therapy could also present infection with MDR organisms [3, 5]. Furthermore, most patients are presented with common clinical symptoms, such as fever, cough, pleuritic chest pain, and breathing difficulty, although these symptoms can be absent in elderly patients. Elderly patients, on the other hand, can also have delirium, abdominal pain, or acute cardiac disorders as part of their clinical presentation [4].

### 2.2. Incidence and risk factors

Despite newer antimicrobial therapy and treatment guidelines, CAP continues to be a significant problem associated with high mortality, morbidity, and cost. In the United States alone, CAP affects approximately 5.6 million patients annually, and it is the sixth cause of death in individuals older than 65 years of age [6, 7]. According to the National Vital Statistics Report of the Centers for Disease Control, pneumonia and influenza were listed as the eighth leading causes of death in the United States in 2011 [8]. As a result, the economic burden of CAP remains significantly high, at more than $17 billion dollars annually in the United States [9].

Several risk factors have been associated with CAP, including age and comorbid diseases [10]. Furthermore, exposure to air pollution and circulating levels of sex hormones also seem to play an important role in the predisposition of some respiratory infections [11, 12]. Although some studies in animals have shown that females are more resistant than males to some bacterial infections [13, 14], others have shown that these patterns are reversed if animals are pre-exposed to environmental pollutants, such as ozone [15–20]. Incidentally, some clinical studies have reported that men are more susceptible to developing CAP and receive more intensive care than women, and show increased risk to die from pneumonia [21]. Moreover, exposure to air pollution has been associated with an increased risk for respiratory disorders due to its negative effects on lung function and immunity [22]. In this regard, long-term exposures to air pollutants, such as ozone, nitric oxide, and particulate matter in older adults have been linked with increased hospitalization rates for CAP [11, 21, 23, 24]. In addition, exposure to diverse environmental agents has been linked to negative lung health outcomes in children and adults (**Table 1**). The mechanisms associated with these clinical outcomes will be discussed in the following sections.

| **Children** | | | **Adults** | | |
|---|---|---|---|---|---|
| Environmental exposure | Health outcome | Sex differences | Environmental exposure | Health outcome | Sex differences |
| Secondhand smoke | Pneumonia (incidence and severity) | N/A | Particulate matter ($PM_{10}$) | Chronic laryngitis | Higher in males |
| Air pollution | Pneumonia, Bronchitis | N/A | House biomass fuel use | Various communicable respiratory disease | Higher in women |
| Household air quality | Pneumonia | Higher in males | Secondhand smoke | Community-acquired pneumonia (elderly) | N/A |
| Air pollution | Outpatient visits for respiratory disease | Higher in females | Air pollution | Outpatient visits for respiratory disease | Higher in males |
| Solid fuel | Pneummonia, Mortality | Higher in females | Air pollution ($PM_{2.5}$, $SO_2$, $NO_2$) | Pneumonia | Higher in males (smokers) Higher in females (never smokers) |
| Environmental tobacco smoking | Pneumonia Chronic bronchitis | N/A | UV radiation, sulfur oxides | Invasive pneumococcal disease | N/A |
| Indoor air pollution (solid fuel cooking, keeping large animals) | Severe pneumonia | N/A | Tobacco smoke | Sinusitis, middle ear infections | Flight attendants |
| $SO_2$, total suspended particles | Pneumonia | N/A | | | |

**Table 1.** Effects of the environment on respiratory tract health in children and adults and observed sex differences.

### 2.3. Pathogenesis of pneumonia

Pneumonia is characterized by a severe inflammation of the peripheral alveolar compartment and abnormal filling with fluid consolidation and exudation caused by infection with viruses, bacteria, and/or pathogen-related molecules. The most common cause of CAP is bacterial infection, but the disease can also be triggered by viral agents (**Table 2**) [6, 25, 26]. Pneumonia-causing microorganisms are classified as typical, atypical (zoonotic and non-zoonotic), Gram-negative, and viruses. *Streptococcus pneumoniae* is the most common cause of pneumonia in adults in the United States. Nevertheless, other typical organisms are also included with some important associations. For example, *Haemophilus influenzae* is found particularly in patients who smoke or have chronic obstructive pulmonary disease (COPD), *Moraxella catarrhalis* and *Staphylococcus aureus* are often found in pneumonia following influenza infection, and in the form of methicillin-resistant *Staphylococcus aureus* (MRSA) [6]. In addition, atypical pneumonia could be produced by zoonotic pathogens, such as *Chlamydia psittaci, Francisella tularensis, Coxiella burnetii* (also known as Q fever) and by non-zoonotic pathogens like *Chlamydia pneumoniae, Mycoplasma pneumoniae,* and *Legionella pneumophila*. Furthermore, patients with these atypical infections have a more frequent presentation of a mild or ambulatory CAP, and also present extrapulmonary manifestations not found in CAP caused by typical pathogens [26]. *S. pneumoniae* colonize the human nasopharynx and can be transmitted from animals in captivity to humans [27]. Differences in strains of *S. pneumoniae* are responsible for differences in virulence and the presence of antigens [27].

Community-acquired pneumonia can also be caused by a variety of viral infections. The most frequent viruses associated with CAP are influenza A and B, and parainfluenza. Less frequently, respiratory syncytial virus (RSV), severe acute respiratory syndrome virus, varicella, hantavirus, and adenovirus, are also responsible for CAP. Furthermore, most of these viral infections present in combination with multiple bacterial pathogens including *S. pneumoniae* and *C. pneumoniae*. However, patients with congestive heart failure (CHF) are at increased risk of acquiring CAP caused by pure viral infections [6, 25]. Gram-negative bacteria (*Pseudomonas aeruginosa, Klebsiella pneumoniae, Escherichia coli, Enterobacter* spp., and *Serratia* spp.) are common in patients with CAP who have had recent contact with health care environments, such as previous hospitalization, probable aspiration, antimicrobial treatment, and pulmonary comorbidities [28]. **Table 2** summarizes common associations of pathogens with clinical factors, history, and environmental factors in patients with CAP [4–6, 25, 26].

| |
|---|
| **Typical** |
| *Streptococcus pneumoniae, Haemophilus influenza, Moraxella catarrhalis, Staphylococcus aureus* |
| **Atypical** |
| **Zoonotic**: *Chlamydia psittaci, Francisella tularensis, Coxiella burnetii* |
| **Non-zoonotic**: *Mycoplasma pneumoniae, Chlamydophila pneumoniae,* and *Legionella pneumophila* |
| **Gram-negative** |
| *Pseudomonas aeruginosa, Klebsiella pneumoniae, Escherichia coli, Enterobacter* spp., *Serratia* spp., *Proteus* spp. |
| **Viruses** |
| *Parainfluenza virus, Influenza virus A* and *B* |
| **Less frequently**: Respiratory syncytial virus (RSV), severe acute respiratory syndrome virus, varicella, hantavirus, and adenovirus |

**Table 2.** Common pathogens in community-acquired pneumonia.

The main mechanism of infection in CAP is micro-aspiration from a previously colonized oropharynx, but inhalation of suspended aerosolized microorganism is the route of infection for viruses and bacterial agents, such as *L. pneumophila* and *Mycobacterium tuberculosis*. However, other factors related to the host immune response, the virulence of the infecting organism, and the size of the inoculum also define the development of the disease [29]. Furthermore, the presence of medical comorbidities, such as chronic respiratory and cardiovascular diseases, cerebrovascular diseases, Parkinson's disease, epilepsy, dementia, dysphagia, HIV infection, and chronic renal, or liver disease can also lead to a defective cough, abnormal mucociliary clearance, and impaired humoral and local immunity that can influence the pathogenesis of pneumonia [30–32]. In addition, lifestyle and social factors including smoking and alcohol consumption, contact with pets, households with more than 10 people, interventions of upper airways, and poor dental health have also been associated with an increased predisposition for the development of CAP [10] (**Table 3**). Smoking affects the respiratory epithelium and the clearance of bacteria from the respiratory tract, increasing the susceptibility to respiratory infections, even in passive smokers [33–35]. Alcoholism has also been linked to alterations in innate and adaptive immunity [36]. Moreover, nutritional deficiencies appear to affect mechanisms of innate immunity, and are associated with the increased risk of CAP development and mortality [37–39].

### 2.4. Gender differences in community-acquired pneumonia

Increasing evidence suggests that sex hormones play a role in the expression of genes involved in the regulation of the immune system, which in turn can impact the individual susceptibility to infectious agents, and incidence of autoimmune diseases [13, 14]. In this regard, patients suffering from systemic autoimmune diseases (including systemic lupus erythematosus, rheumatoid arthritis, systemic sclerosis, polymyositis/dermatomyositis, Sjögren's syndrome, and others) are at increased risk of developing pulmonary infection, aspiration pneumonia, and bronchiolitis obliterans organizing pneumonia [40]. Furthermore, studies have shown that androgens in males can affect the immune system leading to an increased susceptibility to infection and disease caused by parasites, fungi, bacteria, and viruses. On the contrary, estrogen leads to an increase of cell-mediated and humoral immune responses in females, making them more resistant to some infectious diseases [41]. However, the role of estrogen in modulating the immune response remains controversial [42, 43].

Remarkably, physiological changes in male and female sex hormone levels (estradiol, testosterone) play important roles in human lung development, and differences in susceptibility to pulmonary infection are also present at an early age [44–47]. Gender disparities are also displayed in expression of surfactant production that appears earlier in female than male during lung development, and in the incidence of neonatal conditions of prematurity, such as respiratory distress syndrome and bronchopulmonary dysplasia [48, 49]. The earlier presence of surfactant in female neonatal lungs helps open the small airways and may contribute to their higher airflow rate observed [50]. Evidence from human studies suggests that male infants are more susceptible to lung infection, with greater associated morbidity and mortality than female infants, but the reverse is applied in children and adolescents [47, 51, 52]. Regarding respiratory tract infections (RTIs), women are more

| CAP pathogens | Environmental associations/comorbidities |
|---|---|
| *Streptococcus pneumoniae, Gram-negative bacilli, Anaerobes, Haemophilus influenzae, Staphylococcus aureus* (including *methicillin-resistant* forms), *Chlamydophila pneumoniae, Mycobacterium tuberculosis* | Nursing home resident |
| *Streptococcus pneumoniae* (including drug-resistant *S. pneumoniae*), *Anaerobes, Gram-negative bacilli* | Alcoholism |
| *Streptococcus pneumoniae, Haemophilus influenzae, Salmonella, Cytomegalovirus, Cryptococcus, Pneumocystis jirovecii, Anaerobes, Mycobacterium tuberculosis* | HIV infection |
| *Streptococcus pneumoniae, Haemophilus influenzae, Moraxella catarrhalis, Legionella* | Chronic obstructive lung disease |
| *Anaerobes, Gram-negative bacilli* | Aspiration, enteric chemical pneumonitis |
| *Anaerobes* | Poor dental hygiene |
| *Pseudomonas aeruginosa, Pseudomonas cepacia, Staphylococcus aureus* | Structural disease of the lung: (bronchiectasis, cystic fibrosis) |
| *Streptococcus pneumoniae, Staphylococcus aureus, Haemophilus influenzae* | Recent influenza infection |
| Drug-resistant *pneumococcus, Pseudomonas aeruginosa, Gram-negative bacilli* | Recent antibiotic therapy |
| *Chlamydophila psittaci, Cryptococcus neoformans, Histoplasma capsulatum* | Exposure to birds |
| *Coxiella burnetii* (Q fever) | Contact with farm animals or parturient cats<br>Exposure to rabbits |
| *Coccidioides immitis* | Travel to southwest USA |
| *Histoplasma capsulatum* | Exposure to bats |
| *Parainfluenza virus, Influenza virus A* and *B, Respiratory syncytial virus* (RSV) | Congestive heart failure, mixed infections |

**Table 3.** Common pathogens in community-acquired pneumonia and environmental associations.

commonly affected by upper RTIs, such as sinusitis, tonsillitis, and otitis externa. On the other hand, men are at higher risk of developing otitis media, croup, and lower RTIs, including CAP [11]. Furthermore, these infections are more severe and show poorer outcomes and more complications in male than female individuals, leading to increased mortality, especially in CAP [21]. To date, the specific contributions of sex hormones or other factors, such as exposure to air pollution, socioeconomic, racial, and/or behavioral factors, obesity, and other comorbidities have only been explored in small studies [24, 53–56]. Several other factors including anatomic differences of the respiratory tract, behavioral, socioeconomic, and lifestyle factors have also been related with differences in incidence and severity of respiratory infections between genders [11, 41]. **Table 1** summarizes epidemiological data on associations of sex and environmental exposures on various lung health outcomes including pneumonia in children and adults [10, 27, 57–72].

http://dx.doi.org/10.5772/intechopen.69627

## 3. Pneumonia in the laboratory: animal models and mechanisms of infection

### 3.1. Animal models of pneumonia

Wide-ranging research is required to understand the mechanisms underlying pulmonary diseases, such as pneumonia. Studies of human populations, *in vitro* experiments, and exploratory infections of species are needed to advance in the development of new treatments for this condition. Animal models have been widely used in the field and have often provided insight into the physiological processes associated with the disease.

A variety of species have been used as animal models of pneumonia. Even though some species, such as *Danio rerio* (zebrafish) and *Caenorhabditis elegans* (roundworm) do not use lungs to acquire oxygen, and do not have similar sexual characteristics when compared to humans, they can be useful models to provide valuable information about host-pathogen interactions in lung disease [73]. Researchers utilize zebrafish as an alternative vertebrate model to study the pathogen's ability to infect the host [74]. Because zebrafish embryos and 3-week old larvae look transparent, it is feasible to follow the evolution of lung infection in real time [74–76]. In addition, zebrafish have a developed adaptive immune system and a high rate of conserved gene orthologs in humans [77, 78]. On the other hand, *C. elegans* is used as a non-vertebrate model for studying lung bacterial agents. Interestingly, the immune system of *C. elegans* and humans has similar signaling cascades in response to infection [79]. Despite anatomical differences, it is possible to recognize pathogen-specific virulence factors in epithelial surfaces of *C. elegans*, making this model ideal for the study of host defense mechanisms. Likewise, insects, such as *Drosophila melanogaster* (fruit fly) are valuable models of infection for the analysis of bacterial pathogenesis and genetic contributions. Insects have an advanced antimicrobial defense mechanism and a complex and conserved immune system [80]. In addition, a large number of genes that encode for proteins in the immune system are found on the X chromosome, which promote a higher activation of toll and immune deficiency signaling in *D. melanogaster* females than males [81]. Together, all these species possess advantages, such as low cost of maintenance, short life span, small size, fast development, and rapid reproduction making them feasible models for the study of infectious diseases. However, most pneumonia studies performed in animals are conducted in mammals because of their anatomical, genetic, and morphological similarities with humans.

Larger mammalian species, such as rabbits, piglets, and primates are ideal for specialized experiments when physiological monitoring and therapies are evaluated [82]. Currently, primates are the only species able to assess primate-specific infectious agents, but due to ethical concerns, piglets are the most frequently used model to study ventilator-associated pneumonia (VAP). Even though large mammalian animals are phylogenetically close to the human species, the disadvantages associated with their use as models is that they are only useful for a limited number of studies, and they are expensive to house and feed, slow to breed, and genetically diverse. For this reason, infections in the lung have primarily been studied in small mammalian species, predominantly rodents. Rodents are small, inexpensive, and highly reproductive.

Inbred strains are preferred to investigate genetically identical groups by facilitating the use of molecular approaches to understand the mechanisms of diseases. Since studies in mice have become popular in scientific research, the creation of new studies benefit from the extensive literature available regarding genetic engineering, immunological responses to pathogens and host defenses.

### 3.2. Strain differences and associated mechanisms

Knowledge of differences among strains of animals in disease models can provide ideal tools for the discovery of mechanisms of disease development [83]. A strain is defined as a group of genetically identical animals. Laboratory mice are often very diverse in behavior and physiology due to a large variety of inbred, outbred, and transgenic strains produced. In laboratory mice, this is developed through inbreeding. Different mouse strains show different responses to lung infection and environmental exposures, and these can also be affected by sex and age [84]. The most common mice strains used for the study of human pneumonia are BALB/c, C57BL/6, DBA/2, 129/Sy, CBA/Ca, C3H, SJL, and A/J. In addition, a recently developed strain, collaborative cross (CC) is derived from an eight-way cross using several founder strains [85].

A study comparing susceptibility to lung infection in mice reported that, after inducing pneumococcus infection in the respiratory track of various strains, BALB/c mice, which have the ability to produce monoclonal antibodies, show no bacteremia and no lethality. Contrarily, C57BL/6 and DBA/2 mice, which are widely used inbred strains with opposite genetic susceptibility, showed 50% lethality and an intermediate response to bacteremia. Moreover, strains, such as CBA/Ca, C3H, and SJL which are highly susceptible to infection, developed acute bacteremia with 100% lethality [86]. In a similar experiment, following pulmonary *Klebsiella* sp. infection, C57BL/6 strain exhibited more susceptibility to bacterial dissemination and lethality than 129/Sy mice, a strain widely used in the production of targeted mutations [87]. When exposed to *Yersinia pestis*, BALB/c and C57BL/6 mice succumbed to disease, whereas C3H mice were significantly more resistant with 80% survival [88]. Other studies of *Pneumocystis carinii*-induced pneumonia revealed severe effects in C3H mice; moderate effects in BALB/c, C57BL/6, B1O.A(2R), AKR/J, and Swiss Webster mice; and mild effects in DBA/2 and DBA/IJ mice [89]. Furthermore, most strains were unable to get infected by *L. pneumophila.* Finally, it was discovered that A/J mice are susceptible to *L. pneumophila*-induced lung infection because of the lack of cells specific to the adaptive immune system in these mice [90, 91].

In all these species, innate immune mechanisms defend the airways from a wide array of infections that enter the lungs and cause pneumonia. Inbred laboratory mouse strains highly differ in their immune response patterns as a result of mutations and polymorphisms. As an overall rule, toll-like receptor 4 (TLR4) mutant mice, such as C3H/HeJ are more susceptible to Gram-negative infections (e.g. *K. pneumoniae*) than other strains [92]. Moreover, some strains including A/J, DBA/2, DBA/1, FVB/NJ, and SWR are more prevalent to develop pneumonia after infection with microorganisms, such as *Bacillus anthracis, Aspergillus fumigatus,* and *Candida albicans.* The latter is due to a mutation in the complement component 5 (C5), which plays a role in the pathogenesis of autoimmune diseases [93, 94]. However, AKR/J mice, which also carry a C5 mutation, are less susceptible to *C. albicans* infection due to the *C. albicans* resistance loci that modifies host responses in these mice. In addition, studies of the *Klra* natural killer (NK) receptors have demonstrated that *Klra15 is* expressed in 129/J mice, and *Klra12* is expressed in CBA/J and C3H/He mice. None of these, however, are expressed in C57BL/6 mice [95].

Following infection, both human and mouse lungs produce immune mediators, such as cytokines, chemokines, and other components of the immune system. A regulator of IL-1β that is also highly expressed in mouse and human lungs after infection is prostaglandin E ($PGE_2$), and its precursor enzyme cyclooxygenase-2 (COX2) [52]. Studies using depletion of alveolar macrophages have demonstrated that these contribute largely to the stimulation of pro-inflammatory cytokines, such as IL-6 and TNFα [48]. Moreover, interleukin-1β (IL-1β) is induced only by strains containing the cholesterol-dependent cytolysin, pneumolysin (PLY), a major virulence factor of pneumococci infection [51]. In addition, the levels of toll-like receptor 2 (TLR2) and toll-like receptor 4 (TLR4) increase after *S. pneumoniae* infection in the Crl:CD1 mouse strain [96]. Both BALB/c mice and human lungs liberate hydrogen peroxide leading to DNA damage and apoptosis in lung cells [50, 97].

Viruses can also lead to pneumonia. Influenza A and B viruses are the most common causes of pneumonia in adults, but other viruses can contribute to the disease development. The susceptibility of mice models to influenza viruses depends on the strain of virus used. The most commonly used strains in research are A/Puerto Rico/8/1934 (H1N1, PR8) or A/WSN/1933 (H1N1, HSN). Researchers also use several pandemic viruses, such as the 1918 H1N1 pandemic strain, highly pathogenic avian influenza (HPAI) viruses of the H5N1 subtype, certain H7 subtype viruses, a subset of low pathogenic avian influenza viruses, and the 2009 H1N1 pandemic strains. After viral infection in mice, several immunomodulatory mediators are released including IL-1β, IL-6, IL-8, MCP-1, MIP-1α/β, interferon-gamma inducible protein (IP-10) and interferon-beta (IFN-β) in a somewhat strain-specific manner [98–100].

Animal research in viral pneumonia employs either BALB/c or C57BL/6 mice [68]. The majority of laboratory mice are vulnerable to disease and death after infection, whereas, wild mice are resistant to exposure. This is due to the lack of the antiviral factor Mx1 protein in inbred strains [72]. On the other hand, it is possible for researchers to adapt strains to mouse models. DBA/2J and A/J mice are more susceptible to diseases, even with viral isolates that were not adapted to mice, than the more frequently used BALB/C and C57BL/6 strains. Even though mouse-adapted strains are important to model seasonal H1N1 and H3N2 virus infections, certain influenza viruses cause disease in mice without prior adaptation [101]. Therefore, the interpretation of research outcomes in a particular strain may not be applicable in other strains and molecular pathways in pneumonic mouse lungs may differ.

Typically, Th1 cells are important in the clearance of intracellular pathogens, whereas Th2 cells are associated with responses to parasites. C57BL/6 mice display a typical Th1-type bias to pathogens, whereas other strains, such as BALB/c, A/J, and DBA/2 mice, tend toward a Th2 response [102]. These variations may also be reflected in the M1 and M2 macrophage responses to antigen stimulation. In addition, the region *D7Mit341* to *D7Mit247* on mouse chromosome 7 has been reported to be a survival trait against illness associated with *S. pneumoniae*. Susceptibility to experimental pneumococcal infection is strain dependent. In this regard, strains from least to most sensitive include BALB/c, DBA/2, C57BL/6, NIH, AKR, FVB/N, CSH/He, SJL, and CBA/Ca [103]. The majority of inbred mouse strains are resistant to infection with *L. pneumophila*, however, A/J mice carry the Lgn1-s allele, making them susceptible to infection [104].

Currently, researchers are taking advantage of the phenotypic and genetic variations available in CC mice. The CC combines the genomes of eight genetically diverse founder strains, such as A/J, C57BL/6 J, 129S1/SvImJ, NOD/LtJ, NZO/HlLtJ, CAST/EiJ, PWK/PhJ, and WSB/EiJ [85]. This genetic combination is a significant element for the study on human-host susceptibility to major diseases, including infections, such as pneumonia [105]. In a recent study, scientists used the CC mouse model to determine whether the host genetic background could impact the risk of morbidity and mortality to pneumonia caused by infection with *P. aeruginosa*. In this study, the CC strain reproduced the responses of disease severity commonly observed in humans during infection, suggesting that variations in morbidity and mortality are highly affected by host genetic factors [105]. Whereas no significant gender differences on disease phenotypes were observed, it is important to note the sample size was small. Similar variations in morbidity and mortality were found in another study where scientists used CC animals to perform a quantitative trait locus mapping of host susceptibility to *Klebsiella* sp. infection in a study where females were found to be less susceptible to infection than males [106]. In summary, animal models with high genetic diversity, and large size and number of independent recombination are emerging as a powerful tool for genomic studies, helping scientists better understand and develop more effective therapies for pneumonia [107].

### 3.3. Sex differences in pneumonia models

It has been known for several years that sex is a contributing factor in the prevalence and development of a number of pulmonary diseases, such as pneumonia [11, 108]. Animal studies also suggest that there is a sexual dimorphism after puberty in innate and adaptive immune response genes in C57BL/6 mice, with innate immune response genes being highly upregulated in postpubertal male mice but not in female mice. In contrast, postpubertal female mice express high levels of adaptive immune response genes, and expression of these genes occurs at lower levels in postpubertal male mice [60].

Several studies in animals have reported that increase in circulating levels of estrogens may lead to reduced innate immunity, as measured by natural killer cell and macrophage activity, and a decrease of cytokine release [109–111]. Animal models of infection are the simplest tool available to study sex differences due to high availability of castrated animals and hormonal replacement therapies. Multiple studies have demonstrated that susceptibility to invasive viral, bacterial, fungal, and parasitic diseases is higher in males than in females in all age groups [57, 61, 112, 113]. The concept that males are more susceptible to lung infection is further sustained by data from mouse models of bacterial infection, such as *Pneumococcal pneumonia* and *Mycobacterium marinum*, where female mice display longer survival than male mice when exposed to severe sepsis [62, 114]. Infection of C57BL/6 mice with *K. pneumoniae* demonstrated a severe effect in male mice, but not in female mice [19]. In contrast, after infection with *P. aeruginosa*, C57BL/6 female mice showed greater weight loss, bacterial load, and higher levels of inflammatory molecules than male mice. In this context, IL-10-deficient male mice exhibited elevated levels of bacteria when compared to C57BL/6 male mice. These results confirm that both C57BL/6 and IL-10-deficient male mice are more resistant to *P. aeruginosa* infection than female mice [115]. Moreover, external administration of estrogen to adult male mice infected with *P. aeruginosa* resulted in an extreme progression of inflammation and fluid infiltration in lung tissue [116].

### 3.4. Sex-specific mechanisms of infection and immunity

Currently, there is limited understanding of the molecular processes that lead to either immune-suppression or stimulation during pneumonia pathogenesis in males and females. In general, females display strong humoral immune responses after infection or vaccination when compared to males [114]. This is partially due to high levels of CD4+ T cells and variations in regulatory T cells (Treg) that regulate immune responses during the menstrual cycle in women [117]. It is known that estrogen influences transcription of specific genes that alter host immunity and promotes the proliferation of Treg during the follicular phase of the ovarian cycle [89, 118]. Because estrogen regulates CD4+ T cell subsets, there is a direct effect on Th1/Th2 equilibrium known to be crucial against bacterial and viral infections. On the other hand, studies indicate that negative outcomes from infectious pulmonary diseases in males is associated with testosterone-induced immunosuppression causing a decrease in T and B cell proliferation, and immunoglobulin and cytokine production after puberty [14]. These alterations in the adaptive immune system could help explain why men are more susceptible than women to some pulmonary diseases caused by infectious agents. However, treatments for pneumonia are standardized for both men and women indicating a general lack of understanding of sex-based differences.

## 4. Sex hormones and lung immunity

### 4.1. Sex hormones and mechanisms of action

Sex and gender differences in clinical disorders are mostly driven by genetics and sex hormones. In order to understand hormonal effects not only in lung diseases, but also in other health conditions, it is essential to recognize their mechanisms of action, signaling pathways, and active metabolites. The major sex steroid hormones, such as estrogen, progesterone, and testosterone are derived from a common lipid precursor, cholesterol, by a complex series of reactions catalyzed by multiple enzymes [119]. In brief, cholesterol is converted to pregnenolone by the cytochrome P450 enzyme. Pregnenolone, which is a precursor and metabolic intermediate in the biosynthesis of the steroid hormones, can be transformed either to progesterone by the action of 3β-hydroxysteroid dehydrogenase (3β-HSD), or alternatively be converted to dehydroepiandrosterone (DHEA) via cytochrome P450c17 action. DHEA can turn into androstenedione via 3β-HSD and consequently testosterone or estrone via 17β-HSD and aromatase, respectively. Estrone may be further converted to estradiol via 17β-HSD. Testosterone can be also transformed into estradiol via aromatase.

Sex steroids are primarily produced by the gonads (ovaries and testes). Significant evidence suggest that production of sex steroids is also found in peripheral tissues of non-reproductive organs, such as the adrenal gland, heart, breast, and lung implying a dependency on the enzymes present in the organs [120, 121]. It is thought that the source of hormone production can affect the metabolism, circulation, regulation, and concentration of local steroid versus that of circulation, which can play a role in the paradoxical effects observed for some sex hormones [43, 122, 123]. One example is the "estrogen paradox", observed in women with pulmonary hypertension. A large number of animal studies have found estrogen to be protective in the coronary circulation with better outcomes in female mice, and exasperation after ovariectomy. Contrarily, there is a higher prevalence of pulmonary hypertension in women. While some studies in humans have suggested that estrogen may increase the risk of portopulmonary hypertension, others have shown that estrogen enhances pulmonary vascular remodeling [124].

Circulating levels of testosterone range from 2 to 15 ng/ml or 6 to 50 nM in males, and less than 1.5 ng/ml or 5 nM in females throughout life. Even though men produce both estrogen and progesterone, the levels of these hormones are significantly higher in women, fluctuating from 20 pg/ml estrogen and 0.3 ng/ml progesterone in the follicular phase in non-pregnant and postmenopausal women, to 40 ng/ml estradiol and 300 ng/ml progesterone in pregnant women [43]. The significance of the oscillations of hormonal levels consists in their contribution to the local level of any sex steroids. For example, the estrogen produced in tissues may become more prominent in postmenopausal women, while the effect of progesterone may decline. At present, there is not much information available on this issue relevant to the lung.

### 4.2. Effect of sex hormones in immune responses and lung development

Currently, there is an increasing evidence for sex differences in incidence, morbidity, and mortality of lung diseases. Whether sex steroids play a role in modulating these differences is currently under investigation.

Estradiol levels in the fetus emerge in week 20 during the canalicular phase of lung development, and rise throughout birth [125]. Differences in estrogen levels have been observed in lung maturation, preservation, and regeneration, alveoli development and surfactant synthesis suggesting an active role of estrogen in sexual dimorphism [126–131]. Moreover, it is known that estrogen plays a complicated immunomodulatory role in humans and in animal models, suppressing inflammation in some states while enhancing it in others [116]. In animal models, estrogen blocks both B and T cell development, increases thymic atrophy, and decreases all developing T cell populations, while it enhances B cell survival in response to antigen [132–134]. In humans, hormone replacement therapy reduced the amount of T cells, while B cells were unaltered or upregulated in postmenopausal women, increasing the risk of developing B cell-dependent autoimmune diseases [123, 135]. Other studies propose that estrogen enriches the accumulation of Th1 CD4+ T cells in response to antigen in female mice [136]. It was also stated that estrogen inhibits the induction of Th1 pro-inflammatory cytokines (IL-12, IFN$\gamma$, and TNF$\alpha$), while it enhances Th2 anti-inflammatory cytokines (IL-4, IL-10, and TGF$\beta$) in female mice [137]. However, little is known about how puberty affects lung diseases later in life and how the changes in estrogen levels contribute to the pathophysiology of pulmonary diseases. This is important because estrogen can cause effects on the immune system by binding to estrogen receptors (ER) expressed by immune cells, such as B cells, T cells, and macrophages [138]. Variations in the expression of ER in the bronchial and alveolar epithelium suggest a role in estrogen signaling, which can contribute to the gender dimorphism seen in males and females [130, 131, 139, 140]. In addition, estrogen has the ability to indirectly stimulate airway and parenchymal responses by acting on airway and alveolar epithelial cells, which are structural cells [141]. In the case of infection with *P. aeruginosa,* researchers found that female mice were more susceptible than males [115]. Furthermore, in a study where chronic infection of cystic fibrosis (CF) airway by *P. aeruginosa* was studied, researchers found that estrogen increased the severity of pneumonia in adult CF male mice, and proposed two potential mechanisms: enrichment of Th17-regulated inflammation and suppression of innate antibacterial defenses [116]. On the contrary, fetal levels of testosterone are found on week 9 of gestation during the pseudoglandular phase [125]. In this context, elevated levels of androgens, which are any hormones that primarily influence the growth and development of the male reproductive system, are found associated with slow fetal lung development [142–144]. In this context, studies have shown that anti-androgen flutamide can produce high levels of surfactant phospholipid in the male fetal lung, however, androgen dihydrotestosterone (DHT) blocks the synthesis of surfactant phospholipid in the female fetal lung [1, 145]. The development of male fetal lungs depends on the expression of the androgen receptors (AR) [46]. Whether testosterone, and/or its receptors, play a role in modulating sex differences in lung diseases, such as pneumonia remains unknown.

## 5. Pneumonia and air pollution: epidemiological and experimental data

### 5.1. Outdoor air pollution and lung health

In the last several decades, an accumulative body of epidemiological, toxicological, and experimental evidence, including various exposure agents, times, doses, and combinations of pollutants, have linked exposure of air pollution to negative cardiovascular and pulmonary health effects [146], and infection rates (**Table 1**). These include increased inflammation, exacerbation of pre-existing inflammatory lung disease (e.g. asthma, wheezing, and COPD) and allergies, altered lung function and immunity, and increased susceptibility to infection and pneumonia. Extensive epidemiological evidence demonstrated inter-individual differences in the susceptibility to environmental exposures, with age, gender, and genetic polymorphisms significantly contributing to its negative health effects [12]. A summary of the most frequently found pollutants and their health effects is summarized in **Table 4**.

Air pollutants are generally present in the environment as a mixture of several gases and particles that are products of combustion of fossil fuels, diesel traffic, wood smoke, and other industrial processes. Some sources of domestic energy used around the world, especially in developing countries, are the result of combustion of fuels, such as wood, dung, and charcoal but also result in the generation of large amounts of indoor pollutants including small particulates ($PM_{10}$), nitrogen dioxide ($NO_2$), carbon monoxide (CO), sulfur dioxide ($SO_2$), and various hydrocarbons [147]. In this context, individuals who spent time at home, such as mothers and their children are at higher risk of developing respiratory infections [148–150]. In addition, particulate air pollution released by burning plantations has also been associated with pneumonia. For example, in Brazil (one of the main sugar cane producers), the incidence of pneumonia-related emergency department visits has found significant increase during sugar cane burning periods [151]. Air pollution in countries with high industry factory activity, such as Taiwan has also been associated with respiratory diseases, with some differences in age and gender of the patients affected. In these studies, NO and $NO_2$ were two of the main air pollutants related to respiratory diseases, followed by $PM_{10}$, $PM_{2.5}$, $O_3$, CO, and $SO_2$. Young patients (0–15 years of age) were the most affected by air pollution and meteorology factors, followed by elder patients (age ≥66 years), and aged 16–65. A closer look at gender differences revealed that women were more affected than men in the young age group and in the eldest group, but men were more sensitive between ages 16 and 65 groups [152–155]. Other studies have also reported both women and elderly people to be more susceptible to die from air pollution than other population groups [153, 156, 157].

One of the reasons that could explain the increased mortality in women is their high vulnerability to autoimmune disorders, some of which are associated with air pollution [158]. Moreover, anatomic and physiologic differences between men and women also seem to play a role in this disparity. In general, men have higher lean body mass and water content than women, which results in an increased distribution volume of soluble substances. On the contrary, women have more relative fat mass than men, which gives them a larger distribution volume for fat-soluble substances, and most of the chemical particles in the environment are highly lipophilic. Furthermore, important sex differences in the metabolism of such substances also exist. For example, most of the CYP enzymes are regulated by sex

| Pollutant | Health effects |
|---|---|
| Ozone | Decreased lung function<br>Increased airway reactivity<br>Increased lung inflammation<br>Increased hospital visits for lung disease<br>Increased mortality |
| Particulate matter | Decreased lung function<br>Increased respiratory symptoms<br>Increased mortality |
| Nitrogen dioxide | Increased airway reactivity<br>Reduced lung function<br>Bronchitis (children) |
| Carbon monoxide | |
| Sulfur dioxide | Increased respiratory mortality<br>Increased hospital visits for lung disease<br>Aggravation of lung disease<br>Increased lung inflammation |

**Table 4.** Common air pollutants and health effects.

steroids. As a result, some substances are metabolized faster in women liver cells than men, and sometimes the end products are more toxic than the original substance, causing a higher toxicity for women due to increased internal exposure [158].

Accumulating epidemiological, clinical, and experimental evidence suggests that exposure to air pollutants can have serious effects in metabolic and endocrine function, particularly in glucose metabolism [159, 160]. Air pollution, especially traffic-related exposures, $NO_2$, tobacco smoke, and particulate matter, have been associated with obesity, type 2 diabetes, and metabolic syndrome with women showing higher susceptibility than men, and children being especially susceptible [161–164]. Studies conducted in several countries, such as Europe, America, and Asia reported strong associations among exposure to air pollutants, insulin resistance, obesity, and diabetes with women overrepresented in the affected groups [165–170]. These findings have also been recapitulated in animal models, where exposure to particulate matter resulted in increased insulin resistance followed by a high-fat diet [171–173], and these effects were associated with inflammation triggered by mechanisms involving pulmonary oxidative stress [174].

### 5.2. Metabolic effects of air pollution and their relationship with pneumonia

The relationship between diabetes, obesity, and susceptibility to lung infection and pneumonia has also been evaluated in several studies [175]. In these, an increased incidence and mortality from pneumococcal pneumonia, influenza, and tuberculosis was strongly associated with diabetes and obesity [176]. In this context, it is important to mention that obesity affects more women than men globally, and that a high body mass index has been directly associated with CAP risk in women [177, 178]. Animal models of bacterial infection using the leptin-deficient obese mouse have also shown higher susceptibility to pneumonia [179, 180]. Finally, an "obesity paradox" in CAP has also been reported extensively, in which obesity is associated with a higher incidence of bacterial pneumonia, but increased body mass index was associated with increased survival in patients hospitalized with CAP [181].

### 5.3. Genetic contributions to pneumonia risk and severity

We mentioned earlier studies reporting gender, racial, and population variability in both pneumonia incidence and outcome. Therefore, it is highly likely that these differences are the result of a complex interplay between both host and pathogen genetic backgrounds together with nongenetic factors, such as those discussed above [182]. With the recent development of fast and affordable high-throughput sequencing techniques, more studies have begun to explore the contributions of host genetics in the context of pneumonia [183–186]. The majority of these have focused on innate immune molecules, such as toll-like receptors and pro-inflammatory cytokines. Several associations of pneumonia susceptibility and severity with single nucleotide polymorphisms in the interleukin-6, interleukin-10, toll-like receptors TLR2, TLR4, and TLR9, C-reactive protein (CRP), and nitric oxide synthase 3 (NOS3) genes were reported [187–191]. We have summarized these in **Table 5**. Interestingly, most polymorphisms found in the cytokine genes are located in regulatory and promoter regions, where they may be affecting binding of transcription factors, such as GATA1-3, SOX, and heat shock proteins [183].

### 5.4. Pollution models of infection and pneumonia

Air pollution has been shown to exacerbate respiratory diseases, such as pneumonia. Air pollutants that reach the respiratory tract are currently responsible for its genesis, especially particulate matter having an aerodynamic diameter equal to or less than 10 μm, sulfur dioxide ($SO_2$), ground level ozone ($O_3$), nitrogen dioxide ($NO_2$), and carbon monoxide (CO) [192, 193]. However, these pollutants may also increase the risk for pneumonia by altering the function of alveolar macrophages, epithelial cells, mucociliary clearance mechanisms, particle transport, and local immunity in the lungs [194]. Because of methodological difficulties and ethical issues, there are a limited number of studies on the effects of controlled pollutant exposure and infection in humans. It has now been almost 50 years since the "infectivity model" has been created. This model is based on the study of the effects of pollutants on pulmonary activity after pollutant exposure with disease and mortality as end-points in animals, particularly rodents [147].

The infectivity model is used by researchers to determine the amount and concentration of pollutants at which the immune system is compromised and disease is developed. This is accomplished by challenging animals with virulent agents either before or after exposure to different concentrations of the pollutant. Exposure to $NO_2$ before and after infectious challenge in mice show significantly higher death rates [195]. Moreover, mice infected with *S. aureus* and then challenged with $NO_2$ displayed a reduction in lung bactericidal capacity [196]. Exposure to varying concentrations of $NO_2$ affects respiratory tract susceptibility, macrophage viability, systemic cell-mediated and humoral responses to viral infection in CD-1 mice inoculated intratracheally with murine cytomegalovirus [197]. Moreover, the number of viral particles capable of generating infection is lower in animals challenged with $NO_2$ than in animals exposed to filtered air. In addition, the risk of reinfection is higher in mice after $NO_2$ exposure indicating damage in the development of virus-specific immunity following a primary infection [198].

| Gene | SNPs |
|---|---|
| C-reactive protein | rs1205 |
| Interleukin-1 beta | rs16944 |
| Interleukin-6 | rs1800797, rs1800795 |
| Interleukin-8 | rs4073 |
| Interleukin-10 | rs1800896, rs1800871, rs1800872, rs5743629 |
| Nitric oxide synthase 3 | rs1799983 |
| Toll-like receptor 2 | rs5743708 |
| Toll-like receptor 4 | rs4986790, rs4986791 |
| Toll-like receptor 9 | rs5743836 |

**Table 5.** Single nucleotide polymorphisms associated with pneumonia.

There are several pollution models of pneumonia infection combined with particulate matter [199], $SO_2$ [200], CO [201], and other common air pollutants. These models generally involve a higher concentration of pollutants than would be normally found in the atmosphere. This is often necessary because a higher dose of most pollutants is required for rodents versus humans to reach comparable concentrations in the distal lung and generating comparable effects on lung function and immunity.

Ozone exposure can impair breathing, induce coughing, reduce lung function, and trigger lung diseases, such as pneumonia. The effect of ozone exposure has been associated with damage of the entire respiratory epithelia and lung immunity [202]. A study showed that mice infected with *K. pneumoniae* following exposure to 2 ppm of $O_3$ decreased the ability of mice to clear bacteria from the lungs, and that ozone-exposed females were more affected and showed higher mortality rates than males [17, 18]. Contrarily, in the absence of ozone-induced oxidative stress, males were more prompted to have a higher level of propagation of infection compared to females. These mechanisms appear to be mediated by surfactant biology and surfactant protein expression [19].

## 6. Conclusion

Regulation of the lung inflammatory response is critical to the successful outcome of pneumonia. Exposure to air pollutants has been linked to negative lung health outcomes, and sex hormones have been shown to mediate the lung immune response, especially during lung infection. The negative impact of air pollution on lung health, both in the short and long term, is now well accepted, and air quality indexes or scales are available to alert individuals when the air quality is at harmful levels. In this chapter, we have discussed experimental and epidemiological evidence on pneumonia infection incidence in different populations, influences of air pollution and environmental exposures, and sex-specific mechanisms involving male and female hormones in the context of lung immunity. This information could help researchers better explain the differences observed in pneumonia susceptibility and lung health outcomes in men versus women. Understanding the biological basis of these differences is critical for the development of more effective prevention and management strategies for pneumonia in men and women, and could help in the development of better treatment options for these patients.

## Author details

Patricia Silveyra*, Nathalie Fuentes and Lidys Rivera

*Address all correspondence to: psilveyra@pennstatehealth.psu.edu

The Pennsylvania State University College of Medicine, Hershey, USA

## References

[1] Card JW, Zeldin DC. Hormonal influences on lung function and response to environmental agents: Lessons from animal models of respiratory disease. Proceedings of the American Thoracic Society. 2009;**6**(7):588-595

[2] Carey MA, Card JW, Voltz JW, Germolec DR, Korach KS, Zeldin DC. The impact of sex and sex hormones on lung physiology and disease: Lessons from animal studies. American Journal of Physiology—Lung Cellular and Molecular Physiology. 2007;**293**(2):L272-L278

[3] Anand N, Kollef MH. The alphabet soup of pneumonia: CAP, HAP, HCAP, NHAP, and VAP. Seminars in Respiratory and Critical Care Medicine. 2009;**30**(1):3-9

[4] Chalmers JD. The modern diagnostic approach to community-acquired pneumonia in adults. Seminars in Respiratory and Critical Care Medicine. 2016;**37**(6):876-885

[5] Brar NK, Niederman MS. Management of community-acquired pneumonia: A review and update. Therapeutic Advances in Respiratory Disease. 2011;**5**(1):61-78

[6] Nair GB, Niederman MS. Community-acquired pneumonia: An unfinished battle. The Medical Clinics of North America. 2011;**95**(6):1143-1161

[7] Mandell LA, Wunderink RG, Anzueto A, Bartlett JG, Campbell GD, Dean NC, et al. Infectious Diseases Society of America/American Thoracic Society consensus guidelines on the management of community-acquired pneumonia in adults. Clinical Infectious Diseases. 2007;**44**(Suppl 2):S27-S72

[8] Kochanek KD, Murphy SL, Xu J. Deaths: Final data for 2011. National Vital Statistics Reports. 2015;**63**(3):1-120

[9] File TM, Jr., Marrie TJ. Burden of community-acquired pneumonia in North American adults. Postgraduate Medicine. 2010;**122**(2):130-141

[10] Almirall J, Bolibar I, Serra-Prat M, Roig J, Hospital I, Carandell E, et al. New evidence of risk factors for community-acquired pneumonia: A population-based study. European Respiratory Journal. 2008;**31**(6):1274-1284

[11] Falagas ME, Mourtzoukou EG, Vardakas KZ. Sex differences in the incidence and severity of respiratory tract infections. Respiratory Medicine. 2007;**101**(9):1845-1863

[12] Silveyra P, Floros J. Air pollution and epigenetics: Effects on SP-A and innate host defence in the lung. Swiss Medical Weekly. 2012;**142**:w13579

[13] Klein SL, Jedlicka A, Pekosz A. The Xs and Y of immune responses to viral vaccines. The Lancet Infectious Diseases. 2010;**10**(5):338-349

[14] Fish EN. The X-files in immunity: Sex-based differences predispose immune responses. Nature Reviews Immunology. 2008;**8**(9):737-744

[15] Durrani F, Phelps DS, Weisz J, Silveyra P, Hu S, Mikerov AN, et al. Gonadal hormones and oxidative stress interaction differentially affects survival of male and female mice after lung *Klebsiella pneumoniae* infection. Experimental Lung Research. 2012;**38**(4):165-172

[16] Mikerov AN, Hu S, Durrani F, Gan X, Wang G, Umstead TM, et al. Impact of sex and ozone exposure on the course of pneumonia in wild type and SP-A (−/−) mice. Microbial Pathogenesis. 2012;**52**(4):239-249

[17] Mikerov AN, Cooper TK, Wang G, Hu S, Umstead TM, Phelps DS, et al. Histopathologic evaluation of lung and extrapulmonary tissues show sex differences in *Klebsiella pneumoniae*-infected mice under different exposure conditions. International Journal of Physiology, Pathophysiology and Pharmacology. 2011;**3**(3):176-190

[18] Mikerov AN, Gan X, Umstead TM, Miller L, Chinchilli VM, Phelps DS, et al. Sex differences in the impact of ozone on survival and alveolar macrophage function of mice after *Klebsiella pneumoniae* infection. Respiratory Research. 2008;**9**:24

[19] Mikerov AN, Haque R, Gan X, Guo X, Phelps DS, Floros J. Ablation of SP-A has a negative impact on the susceptibility of mice to *Klebsiella pneumoniae* infection after ozone exposure: Sex differences. Respiratory Research. 2008;**9**:77

[20] Mikerov AN, Umstead TM, Gan X, Huang W, Guo X, Wang G, et al. Impact of ozone exposure on the phagocytic activity of human surfactant protein A (SP-A) and SP-A variants. American Journal of Physiology—Lung Cellular and Molecular Physiology. 2008;**294**(1):L121-L130

[21] Kaplan V, Angus DC, Griffin MF, Clermont G, Scott Watson R, Linde-Zwirble WT. Hospitalized community-acquired pneumonia in the elderly: Age- and sex-related patterns of care and outcome in the United States. American Journal of Respiratory and Critical Care Medicine. 2002;**165**(6):766-772

[22] Pope CA. Particulate air pollution and lung function. American Journal of Respiratory and Critical Care Medicine. 2014;**190**(5):485-486

[23] Zanobetti A, Woodhead M. Air pollution and pneumonia: The "old man"; has a new "friend". American Journal of Respiratory and Critical Care Medicine. 2010;**181**:5-6; United States

[24] Neupane B, Jerrett M, Burnett RT, Marrie T, Arain A, Loeb M. Long-term exposure to ambient air pollution and risk of hospitalization with community-acquired pneumonia in older adults. American Journal of Respiratory and Critical Care Medicine. 2010;**181**(1):47-53

[25] de Roux A, Marcos MA, Garcia E, Mensa J, Ewig S, Lode H, et al. Viral community-acquired pneumonia in nonimmunocompromised adults. Chest. 2004;**125**(4):1343-1351

[26] Cunha BA. The atypical pneumonias: clinical diagnosis and importance. Clinical Microbiology and Infection. 2006;**12**(Suppl 3):12-24

[27] Bassani DG, Jha P, Dhingra N, Kumar R. Child mortality from solid-fuel use in India: A nationally-representative case-control study. BMC Public Health. 2010;**10**:491

[28] Arancibia F, Bauer TT, Ewig S, Mensa J, Gonzalez J, Niederman MS, et al. Community-acquired pneumonia due to gram-negative bacteria and *Pseudomonas aeruginosa*: Incidence, risk, and prognosis. Archives of Internal Medicine. 2002;**162**(16):1849-1858

[29] Wunderink RG, Waterer GW. Community-acquired pneumonia: Pathophysiology and host factors with focus on possible new approaches to management of lower respiratory tract infections. Infectious Disease Clinics of North America. 2004; **18**(4):743-759, vii

[30] Torres A, Peetermans WE, Viegi G, Blasi F. Risk factors for community-acquired pneumonia in adults in Europe: A literature review. Thorax. 2013;**68**(11):1057-1065

[31] Shea KM, Edelsberg J, Weycker D, Farkouh RA, Strutton DR, Pelton SI. Rates of pneumococcal disease in adults with chronic medical conditions. Open Forum Infectious Diseases. 2014;**1**(1):ofu024

[32] Pelton SI, Shea KM, Weycker D, Farkouh RA, Strutton DR, Edelsberg J. Rethinking risk for pneumococcal disease in adults: The role of risk stacking. Open Forum Infectious Diseases. 2015;**2**(1):ofv020

[33] Dye JA, Adler KB. Effects of cigarette smoke on epithelial cells of the respiratory tract. Thorax. 1994;**49**(8):825-834

[34] Almirall J, Blanquer J, Bello S. Community-acquired pneumonia among smokers. Archivos de Bronconeumología. 2014;**50**(6):250-254

[35] Almirall J, Serra-Prat M, Bolíbar I, Palomera E, Roig J, Hospital I, et al. Passive smoking at home is a risk factor for community-acquired pneumonia in older adults: A population-based case–control study. BMJ Open. 2014;**4**(6):e005133

[36] Nelson S, Kolls JK. Alcohol, host defence and society. Nature Reviews Immunology. 2002;**2**(3):205-209

[37] Rodriguez-Pecci MS, Carlson D, Montero-Tinnirello J, Parodi RL, Montero A, Greca AA. Nutritional status and mortality in community acquired pneumonia. Medicina (B Aires). 2010;**70**(2):120-126

[38] Leow L, Simpson T, Cursons R, Karalus N, Hancox RJ. Vitamin D, innate immunity and outcomes in community acquired pneumonia. Respirology. 2011;**16**(4):611-616

[39] Orlov AM, Bakulin IG, Mazo VK. Deficiency of selenium in pneumonia: An accident or regularity? Problem of Nutriciology and Gastroenterology. Eksp Klin Gastroenterol. 2013;(2):20-27

[40] Cojocaru M, Cojocaru IM, Silosi I, Vrabie CD. Pulmonary manifestations of systemic autoimmune diseases. Maedica (Buchar). 2011;**6**(3):224-229

[41] Klein SL. The effects of hormones on sex differences in infection: From genes to behavior. Neuroscience & Biobehavioral Reviews. 2000;**24**(6):627-638

[42] Townsend EA, Miller VM, Prakash YS. Sex differences and sex steroids in lung health and disease. Endocrine Reviews. 2012;**33**(1):1-47

[43] Sathish V, Martin YN, Prakash YS. Sex steroid signaling: Implications for lung diseases. Pharmacology and Therapeutics. 2015;**150**:94-108

[44] Pasqualini JR. Enzymes involved in the formation and transformation of steroid hormones in the fetal and placental compartments. Journal of Steroid Biochemistry and Molecular Biology. 2005;**97**(5):401-415

[45] Milewich L, Kaimal V, Shaw CB, Johnson AR. Androstenedione metabolism in human lung fibroblasts. Journal of Steroid Biochemistry. 1986;**24**(4):893-897

[46] Silveyra P. Chapter 9: Developmental lung disease. In: Hemnes AR, editor. Gender, Sex Hormones and Respiratory Disease A Comprehensive Guide; Springer International Publishing, Switzerland. 2016; p. 243

[47] Tettelin H, Nelson KE, Paulsen IT, Eisen JA, Read TD, Peterson S, et al. Complete genome sequence of a virulent isolate of *Streptococcus pneumoniae*. Science. 2001;**293**(5529):498-506

[48] Xu F, Droemann D, Rupp J, Shen H, Wu X, Goldmann T, et al. Modulation of the inflammatory response to *Streptococcus pneumoniae* in a model of acute lung tissue infection. American Journal of Respiratory Cell and Molecular Biology. 2008;**39**(5):522-529

[49] May C, Patel S, Kennedy C, Pollina E, Rafferty GF, Peacock JL, et al. Prediction of bronchopulmonary dysplasia. Archives of Disease in Childhood-Fetal and Neonatal Edition. 2011;**96**(6):F410-F416

[50] Rai P, Parrish M, Tay IJ, Li N, Ackerman S, He F, et al. *Streptococcus pneumoniae* secretes hydrogen peroxide leading to DNA damage and apoptosis in lung cells. Proceedings of the National Academy of Sciences of the United States of America. 2015;**112**(26):E3421-E3430

[51] Fatykhova D, Rabes A, Machnik C, Guruprasad K, Pache F, Berg J, et al. Serotype 1 and 8 pneumococci evade sensing by inflammasomes in human lung tissue. PLoS One. 2015;**10**(8):e0137108

[52] Szymanski KV, Toennies M, Becher A, Fatykhova D, N'Guessan PD, Gutbier B, et al. *Streptococcus pneumoniae*-induced regulation of cyclooxygenase-2 in human lung tissue. European Respiratory Journal. 2012;**40**(6):1458-1467

[53] Haenle MM, Brockmann SO, Kron M, Bertling U, Mason RA, Steinbach G, et al. Overweight, physical activity, tobacco and alcohol consumption in a cross-sectional random sample of German adults. BMC Public Health. 2006;**6**:233

[54] Rosenberg HM, Maurer JD, Sorlie PD, Johnson NJ, MacDorman MF, Hoyert DL, et al. Quality of death rates by race and Hispanic origin: A summary of current research, 1999. Vital and Health Statistics Series 2. 1999;(128):1-13

[55] Wiese AD, Grijalva CG, Zhu Y, Mitchel EF, Griffin MR. Changes in childhood pneumonia hospitalizations by race and sex associated with pneumococcal conjugate vaccines. Emerging Infectious Disease. 2016;**22**(6):1109

[56] Pathak EB. Mortality among black men in the USA. Journal of Racial and Ethnic Health Disparities. 2017;**4**:1-12

[57] Jensen-Fangel S, Mohey R, Johnsen SP, Andersen PL, Sørensen HT, Ostergaard L. Gender differences in hospitalization rates for respiratory tract infections in Danish youth. Scandinavian Journal of Infectious Diseases. 2004;**36**(1):31-36

[58] Fleisher B, Kulovich MV, Hallman M, Gluck L. Lung profile: Sex differences in normal pregnancy. Obstetrics & Gynecology. 1985;**66**(3):327-330

[59] Doershuk CF, Fisher BJ, Matthews LW. Specific airway resistance from the perinatal period into adulthood. Alterations in childhood pulmonary disease. American Review of Respiratory Diseases. 1974;**109**(4):452-457

[60] Lamason R, Zhao P, Rawat R, Davis A, Hall JC, Chae JJ, et al. Sexual dimorphism in immune response genes as a function of puberty. BMC Immunology. 2006;**7**:2

[61] Offner PJ, Moore EE, Biffl WL. Male gender is a risk factor for major infections after surgery. Archives of Surgery. 1999;**134**(9):935-938; discussion 8-40

[62] Marriott I, Huet-Hudson YM. Sexual dimorphism in innate immune responses to infectious organisms. Immunologic Research. 2006;**34**(3):177-192

[63] Katanoda K, Sobue T, Satoh H, Tajima K, Suzuki T, Nakatsuka H, et al. An association between long-term exposure to ambient air pollution and mortality from lung cancer and respiratory diseases in Japan. Journal of Epidemiology. 2011;**21**(2):132-143

[64] White AN, Ng V, Spain CV, Johnson CC, Kinlin LM, Fisman DN. Let the sun shine in: Effects of ultraviolet radiation on invasive pneumococcal disease risk in Philadelphia, Pennsylvania. BMC Infectious Diseases. 2009;**9**:196

[65] Suzuki M, Thiem VD, Yanai H, Matsubayashi T, Yoshida LM, Tho LH, et al. Association of environmental tobacco smoking exposure with an increased risk of hospital admissions for pneumonia in children under 5 years of age in Vietnam. Thorax. 2009;**64**(6):484-489

[66] Ebbert JO, Croghan IT, Schroeder DR, Murawski J, Hurt RD. Association between respiratory tract diseases and secondhand smoke exposure among never smoking flight attendants: A cross-sectional survey. Environmental Health. 2007;**6**:28

[67] Mahalanabis D, Gupta S, Paul D, Gupta A, Lahiri M, Khaled MA. Risk factors for pneumonia in infants and young children and the role of solid fuel for cooking: A case-control study. Epidemiology and Infection. 2002;**129**(1):65-71

[68] Zanobetti A, Schwartz J, Gold D. Are there sensitive subgroups for the effects of airborne particles? Environmental Health Perspectives. 2000;**108**(9):841-845

[69] Kramer U, Behrendt H, Dolgner R, Ranft U, Ring J, Willer H, et al. Airway diseases and allergies in East and West German children during the first 5 years after reunification: Time trends and the impact of sulphur dioxide and total suspended particles. International Journal of Epidemiology. 1999;**28**(5):865-873

[70] Gergen PJ, Fowler JA, Maurer KR, Davis WW, Overpeck MD. The burden of environmental tobacco smoke exposure on the respiratory health of children 2 months through 5 years of age in the United States: Third National Health and Nutrition Examination Survey, 1988 to 1994. Pediatrics. 1998;**101**(2):E8

[71] Lopez Bravo IM, Sepulveda H, Valdes I. Acute respiratory illnesses in the first 18 months of life. Revista Panamericana de Salud Pública. 1997;**1**(1):9-17

[72] Staeheli P, Grob R, Meier E, Sutcliffe JG, Haller O. Influenza virus-susceptible mice carry Mx genes with a large deletion or a nonsense mutation. Molecular and Cellular Biology. 1988;**8**(10):4518-4523

[73] Mizgerd JP, Skerrett SJ. Animal models of human pneumonia. American Journal of Physiology—Lung Cellular and Molecular Physiology. 2008;**294**(3):L387-L398

[74] López Hernández Y, Yero D, Pinos-Rodríguez JM, Gibert I. Animals devoid of pulmonary system as infection models in the study of lung bacterial pathogens. Frontiers in Microbiology. 2015;**6**:38

[75] Ali S, Champagne DL, Spaink HP, Richardson MK. Zebrafish embryos and larvae: A new generation of disease models and drug screens. Birth Defects Research. Part C, Embryo Today. 2011;**93**(2):115-133

[76] Redd MJ, Kelly G, Dunn G, Way M, Martin P. Imaging macrophage chemotaxis in vivo: Studies of microtubule function in zebrafish wound inflammation. Cell Motility and the Cytoskeleton. 2006;**63**(7):415-422

[77] Meeker ND, Trede NS. Immunology and zebrafish: Spawning new models of human disease. Developmental & Comparative Immunology. 2008;**32**(7):745-757

[78] Meijer AH, Spaink HP. Host-pathogen interactions made transparent with the zebrafish model. Current Drug Targets. 2011;**12**(7):1000-1017

[79] Alper S, McElwee MK, Apfeld J, Lackford B, Freedman JH, Schwartz DA. The *Caenorhabditis elegans* germ line regulates distinct signaling pathways to control lifespan and innate immunity. Journal of Biological Chemistry. 2010;**285**(3):1822-1828

[80] Lemaitre B, Hoffmann J. The host defense of *Drosophila melanogaster*. Annual Review of Immunology. 2007;**25**:697-743

[81] Klein SL, Flanagan KL. Sex differences in immune responses. Nature Reviews Immunology. 2016;**16**(10):626-638

[82] Hraiech S, Papazian L, Rolain JM, Bregeon F. Animal models of polymicrobial pneumonia. Drug Design, Development and Therapy. 2015;**9**:3279-3292

[83] Davis JK, Parker RF, White H, Dziedzic D, Taylor G, Davidson MK, et al. Strain differences in susceptibility to murine respiratory mycoplasmosis in C57BL/6 and C3H/HeN mice. Infection and Immunity. 1985;**50**(3):647-654

[84] Vancza EM, Galdanes K, Gunnison A, Hatch G, Gordon T. Age, strain, and gender as factors for increased sensitivity of the mouse lung to inhaled ozone. Toxicological Sciences. 2009;**107**(2):535-543

[85] Churchill GA, Airey DC, Allayee H, Angel JM, Attie AD, Beatty J, et al. The Collaborative Cross, a community resource for the genetic analysis of complex traits. Nature Genetics. 2004;**36**(11):1133-1137

[86] Gingles NA, Alexander JE, Kadioglu A, Andrew PW, Kerr A, Mitchell TJ, et al. Role of genetic resistance in invasive pneumococcal infection: Identification and study of susceptibility and resistance in inbred mouse strains. Infection and Immunity. 2001;**69**(1):426-434

[87] Schurr JR, Young E, Byrne P, Steele C, Shellito JE, Kolls JK. Central role of toll-like receptor 4 signaling and host defense in experimental pneumonia caused by Gram-negative bacteria. Infection and Immunity. 2005;**73**(1):532-545

[88] Lee-Lewis H, Anderson DM. Absence of inflammation and pneumonia during infection with nonpigmented Yersinia pestis reveals a new role for the pgm locus in pathogenesis. Infection and Immunity. 2010;**78**(1):220-230

[89] Walzer PD, Powell RD, Yoneda K. Experimental Pneumocystis carinii pneumonia in different strains of cortisonized mice. Infection and Immunity. 1979;**24**(3):939-947

[90] Brieland J, Freeman P, Kunkel R, Chrisp C, Hurley M, Fantone J, et al. Replicative *Legionella pneumophila* lung infection in intratracheally inoculated A/J mice. A murine model of human Legionnaires' disease. American Journal of Pathology. 1994;**145**(6):1537-1546

[91] De Vooght V, Vanoirbeek JA, Luyts K, Haenen S, Nemery B, Hoet PH. Choice of mouse strain influences the outcome in a mouse model of chemical-induced asthma. PLoS One. 2010;**5**(9):e12581

[92] Wieland CW, van Lieshout MH, Hoogendijk AJ, van der Poll T. Host defence during *Klebsiella pneumonia* relies on haematopoietic-expressed Toll-like receptors 4 and 2. European Respiratory Journal. 2011;**37**(4):848-857

[93] Wetsel RA, Fleischer DT, Haviland DL. Deficiency of the murine fifth complement component (C5). A 2-base pair gene deletion in a 5′-exon. Journal of Biological Chemistry. 1990;**265**(5):2435-2440

[94] Sellers RS, Clifford CB, Treuting PM, Brayton C. Immunological variation between inbred laboratory mouse strains: Points to consider in phenotyping genetically immunomodified mice. Veterinary Pathology. 2012;**49**(1):32-43

[95] Makrigiannis AP, Anderson SK. The murine Ly49 family: Form and function. Archivum Immunologiae et Therapiae Experimentalis (Warsz). 2001;**49**(1):47-50

[96] Tokairin Y, Shibata Y, Sata M, Abe S, Takabatake N, Igarashi A, et al. Enhanced immediate inflammatory response to *Streptococcus pneumoniae* in the lungs of mice with pulmonary emphysema. Respirology. 2008;**13**(3):324-332

[97] Kadioglu A, Weiser JN, Paton JC, Andrew PW. The role of *Streptococcus pneumoniae* virulence factors in host respiratory colonization and disease. Nature Reviews Microbiology. 2008;**6**(4):288-301

[98] Knepper J, Schierhorn KL, Becher A, Budt M, Tönnies M, Bauer TT, et al. The novel human influenza A(H7N9) virus is naturally adapted to efficient growth in human lung tissue. MBio. 2013;**4**(5):e00601-e00613

[99] Weinheimer VK, Becher A, Tönnies M, Holland G, Knepper J, Bauer TT, et al. Influenza A viruses target type II pneumocytes in the human lung. Journal of Infectious Diseases. 2012;**206**(11):1685-1694

[100] Wu W, Zhang W, Booth JL, Metcalf JP. Influenza A(H1N1)pdm09 virus suppresses RIG-I initiated innate antiviral responses in the human lung. PLoS One. 2012;**7**(11):e49856

[101] Bogaert D, De Groot R, Hermans PW. *Streptococcus pneumoniae* colonisation: The key to pneumococcal disease. Lancet Infectious Diseases. 2004;**4**(3):144-154

[102] Mills CD, Kincaid K, Alt JM, Heilman MJ, Hill AM. M-1/M-2 macrophages and the Th1/Th2 paradigm. Journal of Immunology. 2000;**164**(12):6166-6173

[103] Denny P, Hopes E, Gingles N, Broman KW, McPheat W, Morten J, et al. A major locus conferring susceptibility to infection by *Streptococcus pneumoniae* in mice. Mammalian Genome. 2003;**14**(7):448-453

[104] Yamamoto Y, Okubo S, Klein TW, Onozaki K, Saito T, Friedman H. Binding of *Legionella pneumophila* to macrophages increases cellular cytokine mRNA. Infection and Immunity. 1994;**62**(9):3947-3956

[105] Lorè NI, Iraqi FA, Bragonzi A. Host genetic diversity influences the severity of *Pseudomonas aeruginosa* pneumonia in the Collaborative Cross mice. BMC Genetics. 2015;**16**:106

[106] Vered K, Durrant C, Mott R, Iraqi FA. Susceptibility to Klebsiella pneumonaie infection in collaborative cross mice is a complex trait controlled by at least three loci acting at different time points. BMC Genomics. 2014;**15**:865

[107] The Collaborative Cross: A powerful systems genetics tool. 2009 [Available from: https://www.jax.org/news-and-insights/2009/april/the-collaborative-cross-a-powerful-systems-genetics-tool]

[108] WHO. Sex, gender and influenza. 2010 [Available from: http://apps.who.int/iris/bitstream/10665/44401/1/9789241500111_eng.pdf]

[109] Kita E, Takahashi S, Yasui K, Kashiba S. Effect of estrogen (17 beta-estradiol) on the susceptibility of mice to disseminated gonococcal infection. Infection and Immunity. 1985;**49**(1):238-243

[110] Pung OJ, Luster MI. *Toxoplasma gondii*: Decreased resistance to infection in mice due to estrogen. Experimental Parasitology. 1986;**61**(1):48-56

[111] Pung OJ, Tucker AN, Vore SJ, Luster MI. Influence of estrogen on host resistance: Increased susceptibility of mice to Listeria monocytogenes correlates with depressed production of interleukin 2. Infection and Immunity. 1985;**50**(1):91-96

[112] Gannon CJ, Pasquale M, Tracy JK, McCarter RJ, Napolitano LM. Male gender is associated with increased risk for postinjury pneumonia. Shock. 2004;**21**(5):410-414

[113] Gutiérrez F, Masiá M, Mirete C, Soldán B, Rodríguez JC, Padilla S, et al. The influence of age and gender on the population-based incidence of community-acquired pneumonia caused by different microbial pathogens. Journal of Infection. 2006;**53**(3):166-174

[114] Kadioglu A, Cuppone AM, Trappetti C, List T, Spreafico A, Pozzi G, et al. Sex-based differences in susceptibility to respiratory and systemic pneumococcal disease in mice. Journal of Infectious Diseases. 2011;**204**(12):1971-1979

[115] Guilbault C, Stotland P, Lachance C, Tam M, Keller A, Thompson-Snipes L, et al. Influence of gender and interleukin-10 deficiency on the inflammatory response during lung infection with *Pseudomonas aeruginosa* in mice. Immunology. 2002;**107**(3):297-305

[116] Wang Y, Cela E, Gagnon S, Sweezey NB. Estrogen aggravates inflammation in *Pseudomonas aeruginosa* pneumonia in cystic fibrosis mice. Respiratory Research. 2010;**11**:166

[117] Leone M, Textoris J, Capo C, Mege J-L. Sex Hormones and Bacterial Infections: IntechOpen. Rijeka, Croatia; 2012

[118] Aronica SM, Katzenellenbogen BS. Stimulation of estrogen receptor-mediated transcription and alteration in the phosphorylation state of the rat uterine estrogen receptor by estrogen, cyclic adenosine monophosphate, and insulin-like growth factor-I. Molecular Endocrinology. 1993;**7**(6):743-752

[119] Payne AH, Hales DB. Overview of steroidogenic enzymes in the pathway from cholesterol to active steroid hormones. Endocrine Reviews. 2004;**25**(6):947-970

[120] Labrie F. Extragonadal synthesis of sex steroids: Intracrinology. Annales d'Endocrinologie (Paris). 2003;**64**(2):95-107

[121] Luu-The V, Labrie F. The intracrine sex steroid biosynthesis pathways. Progress in Brain Research. 2010;**181**:177-192

[122] Foderaro A, Ventetuolo CE. Pulmonary arterial hypertension and the sex hormone paradox. Current Hypertension Reports. 2016;**18**(11):84

[123] Straub RH. The complex role of estrogens in inflammation. Endocrine Reviews. 2007;**28**(5):521-574

[124] Umar S, Rabinovitch M, Eghbali M. Estrogen paradox in pulmonary hypertension: Current controversies and future perspectives. American Journal of Respiratory and Critical Care Medicine. 2012;**186**(2):125-131

[125] Seaborn T, Simard M, Provost PR, Piedboeuf B, Tremblay Y. Sex hormone metabolism in lung development and maturation. Trends in Endocrinology and Metabolism. 2010;**21**(12):729-738

[126] Massaro GD, Mortola JP, Massaro D. Sexual dimorphism in the architecture of the lung's gas-exchange region. Proceedings of the National Academy of Sciences of the United States of America. 1995;**92**(4):1105-1107

[127] Massaro GD, Mortola JP, Massaro D. Estrogen modulates the dimensions of the lung's gas-exchange surface area and alveoli in female rats. American Journal of Physiology. 1996;**270**(1 Pt 1):L110-L114

[128] Massaro D, Massaro GD. Estrogen regulates pulmonary alveolar formation, loss, and regeneration in mice. American Journal of Physiology—Lung Cellular and Molecular Physiology. 2004;**287**(6):L1154-L1159

[129] Massaro D, Clerch LB, Massaro GD. Estrogen receptor-alpha regulates pulmonary alveolar loss and regeneration in female mice: Morphometric and gene expression studies. American Journal of Physiology - Lung Cellular and Molecular Physiology. 2007;**293**(1):L222-L228

[130] Patrone C, Cassel TN, Pettersson K, Piao YS, Cheng G, Ciana P, et al. Regulation of postnatal lung development and homeostasis by estrogen receptor beta. Molecular and Cellular Biology. 2003;**23**(23):8542-8552

[131] Liu D, Hinshelwood MM, Giguère V, Mendelson CR. Estrogen related receptor-alpha enhances surfactant protein-A gene expression in fetal lung type II cells. Endocrinology. 2006;**147**(11):5187-5195

[132] Lang TJ. Estrogen as an immunomodulator. Clinical Immunology. 2004;**113**(3):224-230

[133] Grimaldi CM, Cleary J, Dagtas AS, Moussai D, Diamond B. Estrogen alters thresholds for B cell apoptosis and activation. Journal of Clinical Investigation. 2002;**109**(12):1625-1633

[134] Grimaldi CM, Hicks R, Diamond B. B cell selection and susceptibility to autoimmunity. Journal of Immunology. 2005;**174**(4):1775-1781

[135] Gompel A, Piette JC. Systemic lupus erythematosus and hormone replacement therapy. Menopause International. 2007;**13**(2):65-70

[136] Maret A, Coudert JD, Garidou L, Foucras G, Gourdy P, Krust A, et al. Estradiol enhances primary antigen-specific CD4 T cell responses and Th1 development in vivo. Essential role of estrogen receptor alpha expression in hematopoietic cells. European Journal of Immunology. 2003;**33**(2):512-521

[137] Salem ML. Estrogen, a double-edged sword: Modulation of TH1- and TH2-mediated inflammations by differential regulation of TH1/TH2 cytokine production. Current Drug Targets. Inflammation and Allergy. 2004;**3**(1):97-104

[138] Cunningham M, Gilkeson G. Estrogen receptors in immunity and autoimmunity. Clinical Reviews in Allergy & Immunology. 2011;**40**(1):66-73

[139] Carvalho O, Gonçalves C. Expression of oestrogen receptors in foetal lung tissue of mice. Anatomia, Histologia, Embryologia. 2012;**41**(1):1-6

[140] Morani A, Warner M, Gustafsson JA. Biological functions and clinical implications of oestrogen receptors alfa and beta in epithelial tissues. Journal of Internal Medicine. 2008;**264**(2):128-142

[141] Draijer C, Hylkema MN, Boorsma CE, Klok PA, Robbe P, Timens W, et al. Sexual maturation protects against development of lung inflammation through estrogen. American Journal of Physiology—Lung Cellular and Molecular Physiology. 2016;**310**(2):L166-L174

[142] Dammann CE, Ramadurai SM, McCants DD, Pham LD, Nielsen HC. Androgen regulation of signaling pathways in late fetal mouse lung development. Endocrinology. 2000;**141**(8):2923-2929

[143] Kimura Y, Suzuki T, Kaneko C, Darnel AD, Akahira J, Ebina M, et al. Expression of androgen receptor and 5alpha-reductase types 1 and 2 in early gestation fetal lung: A possible correlation with branching morphogenesis. Clinical Science (London). 2003;**105**(6):709-713

[144] Volpe MV, Ramadurai SM, Mujahid S, Vong T, Brandao M, Wang KT, et al. Regulatory interactions between androgens, Hoxb5, and TGF β signaling in murine lung development. BioMed Research International. 2013;**2013**:320249

[145] Bresson E, Seaborn T, Côté M, Cormier G, Provost PR, Piedboeuf B, et al. Gene expression profile of androgen modulated genes in the murine fetal developing lung. Reproductive Biology and Endocrinology. 2010;**8**:2

[146] WHO. Ambient (outdoor) air quality and health. 2016 [Available from: http://www.who.int/mediacentre/factsheets/fs313/en/]

[147] Chauhan AJ, Johnston SL. Air pollution and infection in respiratory illness. British Medical Bulletin. 2003;**68**:95-112

[148] Collings DA, Sithole SD, Martin KS. Indoor woodsmoke pollution causing lower respiratory disease in children. Tropical Doctor. 1990;**20**(4):151-155

[149] Pandey MR. Domestic smoke pollution and chronic bronchitis in a rural community of the Hill Region of Nepal. Thorax. 1984;**39**(5):337-339

[150] Armstrong JR, Campbell H. Indoor air pollution exposure and lower respiratory infections in young Gambian children. International Journal of Epidemiology. 1991;**20**(2):424-429

[151] Arbex MA, Pereira LA, Carvalho-Oliveira R, Saldiva PH, Braga AL. The effect of air pollution on pneumonia-related emergency department visits in a region of extensive sugar cane plantations: A 30-month time-series study. Journal of Epidemiology & Community Health. 2014;**68**(7):669-674

[152] Wang KY, Chau TT. An association between air pollution and daily outpatient visits for respiratory disease in a heavy industry area. PLoS One. 2013;**8**(10):e75220

[153] Makri A, Stilianakis NI. Vulnerability to air pollution health effects. International Journal of Hygiene and Environmental Health. 2008;**211**(3-4):326-336

[154] Ostro B, Lipsett M, Reynolds P, Goldberg D, Hertz A, Garcia C, et al. Long-term exposure to constituents of fine particulate air pollution and mortality: Results from the California Teachers Study. Environmental Health Perspectives. 2010;**118**(3):363-369

[155] Wen M, Gu D. Air pollution shortens life expectancy and health expectancy for older adults: The case of China. Journals of Gerontology. Series A, Biological Sciences and Medical Sciences. 2012;**67**(11):1219-1229

[156] Oiamo TH, Luginaah IN. Extricating sex and gender in air pollution research: A community-based study on cardinal symptoms of exposure. International Journal of Environmental Research and Public Health. 2013;**10**(9):3801-3817

[157] Westergaard N, Gehring U, Slama R, Pedersen M. Ambient air pollution and low birth weight—Are some women more vulnerable than others? Environment International. 2017

[158] Butter ME. Are women more vulnerable to environmental pollution? Journal of Human Ecology: Kamla-Raj. 2006;**20**:221-336

[159] Rajagopalan S, Brook RD. Air pollution and type 2 diabetes: Mechanistic insights. Diabetes. 2012;**61**(12):3037-3045

[160] Kodavanti UP. Air pollution and insulin resistance: Do all roads lead to Rome? Diabetes. 2015;**64**(3):712-714

[161] Rao X, Montresor-Lopez J, Puett R, Rajagopalan S, Brook RD. Ambient air pollution: An emerging risk factor for diabetes mellitus. Current Diabetes Reports. 2015;**15**(6):603

[162] Brook RD, Cakmak S, Turner MC, Brook JR, Crouse DL, Peters PA, et al. Long-term fine particulate matter exposure and mortality from diabetes in Canada. Diabetes Care. 2013;**36**(10):3313-3320

[163] Alderete TL, Habre R, Toledo-Corral CM, Berhane K, Chen Z, Lurmann FW, et al. Longitudinal associations between ambient air pollution with insulin sensitivity, β-cell function, and adiposity in Los Angeles Latino children. Diabetes. 2017. In press

[164] Meo SA, Memon AN, Sheikh SA, Rouq FA, Usmani AM, Hassan A, et al. Effect of environmental air pollution on type 2 diabetes mellitus. European Review for Medical and Pharmacological Sciences. 2015;**19**(1):123-128

[165] Brook RD, Jerrett M, Brook JR, Bard RL, Finkelstein MM. The relationship between diabetes mellitus and traffic-related air pollution. Journal of Occupational and Environmental Medicine. 2008;**50**(1):32-38

[166] Krämer U, Herder C, Sugiri D, Strassburger K, Schikowski T, Ranft U, et al. Traffic-related air pollution and incident type 2 diabetes: Results from the SALIA cohort study. Environmental Health Perspectives. 2010;**118**(9):1273-1279

[167] Pearson JF, Bachireddy C, Shyamprasad S, Goldfine AB, Brownstein JS. Association between fine particulate matter and diabetes prevalence in the U.S. Diabetes Care. 2010;**33**(10):2196-2201

[168] Puett RC, Hart JE, Schwartz J, Hu FB, Liese AD, Laden F. Are particulate matter exposures associated with risk of type 2 diabetes? Environmental Health Perspectives. 2011;**119**(3):384-389

[169] Andersen ZJ, Raaschou-Nielsen O, Ketzel M, Jensen SS, Hvidberg M, Loft S, et al. Diabetes incidence and long-term exposure to air pollution: A cohort study. Diabetes Care. 2012;**35**(1):92-98

[170] Jerrett M, Brook R, White LF, Burnett RT, Yu J, Su J, et al. Ambient ozone and incident diabetes: A prospective analysis in a large cohort of African American women. Environment International. 2017;**102**:42-47

[171] Sun Q, Yue P, Deiuliis JA, Lumeng CN, Kampfrath T, Mikolaj MB, et al. Ambient air pollution exaggerates adipose inflammation and insulin resistance in a mouse model of diet-induced obesity. Circulation. 2009;**119**(4):538-546

[172] Goettems-Fiorin PB, Grochanke BS, Baldissera FG, Dos Santos AB, Homem de Bittencourt PI, Ludwig MS, et al. Fine particulate matter potentiates type 2 diabetes development in high-fat diet-treated mice: Stress response and extracellular to intracellular HSP70 ratio analysis. Journal of Physiology and Biochemistry. 2016;**72**(4):643-656

[173] Zhong J, Allen K, Rao X, Ying Z, Braunstein Z, Kankanala SR, et al. Repeated ozone exposure exacerbates insulin resistance and activates innate immune response in genetically susceptible mice. Inhalation Toxicology. 2016;**28**(9):383-392

[174] Haberzettl P, O'Toole TE, Bhatnagar A, Conklin DJ. Exposure to fine particulate air pollution causes vascular insulin resistance by inducing pulmonary oxidative stress. Environmental Health Perspectives. 2016;**124**(12):1830-1839

[175] Fisher-Hoch SP, Mathews CE, McCormick JB. Obesity, diabetes and pneumonia: The menacing interface of non-communicable and infectious diseases. Tropical Medicine & International Health. 2013;**18**(12):1510-1519

[176] Falagas ME, Kompoti M. Obesity and infection. Lancet Infectious Diseases. 2006;**6**(7): 438-446

[177] Baik I, Curhan GC, Rimm EB, Bendich A, Willett WC, Fawzi WW. A prospective study of age and lifestyle factors in relation to community-acquired pneumonia in US men and women. Archives of Internal Medicine. 2000;**160**(20):3082-3088

[178] Jedrychowski W, Maugeri U, Flak E, Mroz E, Bianchi I. Predisposition to acute respiratory infections among overweight preadolescent children: An epidemiologic study in Poland. Public Health. 1998;**112**(3):189-195

[179] Moore SI, Huffnagle GB, Chen GH, White ES, Mancuso P. Leptin modulates neutrophil phagocytosis of *Klebsiella pneumoniae*. Infection and Immunity. 2003;**71**(7):4182-4185

[180] Mancuso P, Gottschalk A, Phare SM, Peters-Golden M, Lukacs NW, Huffnagle GB. Leptin-deficient mice exhibit impaired host defense in Gram-negative pneumonia. Journal of Immunology. 2002;**168**(8):4018-4024

[181] Corrales-Medina VF, Valayam J, Serpa JA, Rueda AM, Musher DM. The obesity paradox in community-acquired bacterial pneumonia. International Journal of Infectious Diseases. 2011;**15**(1):e54-e57

[182] Salnikova LE, Smelaya TV, Moroz VV, Golubev AM, Rubanovich AV. Host genetic risk factors for community-acquired pneumonia. Gene. 2013;**518**(2):449-456

[183] Smelaya TV, Belopolskaya OB, Smirnova SV, Kuzovlev AN, Moroz VV, Golubev AM, et al. Genetic dissection of host immune response in pneumonia development and progression. Scientific Reports. 2016;**6**:35021

[184] Salnikova LE, Smelaya TV, Vesnina IN, Golubev AM, Moroz VV. Genetic susceptibility to nosocomial pneumonia, acute respiratory distress syndrome and poor outcome in patients at risk of critical illness. Inflammation. 2014;**37**(2):295-305

[185] Salnikova LE, Smelaya TV, Golubev AM, Rubanovich AV, Moroz VV. CYP1A1, GCLC, AGT, AGTR1 gene-gene interactions in community-acquired pneumonia pulmonary complications. Molecular Biology Reports. 2013;**40**(11):6163-6176

[186] Salnikova LE, Smelaya TV, Moroz VV, Golubev AM, Rubanovich AV. Functional polymorphisms in the CYP1A1, ACE, and IL-6 genes contribute to susceptibility to community-acquired and nosocomial pneumonia. International Journal of Infectious Diseases. 2013;**17**(6):e433-e442

[187] Azab SF, Abdalhady MA, Elsaadany HF, Elkomi MA, Elhindawy EM, Sarhan DT, et al. Interleukin-10 -1082 G/A gene polymorphisms in Egyptian children with CAP: A case-control study. Medicine (Baltimore). 2016;**95**(26):e4013

[188] Zhao J, Zhang W, Shen L, Yang X, Liu Y, Gai Z. Association of the ACE, GSTM1, IL-6, NOS3, and CYP1A1 polymorphisms with susceptibility of *Mycoplasma pneumoniae* pneumonia in Chinese children. Medicine (Baltimore). 2017;**96**(15):e6642

[189] Hayden LP, Cho MH, McDonald MN, Crapo JD, Beaty TH, Silverman EK, et al. Susceptibility to childhood pneumonia: A genome-wide analysis. American Journal of Respiratory Cell and Molecular Biology. 2017;**56**(1):20-28

[190] Chou SC, Ko HW, Lin YC. CRP/IL-6/IL-10 Single-nucleotide polymorphisms correlate with the susceptibility and severity of community-acquired pneumonia. Genetic Testing and Molecular Biomarkers. 2016;**20**(12):732-740

[191] Mao ZR, Zhang SL, Feng B. Association of IL-10 (−819 T/C, −592A/C and −1082A/G) and IL-6 -174G/C gene polymorphism and the risk of pneumonia-induced sepsis. Biomarkers. 2017;**22**(2):106-112

[192] Nascimento LF, Pereira LA, Braga AL, Módolo MC, Carvalho JA. Effects of air pollution on children's health in a city in Southeastern Brazil. Revista de Saúde Pública. 2006;**40**(1):77-82

[193] Arbex MA, Santos UeP, Martins LC, Saldiva PH, Pereira LA, Braga AL. Air pollution and the respiratory system. Jornal Brasileiro de Pneumologia. 2012;**38**(5):643-655

[194] Negrisoli J, Nascimento LF. Atmospheric pollutants and hospital admissions due to pneumonia in children. Revista Paulista de Pediatria. 2013;**31**(4):501-506

[195] Ehrlich R. Effect of nitrogen dioxide on resistance to respiratory infection. Bacteriological Reviews. 1966;**30**(3):604-614

[196] Jakab GJ. Modulation of pulmonary defense mechanisms against viral and bacterial infections by acute exposures to nitrogen dioxide. Research Report. Health Effects Institute. 1988;(20):1-38

[197] Rose RM, Fuglestad JM, Skornik WA, Hammer SM, Wolfthal SF, Beck BD, et al. The pathophysiology of enhanced susceptibility to murine cytomegalovirus respiratory infection during short-term exposure to 5 ppm nitrogen dioxide. American Review of Respiratory Diseases. 1988;**137**(4):912-917

[198] Rose RM, Pinkston P, Skornik WA. Altered susceptibility to viral respiratory infection during short-term exposure to nitrogen dioxide. Research Report. Health Effects Institute. 1989;(24):1-24

[199] Finnerty K, Choi JE, Lau A, Davis-Gorman G, Diven C, Seaver N, et al. Instillation of coarse ash particulate matter and lipopolysaccharide produces a systemic inflammatory response in mice. Journal of Toxicology and Environmental Health. Part A. 2007;**70**(23):1957-1966

[200] Lebowitz MD, Fairchild GA. The effects of sulfur dioxide and A2 influenza virus on pneumonia and weight reduction in mice: An analysis of stimulus-response relationships. Chemico-Biological Interactions. 1973;**7**(5):317-326

[201] Ameredes BT, Otterbein LE, Kohut LK, Gligonic AL, Calhoun WJ, Choi AM. Low-dose carbon monoxide reduces airway hyperresponsiveness in mice. American Journal of Physiology—Lung Cellular and Molecular Physiology. 2003;**285**(6):L1270-L1276

[202] Hollingsworth JW, Kleeberger SR, Foster WM. Ozone and pulmonary innate immunity. Proceedings of the American Thoracic Society. 2007;**4**(3):240-246

Chapter 2

# Pneumonia: A Challenging Health Concern with the Climate Change

Jean-Marie Ntumba Kayembe and
Harry-César Ntumba Kayembe

Additional information is available at the end of the chapter

http://dx.doi.org/10.5772/intechopen.71609

**Abstract**

Pneumonia is still a global health concern with high mortality rate, mainly among children under 5 years and adults over 65 years. In addition to pathogen virulence, immunoevasion capacity, and drug resistance ability, risk factors for the patient include aging, comorbidities, malnutrition, and all causes affecting the immune system. The extent to which environmental disorders affect the respiratory health is established for chronic diseases such as asthma, COPD, and cardiovascular diseases, but less is known about the underlying mechanisms of their impact on infectious diseases of the respiratory system. This chapter aims to recall the epidemiology, diagnosis, and treatment of pneumonia, with a focus on the impact of climate change and related risk factors on acute low tract respiratory infections.

**Keywords:** pneumonia, risk factors, climate change

## 1. Introduction

Pneumonia is a challenging health concern worldwide and more acutely in developing world, where healthcare facilities are less available. It is a leading cause of mortality due to infectious agents. Insufficient or inappropriate treatment contributes to the emergence of pathogen resistance to antibiotic or increased mortality. A recent report from UNICEF shows 1.4 million deaths per year among children attributable to pneumonia and diarrhea [1]. Both killers remain major contributors to child mortality worldwide, and could be fueled by climate change and related environmental deleterious effects. Pneumonia, a common lower respiratory infection accounted for 2.7 million deaths worldwide [2]; being the leading cause in children under 5 years, adults over 65 years, and immunocompromised subjects [3].

INTECH
open science | open minds

© 2017 The Author(s). Licensee InTech. This chapter is distributed under the terms of the Creative Commons Attribution License (http://creativecommons.org/licenses/by/3.0), which permits unrestricted use, distribution, and reproduction in any medium, provided the original work is properly cited. (cc) BY

According to the setting of occurrence, pneumonia is characterized as community acquired (CAP) or nosocomial, the latter occurring in the hospital after at least 48 h of admission or in a patient who has been hospitalized within the last 3–6 months and received antimicrobial treatment. Hospital-acquired pneumonia (HAP) includes really hospital acquired, ventilator-acquired pneumonia (VAP), and healthcare-associated pneumonia (HCAP) with extension to disease affecting patients in nursing homes and in dialysis services [4].

CAP represents a disease contracted out of the hospital, in the community. Clinical features allow the categorization in classic pneumonia due to bacteria such as *Streptococcus pneumoniae, Haemophilus influenzae* type b, *Staphylococcus aureus,* and viruses such as respiratory syncytial virus (29%) and influenza virus (17%); most prevalent in children and influenza virus most common in adults [4]. Atypical pneumonia results from the infection with intracellular bacteria such as Chlamydia and Mycoplasma. Nosocomial pneumonia may affect ventilated patients or not and the former group is identified as ventilator-associated pneumonia (VAMP) with a greater risk of multidrug resistance and subsequent poor prognosis. Pneumonia in the immunosuppressed host is a severe form of the disease, which may affect individual whatever the setting, with a poorer prognosis due to the underlying immune status.

Many traditional risk factors have been previously identified including extreme age (children under 60 months and adults aged ≥65 years), poverty, and comorbidities. Malnutrition, low birth weight, nonexclusive breast-feeding, lack of measles vaccination, outdoor and indoor air pollution and crowding, mother's education, parental smoking, vitamin A and/or zinc deficiencies are thought to influence children susceptibility to infections in developing countries. Possible additional risk factors thought to increase the susceptibility to respiratory infections and allergic diseases include climate change with the potential of affecting dispersion, timing, and quality of aeroallergens and the lifecycle of some vectors of diseases, high altitude, humidity, and concomitant diseases [5, 6].

This chapter aims to recall the epidemiology, diagnosis, and treatment of pneumonia, with a focus on the impact of climate change and related risk factors on acute low tract respiratory infection (ALTRI).

## 2. Climate change and respiratory health

The extent to which outdoor and indoor environments affect the respiratory health is established for chronic diseases such as asthma, COPD, and cardiovascular diseases, but less is known about the underlying mechanisms of their impact on infectious diseases of the respiratory system. Climate change is claimed to be a great global health concern. The impact of industrialization and anarchic urbanization in developing countries contributes to high production of greenhouse gases, carbon dioxide ($CO_2$), methane ($CH_4$), etc., which affect the earth temperature. The monthly average temperature is increasing leading to many weather-related events such as heat waves, humidity, precipitations, floods, storms, dry conditions, and wildfires, which affect differently the environment and human health between temperate and tropical regions [7, 8]. The increased morbidity and mortality due to ALRTI in children and adults over 65 years are linked to many risk factors, the additional effect of weather change could be powered by the inadaptability of the metabolism of these vulnerable populations to heat stress and temperature variations; emphasizing the need for further research addressing health effects of climate variations. Strategies addressing climate change are getting more and more relevant to give strong support to clean environment. There is a need to better understand the underlying mechanisms of the human, animal, or plant reactions to the changing weather to develop appropriate policies with a real impact on the susceptibility of humans to deleterious effects of the phenomenon. New technologies are underdeveloped to address the physiological responses of human and animal to the environmental-induced stress and survival, relaying on DNA/RNA sequencing as reported by Biggar et al. [9]. Stress biology research will allow implementation of targeted responses to the health effects of climate change. Direct or indirect health effects act through warming temperatures with increase in atmospheric ozone, nitrogen oxide, particulate matter (PM), sulfur dioxide, and ultraviolet (UV) radiation, resulting in many conditions such as: exacerbations of chronic respiratory diseases (asthma, COPD) and respiratory infections, as well as nonrespiratory diseases including heat stress, water-borne diseases, transmittable diseases (malaria), and malnutrition.

Heat waves, floods, wildfires may influence the incidence of respiratory infection through the shift in the epidemiology of climate sensitive pathogens. The threat on global health are highlighted by many previous studies such as one report from Australia about an increased incidence in childhood pneumonia associated with sharp temperature drops from 1 day to the next [10], or the outbreak of Hantavirus, which occurred in Panama in 2000, linked to the increase in rodent population attributed to a substantial increase in rainfall [11]. A report from Japan about aspergillosis among survivors of tsunami in 2011 is one more illustration of the link between climate change and respiratory health [12].

Respiratory infection results from inhaled aerosols or hematogenous spread of pathogens. Pathogen-related compounds (virulence, concentration, survival) or host related (immunity, comorbidities, aging) play a key role in the incidence and severity of the illness. Climate alterations could impact the disease by affecting the vectors or the host immunity [13]. The seasonality of respiratory infections has been demonstrated for influenza and streptococcal pneumonia during winter months in temperate climate [14, 15]. The later study reported a 2% incidence of CAP for all overnight hospital admissions, with a significantly higher rate during winter and spring, mainly in December and January [15].

Possible explanations of the seasonality seem to be the closer contact as a result of indoor crowding, lower humidity, induced variations in the human immune responses, indoor air pollution, low exposition to sunlight and ultraviolet (UV) radiation, keeping in mind the bactericidal effect of the latter [16]. In tropical regions, climate change also affects the pattern and seasonability of infections. Temperature, moisture and dehydration, and UV light greatly influence the pathogen cycle and survival in the environment and act on the transmission of air-borne aerosols. Dry air and wind-driven atmospheric pollutants could act on mucociliary escalator of the respiratory mucosa, impairing its defense mechanisms [17], and there is evidence from animal and human studies for the induced weaknesses of the immune system during winter [18]. Immune system is also under influence of adrenocortical hormones known to be more expressed during winter season than summer, and increased secretion of steroids is associated with immunodeficiency [19]. The rainy period is more prone to water-borne diseases such as cholera following floods and storms. The changing pattern in vector and pathogen infectivity, the low exposure to sunlight during rainy seasons, people spending more time indoor in crowded environment, with subsequent seasonal variations in vitamin D levels could explain the seasonability of infectious diseases. The deficiency in vitamin D linked to the reduced exposure of skin surface to sunlight has harmful effect on human immunity [20, 21] and could increase the vulnerability to infections, mainly in people at extreme ages.

Previous studies have emphasized the harmful role of ambient air pollution and particulate matter and the heat effect of high temperature on daily mortality [22, 23]. Climate change stands as a new health challenge for the increasing morbidity due to respiratory and cardiovascular diseases worldwide. These changes affect physical and biological systems through environmental conditions including air and water pollution, water heating, increasing the risk of transmission of water-borne pathogens. The impact of air pollution on chronic respiratory diseases such as asthma and COPD is well established. The extent to which weather patterns could influence respiratory infections is still debatable. Heat, air pollution, change in quantity and quality of aeroallergens, and shift in infectious diseases linked to changing ecology of the pathogens have been previously reported as strong risk factors affecting respiratory health. Direct health effects of climate changes include heat-related illness, exacerbations of chronic cardiorespiratory diseases such as COPD and asthma due to the changing pattern of environmental exposure [24]. Previous epidemiological studies suggest the seasonal variability of respiratory infections, but the pathobiology of this link is far from being clearly assessed. Cold and dry conditions in temperate regions power the transmission of influenza and respiratory syncytial viruses, while the wet conditions of the tropics seem to reduce the aerosol transmission of the influenza virus [25]. Studies addressing the link between climate change and pneumonia still need to be conducted worldwide, mainly in poor resource countries and also in the most affected by lack of hygiene and unpreparedness. Lower respiratory tract infections seem to be more frequent during winter in temperate areas and during rainy season in tropical regions [25, 26]. Studies in Hong Kong [27] and China [28], respectively support the impact of the changing weather pattern on the magnitude of respiratory infection and the seeking of emergency healthcare. The pattern of seasonality on viral respiratory infections has clearly been reported in temperate countries, but data from tropical regions are sparse [29]. The vulnerability of children under the tropics could be emphasized by poverty-related conditions such as malnutrition and helminth infections as well as poor access to healthcare facilities. Chronic helminth infections stimulate the T-cells to produce more Th2 type cytokines (IL-3, IL-5, IL-13) than Th-1 profile (IL-2, IFN-gamma). This imbalance could be a possible explanation for the increased susceptibility to bacterial infections in affected individuals. Lozano et al. have illustrated the negative role of air and water pollution linked to storms and floods affecting agricultural products. These authors reported an increase in pneumonia deaths in children under 5 years due to malnutrition [30]. Malnutrition predisposes to immunosuppression through lack of many elements or oligo-elements such as zinc and cupper, involved in the functionality of many components of the immune system.

Biggar et al. have illustrated the relevance of studying stress biology to characterize human responses to environmental challenges [9]; the way we will act to reduce greenhouse gas emissions will really benefit to global health.

How the climate change could impact on the transmission and outcome of infectious diseases needs to be elucidated for appropriate preparedness of the healthy systems around the world. Health effects of air pollution are of concern; atmospheric pollutants in gaseous (mainly carbon dioxide, methane, nitrous oxide) or particulate forms may affect respiratory system according to their physical properties (solubility), their concentration, and the rate and depth of the ventilation of the subject. Use of biomass fuel for cooking in many developing countries increases the risk of exposure to outdoor or indoor pollution. Biologic agents such as fungi in indoor air could trigger the respiratory system through direct toxicity, infection, or induced immune hyperresponsiveness. Smith et al. have described the risk for pneumococcal infection in children living in a low air exchange rate environment in developing countries [31]. There is a body of evidence for the association between the increasing global main temperature and increasing global mortality [32]. The heat-related risk of mortality for respiratory diseases needs to be addressed for relevant environmental measures focusing on the one health concept. Evidence of associations between outdoor heat and respiratory hospitalizations has been reported in previous studies in developed countries, but data are lacking on the harmful effects of climate change on health in developing regions, where global warming and progressive population aging are expected with the improved accessibility to ARVs and anti-tuberculosis treatments resulting in the reduction of the mortality linked to both killers. The role of sociodemographic components and low education as well as poor accessibility to healthcare in general are strong modifiers of treatment outcomes suggesting the relevance of their regular assessment as risk factors of respiratory illnesses. Along with the changing warming climate, the role of air pollution, evidenced in respiratory exacerbations of chronic diseases such as asthma, COPD, and cardiovascular diseases, following the inhalation of ozone, $SO_2$, $CO_2$, $CH_4$, and particulate matters (PM10) (from increased forest fires, wild urbanization, desertification) with aerodynamic diameters <10 μm is reported in many studies [32, 33]. Greenhouse gas emissions generated by human activity are pointed as the main provider of the changing Earth's climate through thermal stress, extreme weather events, and changing pattern of infectious diseases, suggesting the urgent need to develop strategies addressing human, animals, and plants health as a whole (one health concept). The climate change is expected to affect mainly vector-borne and water-borne infectious diseases, with a potential of increasing the range in case of nonadopting early preventive and warning measures [34]. Indirect effects of increased warming include shifts in vector-borne illness, increase in allergen concentration, loss of biodiversity, degradation of ecosystem, desertification, all with a negative impact on human health. Among realistic measures to reduce climate change-related respiratory morbidity, green structures development has been considered. Whiitford et al. [35] and Burgess et al. [36] have reported the environmental benefits of green spaces on the stabilization of ecological system and the reduction of the risk of respiratory mortality. These authors showed that largest patch percentage of green structures reduces the mortality of pneumonia and lower respiratory diseases through the reduction of primary and secondary air pollutants; while their fragmentation has deleterious effect by increasing the temperature and the air pollutants. Green spaces are shown to block secondary air pollutants (ozone and PM 2.5). Rationale management of green structures needs to be encouraged in the urbanization policies among other preventive measures to improve respiratory health [37–39].

## 3. Community-acquired pneumonia (CAP): epidemiology, clinical feature, and treatment

### 3.1. CAP: epidemiology

Community-acquired pneumonia (CAP) is still the leading cause of death attributable to infectious diseases, and epidemiological data show that its attributable mortality rate remains static or is rising, while declining for cardiovascular diseases and many cancers in developed countries [40]. Mortality in European adults varies from country to country and based on the age, it ranges from 4.5 to 5 per 100,000 in turkey and Georgia to 30 to 35 per 100,000 in Portugal and UK [41]. Near a half of under-five deaths worldwide are due to preventable diseases including pneumonia, diarrhea, and malaria with 2.2 million deaths in children under 5 years in 2012, in Nigeria, Democratic Republic of Congo, India, Pakistan, and China [42]. The overall prevalence of CAP in Africa is unknown, due to the lack of standardized protocols and reporting. A study in Uganda reported *Klebsiella pneumoniae* as the prevalent pathogen in neonates and *S. pneumoniae* was the most common etiological agent in those aged between 3 months and 5 years [43–45].

Outcome of pneumonia is still a health concern, mainly in developing countries, despite the development of new antibacterial agents. This phenomenon relays on the emerging antibiotic resistance of the pathogen on one hand and on host-related factors (impaired immunity, poor hygiene, age, malnutrition, comorbidities) on the other. Innovative approaches through better understanding of pathophysiology of the disease and environmental changes, early diagnosis techniques, multidisciplinary approach, and host-driven measures (behavior, accessibility to health facilities) need to be developed to improve the control of respiratory mortality.

Community-acquired pneumonias is the leading cause of death due to the infectious disease in both developed and developing world [22]. Developing countries are also the most affected due to many additional conditions such as poverty, low economic access to healthcare, lack of appropriate tools for early diagnosis, many socio-cultural barriers, and the unpreparedness against environmental changes. A study from Tanzania has identified the negative role of difficult diagnoses and comorbidities in the prognosis of CAP [46]. Children under 5 years and elderly are the most vulnerable population, and 30-day mortality has not been improved since the 1950s, despite the availability of new antibiotics [47]. CAP occurs in almost 1–10 per 1000 of the adult population each year and more commonly in extreme ages. According to the WHO European region report in 2010, lower respiratory tract infections ranked fifth in the global burden disease study [30]. The same report identified infectious diseases, childhood illnesses, and maternal causes of death as accounting for 70% of the burden of diseases in sub-Saharan Africa, while representing <20% in all others countries. Even reduced compared to two decades ago, the rate of mortality caused by diarrheal and low tract infection diseases remains high and the major cause of early deaths in the country. The big five, COPD, asthma, low respiratory tract infections, TB, and lung cancer are among the most common causes of severe illness death worldwide.

The lack of standardized protocols and regular statistic reports does not allow the assessment of accurate incidence rate of CAP across the sub-Saharan region. In Europe, this incidence rate in adults is between 1.07 and 1.2 per 1000 person year and 1.54 and 1.7 per 1000 population according to a report by Torres et al. [48]. Older age and underlying comorbidities including COPD, cardiovascular and liver diseases, diabetes, cancers as well as all causes of immunosuppression (steroids treatment, malnutrition, HIV-AIDS) affect the prognosis of the disease and this is highlighted by the CURB 65 criteria in use for assessing the severity of CAP. There is a regular increase in the incidence of CAP worldwide, may be associated to demographic changes, increasingly aging population, growing poverty, low accessibility to healthcare facilities, precarity and war displacements, smoking and alcohol consumption. It is more and more clear that air pollution and climate change play important roles in the rising morbidity and mortality related to respiratory diseases. The heat stress linked to the warming of the climate induces environmental changes allowing the emergence of new pathogens worldwide. The real involvement of these ecological modifications needs to be addressed.

### 3.2. Pathophysiology

Pneumonia could result from infectious pathogens including bacteria, viruses, fungi, and parasites, or from noninfectious agents, of physical or chemical nature (aspiration pneumonia, gas inhalation). The main route for bacterial contamination is bronchogenic dissemination following microaspiration of pharyngeal secretions. Hematogenous spread follows bloodstream invasion by pathogens; and infection could also spread from contiguous tissues. In the alveolar space, host local defenses through humoral or cellular-mediated immune responses or mechanical processes (mucociliary escalator, cough reflex) when overwhelmed, allow the infection onset. The inflammation in the lung structures results in the release of mediators and accumulation of an exudate impairing the local immune system. The thickening of the alveolocapillary membrane alters the gas diffusion, inducing hypoxemia. The mismatch in the ventilation-perfusion ratio due to the reduced minute-ventilation increases the hypoxemia. Pneumococcal carriage in the posterior nasopharynx is a prerequisite for the development of pneumonia due to *S. pneumoniae*. Human to human transmission occurs through inhaled aerosols or close contact. The virulence of the pathogen is carried by factors allowing adhesion to the respiratory epithelium and released virulence factors such as pneumolysin and neuraminidase, which can damage the lung structures. The concentration of the pathogens is also a requirement for the onset of disease. Host immunity through humoral- and cell-mediated immunity is the main way of defense. Airway epithelium secretes also lactoferrin with the potential of deprecating the pathogen from iron, and then impairing the growth of the bacteria. Lysozyme and human defensins are along with cathelicidin-related antimicrobial peptides LL-37, also involved in the lysis of bacteria [49]. The classic evolution of acute pulmonary inflammatory response will turn in red hepatization, gray hepatization, and resolution. Main causes of CAP are *S. pneumoniae*, *M. pneumoniae*, *H. influenzae*, *C. pneumoniae*, *Legionella* sp., or respiratory virus with influenza A and B, respiratory syncytial (RSV), rhinovirus, and parainfluenza as the most encountered. Fungal infection mainly affects immunocompromised patients and parasitic infections are mainly endemic [50]. Clinical syndrome of condensation and radiological alveolar syndrome occur in few days. Pathogens implicated in nosocomial infection include a larger panel with methicillin-resistant staphylococcus aureus (MRSA), Enterobacteriaceae, and different types with a potential of resistance and difficult to treat infections.

### 3.3. Diagnosis of CAP

Patient with CAP mainly complaints of cough, fever, shivers, pleuritic chest pain of abrupt onset. Dyspnea may occur when the involved pulmonary sector is large. Sputum production is not rare, of purulent aspect or blood stained. Physical examination may reveal a condensation syndrome with focal crackles. It is of great importance to consider also extrathoracic signs (mouth, nose, ear).

History should be extended to demographic and behavioral considerations (age, gender, style and site of living) and comorbidities. CRB65, which is a clinical score for assessment of CAP is recommended in many guidelines. It includes data about confusion, respiratory rate, blood pressure, and age $\geq 65$ years. A CRB65n score of 0 seems a patient at low risk of death and not normally requiring hospitalization.

Additional investigations are required to guide the diagnosis setting, such as inflammatory markers (leukocytosis and differential counts, ESR, CRP) and etiological identification of pathogens through conventional microbiological analyses of samples (sputum, nasotracheal aspirates, bronchoalveolar lavage), the latter could be positive in only 15% of cases. The quality of the specimen to be examined by gram stain is a prerequisite, and the sputum should contain more than 10–25 polymorphonuclear cells by microscopic screening to be suitable. Culture-based techniques are widely used for the diagnosis of pneumonia. That is the case of blood, sputum cultures, or endotracheal aspirates, which can allow pathogen identification and antibiotic sensitivity tests. Urinary antigen tests are helpful for *S. pneumoniae* and *L. pneumophila*. Molecular diagnosis tools are currently more and more used for diagnosis of infectious diseases. CRP, an acute-phase protein during acute inflammation has not proven to be accurate in differential diagnosis between bacterial or viral infections; it is nevertheless an indicator of response to the treatment. Other biomarkers are being developed, such as procalcitonin, a prohormone elevated in response to bacterial infections. Studies using this biomarker have not provided sufficient probes for large clinical use [51]. Otherwise, both biomarkers are useful in the assessment of response to treatment and suitability of the antibiotic prescribed.

Serological tests find applicability in the diagnosis of pneumonia due to atypical pathogens such as Chlamydia, Mycoplasma, and viral infections, not easy to identify by current culture-based techniques.

Molecular techniques are now developed ensuring an early diagnosis and sensitivity tests for resistance to treatment. Dried blood spots have been used for bacterial identification and have proven to be a useful and easily accessible tool for molecular diagnosis in poor resources countries [46]. Urinary antigen tests are available for *S. pneumoniae* and *L. pneumophila*.

Bronchoscopic aspirations are more relevant than sputum samples culture to minimize the likelihood of commensal flora.

Chest radiograph demonstrating a peripheral airspace consolidation pattern is relevant in the diagnosis of pneumonia. Lung shadowing of lobar pattern associated to air bronchogram is common, while centrilobular and peribronchiolar opacity are defining the bronchopneumonia pattern. The lower lobes are most commonly affected. Recent literature illustrates the relevance of lung ultrasound in the diagnosis of CAP. A multicenter study in 14 European centers has shown a sensitivity of 93.4% and a specificity of 97.7% in the confirmation of the diagnosis [52].

The differential diagnosis should consider all illness expressed with dyspnea such as pulmonary embolism, COPD exacerbations, bronchiectasis, exacerbation of fibrosis, or with cough and associated fever such as acute bronchitis.

### 3.4. Complications of CAP and prevention

CAP mortality remains high despite the development of new antibiotics and new tools for early-onset diagnosis. Main complications are sepsis and respiratory failure, but about 50% of CAP mortality in the first month is due to comorbidities [53]. Respiratory infections through hypoxemia and oxidative stress are a potential determinant of cardiovascular adverse events. The underlying atherosclerosis as shown by the increased rate of inflammatory biomarkers (fibrinogen, CRP, cytokines) in infectious status may impact on prothrombotic vascular conditions and subsequent cardiovascular ischemic diseases [54, 55]. The prognosis of acute myocardial infarction, cardiac arrhythmias, and heart failure is often worsened by respiratory infections according to few previous studies [55–57].

CAP is not simply a local but systemic inflammatory response as expressed by the measurable increase in serum biomarkers such as IL-6, IL-8, and TNF-alpha. To improve patients' outcomes, preventive measures are strongly recommended such as smoking cessation interventions and accurate screening of comorbidities. About a half of CAP mortality within the first month is due to the comorbidities such as cardiovascular complications, cancer, chronic lower respiratory diseases renal failure, and infections, mainly involving the elderly [58, 59]. Cardiovascular mortality contributes for almost 30% of deaths after CAP; that is the case of myocardial infarction in a multicenter study by Lichtman et al. reporting a 7.2% of CAP in patients admitted to the hospital with an acute myocardial infarction [60]. Cardiac arrhythmias are also observed sometimes induced by the use of macrolides alone or in combination therapy [61]. Respiratory infections were more frequent (19 vs. 6%) in a comparison study of stroke patients and control [62], suggesting the comorbidity of this condition.

Empyema is a harmful complication of pneumonia occurring mostly in more vulnerable subjects (comorbidities, immune disorders).

Preventive measures through behavioral changes such as smoking cessation and vaccination in vulnerable populations such as drepanocytosis patients, COPD, renal insufficiency patients with influenza, and pneumococcal vaccines need to be largely implemented to reduce the mortality rate.

### 3.5. Treatment of CAP

Severity assessment is a prerequisite to an accurate decision for the place of care (ICU or not). Empirical antibiotic therapy is widely used in the treatment of CAP and should include pneumococcal coverage. The promptitude of the treatment (less than 8 h from diagnosis) has been shown to improve mortality rate. Few recommendations by the American Thoracic Society (ATS) emphasize the relevance of some conditions such as the severity of the pneumonia, the previous health status of the patient, the comorbidities, and a previous use of antibiotic therapy less than 3 months. The combination therapy or the monotherapy is regularly questioned, but evidence shows the superiority of the combination therapy in severe patients [57, 63, 64]. The use of pneumonia severity index and CURB 65 will help to improve the outcomes of CAP, by a relevant orientation of the patients. In ambulatory patients with mild to moderate disease, monotherapy, and mainly by oral route is a common practice. The empirical choice is the class of β-lactamases (amoxicillin) or macrolides in case of allergy to the former. Fluoroquinolones in monotherapy, even recommended in some developed countries such as the North America should be discouraged in the settings where TB is a great concern, because of the influence of these drugs on the delay of TB diagnosis and the lack of alternative diagnosis tools for smear-negative tuberculosis. Macrolides and doxycycline are suitable when mycoplasma or chlamydia are the suspected etiologic agents. A previous history of antibiotic therapy in the latter 3 months guides the choice for a not yet used antibiotic by the patient. This is to minimize the emergence of resistance to antibiotics. In hospitalized patients, a part from taking care of the comorbidities, monotherapy using amoxicillin-clavulanic acid may be a choice according to the severity of the illness; combination therapy of the latter with advanced macrolides (clarithromycin, azithromycin) is often recommended. In case of a risk of aspiration pneumonia (Dementia, Alzheimer, Diphtheria), the clindamycin should be added. Patients admitted in ICU need combination therapy as first choice and G3-cephalosporins; or carbapenems are regularly prescribed. The emergence of resistance is nevertheless a threat in these critically ill subjects. Adjunctive therapies in hospitalized patients include oxygen suppliance if necessary, low doses corticosteroids in suspected adrenal insufficiency following the bacteremia phase may be added to improve outcomes. Nonsevere CAP could be treated ambulatory with a 7-day monotherapy with oral antibiotics. The use of pneumonia severity index and CURB 65 or serum biomarkers may improve the prognosis of the illness. Among the biomarkers, the procalcitonin has been assessed in the decision of initiation or discontinuation of antibiotic therapy in adults. The discontinuation may be applied if the PCT level after 3 days is lower than 0.25 ng/mL or as decreased by more than 80–90% relative to the initial value [65].

## 4. Conclusion

Pneumonia remains a global threat despite the development of newer antibiotics. Early diagnosis tools need to be widely available, including easily accessible molecular analyzes. The empirical antibiotic treatment should relay on site of care, severity index of the disease, comorbidities, cost effectiveness, but also on identifications of new risk factors challenging the outcomes of patients such as climate changes.

## Author details

Jean-Marie Ntumba Kayembe[1]* and Harry-César Ntumba Kayembe[2]

*Address all correspondence to: dr12jmkayembe@yahoo.com

1 Pneumology Unit, Department of Internal Medicine, Faculty of Medicine, University of Kinshasa, DR Congo

2 Ecom-Alger, University of Kinshasa, DR Congo

## References

[1] UNICEF The State of the World's Children 2016. Available from: https://www.unicef.org/publications/files/UNICEF_SOWC_2016.pdf [Accessed: 2017-07-01]

[2] GBD Collaborators. Global, regional and national levels of age-specific mortality and 240 causes of death. 1990-2013: A systematic analysis for the Global burden of Disease Study 2013. Lancet. 2015;**385**:1990-2013

[3] Tong N. Background Paper 6.22 Pneumonia 2013. http://www.who.int/medicines/BP622Pneumo.pdf [Accessed: January 16, 2016]

[4] Marcos MA, Esperatti M, Torres A. Viral pneumonia. Current Opinion in Infectious Diseases. 2009;**22**:143-147

[5] Rudan I, Boschi-Pinto C, Biloglav Z, et al. Epidemiology and etiology of childhood pneumonia. Bulletin of the World Health Organization. 2008;**86**:408-416. DOI: 10.2471/BLT.07.048769

[6] Boloursaz MR, Lotfian F, Aghahosseini F, et al. Epidemiology of lower respiratory tract infections in children. Journal of Comprehensive Pediatrics. 2013;**4**:93-98. DOI: 10.17795/compreped-10273

[7] Overpeck JT, Otto-Bliesner BL, Miller GH, Muhs DR, Alley RB, Kiehl JT. Paleoclimatic evidence for future ice-sheet instability and rapid sea-level rise. Science. 2006;**311**:1747-1750

[8] Alley RB, Clark PU, Huybrechts P, Joughin I. Ice-sheet and see-level changes. Science. 2005;**310**:456-460

[9] Biggar KK, Storey KB. New approaches to comparative and animal stress biology research in the post-genomic era: A contextual overview. Computational and Structural Biotechnology Journal. 2014;**30**:138-146. DOI: 10.1016/j. csbj.2014.09.006 eCollection 2014 Sep

[10] Mirsaeidi M, Motahari H, Khamesi MT, Sharif A, Campos M, Schraufnagel DE. Climate change and respiratory infections. Annals of the American Thoracic Society. 2016;**13**(8):1223-30. DOI: 10.1513/AnnalsATS.201511-729PS

[11] Bayard V, Kitsutani PT, Barria EO, Rueda LA, Tinnin DS, Mnoz C, de Mosca IB, Guerrero G, Kant R, Garcia A, *et al*. Outbreak of hantavirus pulmonary syndrome, Los Santos, Panama,1999-2000. Emerging Infectious Diseases. 2004;**10**:1635-1642

[12] Kawakami Y, Tagami T, Kusakabe T, Kido N, Kawaguchi T, Omura M, Tosa R. Disseminated aspergillosis associated with tsunami lung. Respiratory Care. 2012;**57**:1674-1678

[13] Dobson A. Climate variability, global change, immunity, and the dynamics of infectious diseases. Ecology. 2009;**90**:920-927

[14] Ben-Shimol S, Greenberg D, Hazan G, Shemer-Avni Y, Givon-Lavi N, Dagan R. Seasonality of both bacteremic and nonbacteremic pneumonia coincides with viral lower respiratory tract infections in early childhood, in contrast to nonpneumonia invasive pneumococcal disease, in the pre-pneumococcal conjugate vaccine era. Clinical Infectious Diseases. 2015;**60**:1384-1387

[15] Murdoch KM, Mitra B, Lambert S, Erbas B. What is the seasonal distribution of community acquired pneumonia over time? A systematic review. Australasian Emergency Nursing Journal. 2014;**17**:30-42

[16] White AN, Ng V, Spain CV, Johnson CC, Kinlin LM, Fisman DN. Let the sun shine in: Effects of ultraviolet radiation on invasive pneumococcal disease risk in Philadelphia, Pennsylvania. BMC Infectious Diseases. 2009;**9**:196

[17] Agius AM, Smallman LA, Pahor AL. Age, smoking and nasalciliary beat frequency. Clinical Otolaryngology and Allied Sciences. 1998;**23**:227-230

[18] Altizer S, Dobson A, Hosseini P, Hudson P, Pascual M, Rohani P. Seasonality and the dynamics of infectious diseases. Ecology Letters. 2006;**9**:467-484

[19] Skwarlo-Sonta K. Functional connections between the pineal gland and immune system. Acta Neurobiologiae Experimentalis. 1996;**56**(1):341-357

[20] Fares A. Factors influencing the seasonal patterns of infectious diseases. International Journal of Preventive Medicine. 2013;**4**:128-132

[21] Yamshchikov AV, Desai NS, Blumberg HM, Ziegler TR, Tangpricha V. Vitamin D for treatment and prevention of infectious diseases: A systematic review of randomized controlled trials. Endocrine Practice. 2009;**15**:438-449

[22] Zanobetti A, Schwartz J, Samoli E, et al. The temporal pattern of respiratory and heart disease mortality in response to air pollution. Environmental Health Perspectives. 2003;**111**(9): 1188-1193

[23] Michelozzi P, Accetta G, De Sario M, et al. High temperature and hospitalizations for cardiovascular and respiratory causes in 12 European cities. American Journal of Respiratory and Critical Care Medicine. 2009;**179**(5):388-383

[24] Takaro TK, Knowlton K, Balmes JR. Climate change and respiratory health: current evidence and knowledge gaps. Expert Review of Respiratory Medicine. 2013;**7**(4):349-361. DOI: 10.1586/17476348.2013.814367

[25] Paynter S. Humidity and respiratory virus transmission in tropical and temperate settings. Epidemiology and Infection. 2015;**143**(6):1110-1118. DOI: 10.1017/S0950268814002702 Epub 2014 Oct 13

[26] Yusuf S, Piedimonte G, Auais A, et al. The relationship of meteorological conditions to the epidemic activity of respiratory syncytial virus. Epidemiology and Infection. 2007;**135**(7): 1077-1090

[27] Chan PK, Mok HY, Lee TC, Chu IM, Lam WY, Sung JJ. Seasonal influenza activity in Hong Kong and its association with meteorological variations. Journal of Medical Virology. 2009;**81**(10):1797-1806

[28] Ge WZ, Xu F, Zhao ZH, Zhao JZ, Kan HD. Association between diurnal temperature range and respiratory tract infections. Biomedical and Environmental Sciences. 2013;**26**(3):222-225

[29] Kamogaki T, Chaw L, Tan Alvin G, Tamaki R, Alday PP, Javier JB, et al. Seasonality of influenza and respiratory syncytial viruses and the effect of climate factors in subtropical- tropical Asia using influenza-like Illnes surveillance data, 2010-2012. PLoS One. 2016;**11**(12): e0167712

[30] Lozano R, Naghavi M, Foreman K, et al. Global and regional mortality from 235 causes of death for 20 age groups in 1990 and 2010: A systematic analysis for the global burden of disease study 2010. Lancet. 2012;**380**(9859):2095-2128

[31] Brooke Anderson G, Dominici F, Wang Y, Meredith C, et al. HEAT-related emergency hospitalizations for respiratory diseases in the medicare population. American Journal of Respiratory and Critical Care Medicine. 2013;**187**(10):1098-1103

[32] McMichael AJ, Wooddruff RE, Hales S. Climate change and human health: Present and future risks. Lancet. 2006;**367**(9513):859-863

[33] Kinney PL. Climate change, air quality, and human health. American Journal of Preventive Medicine. 2008;**35**(5):459-467

[34] Shuman EK. Global climate change and infectious diseases. The International Journal of Occupational and Environmental Medicine. 2011;**2**(1):11-19

[35] Whiitford V, Ennos AR, Handley JF. City form and natural process–indicators for the ecological performance of urban areas and their application to Mersseyside, UK. Landscape and Urban Planning. 2001;**57**:91-103. DOI: 10.1016/s0169-2046(01)00192-x

[36] Burgess J, Harrison CM, Limb M. People, parks and urban green: A study of popular meanings and values for open spaces in the city. Urban Studies. 1988;**25**:455-473. DOI: 10.1080/00420988820080631

[37] Jim CY, Chen WY. Assessing the ecosystem service of air pollutant removal by urban trees in Guanzhou (China). Journal of Environmental Management. 2008;**88**:665-676. DOI: 10.1016/j.jenvman.2007.03.035

[38] Jo H-k. Impacts of urban greenspace on offsetting carbon emissions for middle Korea. Journal of Environmental Management. 2002;**64**:115-126. DOI: 10.1006/jema.2001.0491

[39] Yang J, McBride J, Zhou J, Sun Z. The urban forest in Beijing and its role in air pollution reduction. Urban Forestry & Urban Greening. 2015;**3**:65-78. DOI: 10.1016/j.scitotenv. 20145.03.1030

[40] Chalmers JD, Plet MW, Aliberti S. Community-Acquired Pneumonia. European Respiratory Monographs. Sheffield: European Respiratory Society; 2014. ISBN: 978-1-849-84049-1

[41] Gibson GJ, Loddenkemper R, Lundba B, Sibille Y. Respiratory health and disease in Europe: the new European Lung White Book. Respiratory Health and Disease in Europe. Sheffield: European Respiratory Society; 2013; **42**:559-563. DOI: 10.1183/09031936.00105513

[42] Guerrera G. Neonatal and pediatric healthcare worldwide: A report from UNICEF. Clinica Chimica Acta. 2015;**451**:4-8

[43] Delport SD, Brisley T. Aetiology and outcome of severe community-acquired pneumonia in children admitted to a paediatric intensive care unit. South African Medical Journal. 2002;**92**:907-911. 12506595

[44] Adegbola RA, Falade AG, Sam BE, Aidoo M, Baldeh I, Hazlett D, Whittle H, Greenwood BM, Mulholland EK. The etiology of pneumonia in malnourished and well-nourished Gambian children. The Pediatric Infectious Disease Journal. 1994;**13**:975-982; PMID:7845751. http://dx.doi.org/10.1097/00006454-199411000-00008

[45] Johnson A-W, Osinusi K, Aderele WI, Gbadero DA, Olaleye OD, Adeyemi-Doro FAB. Etiologic agents and outcome determinants of community-acquired pneumonia in urban children: A hospital-based study. Journal of the National Medical Association. 2008;**100**:370-385; PMID:18481475. http://dx.doi.org/10.1016/S0027-9684(15)31269-4

[46] Caggiano S, Ullmann N, De Vitis E, Trivelli M, Mariani C, Podagrosi M, Ursitti F, et al. Factors that negatively affect the prognosis of pediatric community-acquired pneumonia in district hospital in Tanzania. International Journal of Molecular Sciences. 2017;**18**:3. DOI: 10.3390/ijms18030623

[47] Shaddock EJ. Pneumonia. Nathan. 2016;**8**:17. DOI: 10.1186/s41479-016-0017-7.eCollection 2016

[48] Torres A, Peetermans WE, Viegi G, et al. Risk factors for community-acquired pneumonia in adults in Europe: A literature review. Thorax. 2013;**68**:105761065

[49] Tecle T, Tripathi S, Hartshor KL. Defensins and cathelicidins in lung immunity. Innate Immunity. 2010; **16**:151-159

[50] Ntumba Jean-Marie Kayembe. Tropical Lung Diseases, Oncogenesis, Inflammatory and Parasitic Tropical Diseases of the Lung, Prof. Jean-Marie Kayembe (Ed.), InTech, 2013. DOI: 10.5772/52371. Available from: https://www.intechopen.com/books/oncogenesis-inflammatory-and-parasitic-tropical-diseases-of-the-lung/tropical-lung-diseases

[51] Holm A, Pedersen SS, Nexoe J, et al. Procalcitonin versus C-reactive protein for predicting pneumonia in adults with lower respiratory tract infection in primary care. The British Journal of General Practice. 2007;**57**:555-560

[52] Reissig A, Copetti R, Mathis G, et al. Lung ultrasound in the diagnosis and follow-up of community-acquired pneumonia: A prospective; multicenter, diagnostic accuracy study. Chest. 2012;**142**:965-972

[53] Mortensen EM, Coley CM, Singer DE, et al. Causes of death for patients with community -acquired pneumonia results from the pneumonia patient outcomes research team cohort study. Archives of Internal Medicine. 2002;**162**:1059-1064

[54] Meier CR, Jick SS, Derby LE, et al. Acute respiratory-tract infection and risk of first time acute myocardial infarction. Lancet. 1998;**351**:146761471

[55] Clayton TC, Thompson M, Meade TW. Recent respiratory infection and risk of cardiovascular disease: Case-control study through a general practice database. European Heart Journal. 2008;**29**:96-103

[56] Spodick DH, Flessas AP, Johson MM. Association of acute respiratory symptoms with onset of acute myocardial infarction, prospective investigation of 150 consecutive patients and matched control patients. The American Journal of Cardiology. 1984;**53**:481-482

[57] Brown RB, Iannini P, Gross P, et al. Impact of initial antibiotic choice on clinical outcomes in community-acquired pneumonia analysis a hospital claims-made database. Chest. 2003;**123**:1503-1511

[58] Bracanti FL, Chow JW, Wagener MM, et al. Is pneumonia really the old man's friend? Two year prognosis after community-acquired pneumonia. Lancet;**342**:30-33

[59] Yende S, D'Angelo G, Kellun JA, et al. Inflammatory markers at hospital discharge predict subsequent mortality after pneumonia and sepsis. American Journal of Respiratory and Critical Care Medicine. 2008;**177**:1242-1247

[60] Lichtman JH, Fathi A, Radford MJ, et al. Acute, severe non cardiac conditions in patients with acute myocardial infarction. American Journal of Medicine. 2006;**119**:843-850

[61] Wayne RA, Murray KT, Hall K, et al. Azithromycin and the risk of cardiovascular death. The New England Journal of Medicine. 2012;**366**:1881-1890

[62] Zurru MC, Alonzo C, Brescacin L, et al. Recent respiratory infection predicts atherothrombotic stroke : Case-control study in a Buenos Aires healthcare system. Stroke. 2009;**40**:1986-19990

[63] Tessmer A, Welte T, Martus P, et al. Impact of intravenous ß-lactam monotherapy on mortality in hospitalized patients with community-acquired pneumonia. The Journal of Antimicrobial Chemotherapy. 2009;**63**:1025-1033

[64] Rodrigo C, Mckeever TM, Woodhead M, et al. Single versus combination antibiotic therapy in adults hospitalized with community acquired pneumonia. Thorax. 2013;**68**:493-495

[65] Quenot JP, Luyt CH-E, Roche N, Chalumeau M, Charles PE, Claessens YE, et al. Role of biomarkers in the management of antibiotic therapy: An expert panel review II: Clinical use of biomarkers for initiation or discontinuation of antibiotic therapy. Annals of Intensive Care. 2013;**3**:21

Section 2

# Drug-Resistant Pneumonia

Chapter 3

# The Emerging Problems of Carbapenem-Resistant Gram-Negative Bacillary Pneumonia

Mihaela Ileana Ionescu

Additional information is available at the end of the chapter

http://dx.doi.org/10.5772/intechopen.69630

**Abstract**

Carbapenem-resistant Gram-negative organisms are increasingly isolated from lower respiratory tract infections. Limited treatment options are the main problems for physicians and clinical microbiologists who have to face such clinical cases. Bacteriological diagnosis, starting with accurate Gram smear performed from properly collected specimens and ending with antibiotic susceptibility testing, is essential. Morphological characters of bacterial cells provide important clues about the nature of infection, prior to bacterial isolation and identification. Attempts to find complementary options for the respiratory contamination and treatment of carbapenem-resistant Gram-negative bacillary pneumonia led us to test the susceptibility of 21 essential oils. Among them, *Thymus vulgaris, Eugenia caryophyllata, Origanum vulgare, Melaleuca alternifolia* and *Aniba rosaeodora* essential oils proved to be efficient against *Acinetobacter baumannii* carbapenem-resistant strain and *Escherichia coli* ATCC 25922. In an attempt to evaluate the magnitude of environmental spreading of the carbapenemase genes, 40 carbapenemase sequences of different organisms were compared. Carbapenemases show striking similarities inside each beta-lactamase class (A, D, and B), no matter their origin—environmental organisms or clinical isolates. Class B carbapenemases are most widely distributed, metallo-beta-lactamases being present in bacteria as well in Archaea.

**Keywords:** carbapenemase producer, nosocomial pneumonia, essential oils, environmental pollution

## 1. Introduction

*Enterobacteriaceae* and nonfermenters Gram-negative bacilli are increasingly isolated from lower respiratory tract infections. In patients in intensive care units (ICUs), the ventilator-associated pneumonia (VAP) is a constant concern for practitioners [1]. Improving the management of bacterial pneumonia led to guidelines for use by health-care personnel.

INTECH
open science | open minds

© 2017 The Author(s). Licensee InTech. This chapter is distributed under the terms of the Creative Commons Attribution License (http://creativecommons.org/licenses/by/3.0), which permits unrestricted use, distribution, and reproduction in any medium, provided the original work is properly cited. (cc) BY

Nosocomial infections caused by Gram-negative bacteria resistant to carbapenems, mostly multiple-resistant, represent a challenge due to limited treatment options [2, 3]. Like other beta-lactamines, the carbapenems are included in preferred treatment regimens for various infectious diseases [4]. Antibiotic-resistant patterns of bacterial isolates from nosocomial infections are continuously changed. Therefore, it is of highest interest in finding alternative methods for preventing contamination with multidrug-resistant strains. Since ancient times, people have had an intuitive feeling that some spices have real benefits not only as air fresheners but also in that era they were the only therapeutic option for many diseases. Thus, they correctly guessed that concentrated lotions/oils are not only more efficient but easy to use and to store. Essential oils (EOs) from natural products proved their positive effects in various clinical conditions. Although the specific mechanisms of their components are not deciphered, many studies demonstrated certain biological activity of some phytochemicals. Terpinen-4-ol found in many EOs are demonstrated to act synergistically with chemotherapeutic agents in digestive malignancies [5]. There are many studies about antibacterial effects of EOs, mainly on supragingival plaque. The results are not constant, for example, some authors do not find a positive effect of tea tree oil on supragingival plaque [6].

Antibiotic-resistance genes are nowadays a constant presence not only in the hospital environment but are also more and more demonstrated in various ecosystems [7–9]. Antibiotic-resistance genes naturally already exist in organisms living in most diverse environments. Surely, antibiotic-resistance genes have an essential role in maintaining of inter-species equilibrium on specific ecosystems [10]. All living things from prokaryotes to eukaryotes are constantly exposed to a huge mixture of organic and inorganic compounds. Even if, nowadays, accurate methods exist to isolate and to characterize antibiotic-resistant microorganisms, it is not possible to calculate the influence of a myriad factors that interfere in every environment. An interesting study demonstrated the utility of transmission electron microscopy for observing of aquatic microorganism structural abnormalities in different environmental conditions [11]. The terrestrial ecosystem is also prone to be reshaped by human activities [12]. Intensive farming implies antibiotics, so the spread of intestinal bacteria which harbor antibiotic-resistance genes is an immediate consequence. This does not imply that once a certain bacteria species is present in a certain geographic area its antibiotic-resistance pattern remains unchanged. Atmospheric conditions, notably rainfalls, could contribute to spreading of contaminants from the soil to groundwater and greatly alter the count of microorganisms. Different bacterial species do not behave the same, antibiotic-resistance patterns differently changed, but certain beta-lactamines could be used as indicators of antibiotic resistance at least for *Escherichia coli* [13]. Consequently, it is not wrong to include antibiotic-resistance genes into the long list of environmental pollutants [14].

The physicians require bacteriological diagnosis on admission of the patients in ICUs and for surveillance of any nosocomial infection. For respiratory infections, Gram smears from sputum, endotracheal aspirate, or bronchoalveolar lavage are mandatory. Very often in ICUs, respiratory infections are due to carbapenem-resistant Gram-negative bacilli. In our opinion, testing volatile EOs, as complementary substances, for prevention of respiratory infections is not a futile idea. Finally, last but not least, wide use of antibiotics alters not only the hospital environment but also disturbs other ecological niches (water and soil). These topics will be our concern in the next sections.

## 2. Carbapenem resistance

The carbapenems are sometimes the last-resort antibiotics for treating of extended spectrum beta-lactamase (ESBL) producing Gram-negative bacteria. But carbapenem resistance is increasingly reported in *Enterobacteriaceae* and nonfermenters like *Acinetobacter* spp. or *Pseudomonadaceae*. Carbapenem resistance is mainly due to carbapenemase (E.C. 3.5.2.6) production. Structural classification of beta-lactamases implies the primary structure (sequence homology) and distinguishes four molecular classes of beta-lactamases—A, C, D (serine beta-lactamases), and B (MBL-metallo beta-lactamase) [15–17]. Functional classifications of beta-lactamases are more closer to clinical issues [18, 19] and recognize three groups of beta-lactamases: Group 1 (Class C) cephalosporinases; Group 2 (Classes A and D) broad-spectrum beta-lactamases, inhibitor-resistant beta-lactamases, extended-spectrum beta-lactamases, serine carbapenemases, and Group 3 metallo-beta-lactamases. So far in this section, we have taken in consideration only different types of beta-lactamases as a resistance mechanism. Besides producing carbapenemases, the reduction of carbapenem influx into the periplasma is commonly observed in clinical isolates. Different mutations in porins significantly contribute to the failing of drug accumulation at appropriate concentration in periplasmic space; therefore, carbapenem resistance is often more complex than one thought at the first sight [20]. Readers, who wish to know further details regarding carbapenem resistance, should consult excellent papers devoted to this particular topic [21–24].

## 3. Microbiological investigations

Microbiological evaluation is mandatory for an adequate therapeutic regimen; accurate identification of the bacterial species is essential to avoid administration of broad-spectrum antibiotics. The optimal recovery of the pathogens ultimately depends on the accuracy of sample collection (sputum, endotracheal aspirate, or bronchoscopically obtained specimens by bronchoalveolar lavage). Bacteriological assessment of lower respiratory tract infections begins with care evaluation of Gram-stained smear performed from respiratory tract specimen. The low-power scanning provides a first sight of the quality of the sample—for sputum more than 10 squamous epithelial cells show oropharyngeal contamination. The examination with the oil immersion provides more details regarding bacterial morphology. The importance of this step in the management of bacterial pneumonia is well recognized. As illustrated in **Figures 1** and **2**, it is possible to anticipate the diagnosis toward a nonfermenter or an *Enterobacteriaceae*. *Acinetobacters* are short Gram-negative nonsporing bacilli but in exponential phase became coccoids often arranged in diplo. Many strains are encapsulated and sometimes retain the methyl violet in Gram's stain. The *Enterobacteriaceae* appear typically as Gram-negative nonsporing bacilli with parallel sides and rounded ends. There are wide ranges of derivatives from this classical appearance, from filamentous rods to coccoids. Some species are encapsulated, for example, *Klebsiella*, sometimes *E. coli.*

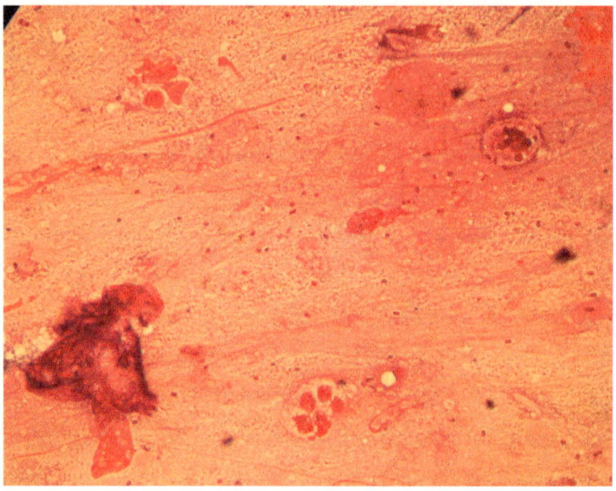

**Figure 1.** High-power examination (1000× magnification). Gram-stained smear of endotracheal aspirate shows Gram-negative coccobacilli isolated or in diplo (*Acinetobacter* spp.).

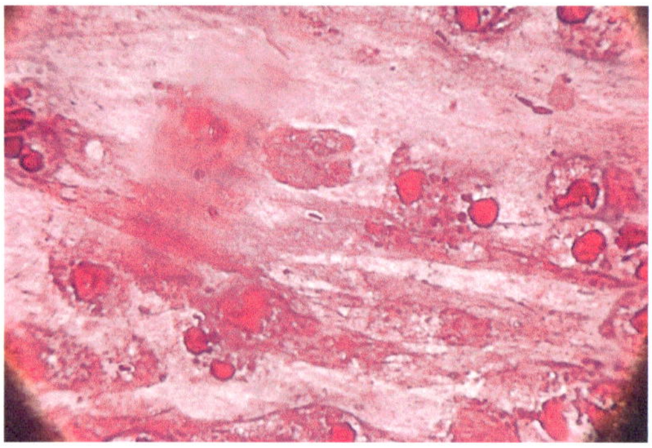

**Figure 2.** High-power examination (1000× magnification). Gram-stained smear of endotracheal aspirate shows Gram-negative capsulate rods.

Since this chapter is not intended to be a highly elaborate description of bacterial diagnosis of Gram-negative bacillary pneumonia, further details about isolation and bacterial identification were not be reviewed. However, the microscopic examination of clinical sample offers essential clues about the nature of bacterial infection. For busy clinicians—in ICUs the physicians have always needed a microbiologic response as quickly as possible—these details, provided in advance, could make the difference.

## 4. Therapeutic issues

### 4.1. Prevention of respiratory contamination

A particular issue of ventilator associated pneumonia (VAPs) is the risk of infection with multidrug-resistant strains and carbapenem-resistant bacilli too. Not surprisingly, severely injured patients—VAPs and burn patients—are most prone to infection with carbapenem-resistant species. The chief question for carbapenem-resistant Gram-negative bacillary pneumonia is how to efficiently prevent them. First of all, could these infections be stopped? In the hospital environment, hand hygiene and alcohol-based disinfection remain, undeniably, the sanitation gold standard. Rigorous monitoring of patients at admission and an accurate history are early stages in identification of patients with documented multidrug-resistant strains for further isolation or, at least clustering separately to prevent the risk of cross-contamination [25, 26]. Respiratory contamination depends on so many circumstances, almost impossible to eliminate, that the specific strategies are designed in order to reduce VAP, rather than to eliminate such infections [27]. What else could be taken in consideration apart from already established strategies? As it was underlined in introduction, from the ancient times, people are aware of the so-called air purification performed intuitively by burning scented substances or widespread use of all sorts of perfumes, plant extracts, or spices.

### 4.2. Antibiotic therapy

Antibiotic regimens of carbapenem-resistant bacillary pneumonia often rely only on few antibiotics. Although there is not an ideal therapeutic regimen for the treatment of pneumonia due to carbapenem-resistant species, Polymixin B, Tigecycline, and Amikacine remain the most valid options [28]. A prerequisite for adequate treatment of VAPs is intravenous administration of the suitable antibiotic. Aerosolized antibiotics delivery has been experimentally studied in order to reduce the side effects of systemic administration of antibiotics. Efficiency of these methods relies on the antibiotics' ability on crossing the alveolar-capillary membrane [29]. An abundant literature is devoted to the issue of carbapenem-resistant strains. Because antibiotic resistance continuously evolved, clinical guidelines rapidly changed, therefore, a unique treatment scheme is almost impossible to establish. Clearly, we must look at the information provided by extensive epidemiological studies to up-date infection control and treatment options [30].

### 4.3. Inhibitory activity of essential oils

In spite of specific protocols implemented in ICUs, it is worthwhile to consider additional methods to prevent respiratory contamination. We should be considering the inhibitory effect of some essential oils (EOs), underlining the efficiency of volatile substances. EOs are more and more regarded as complementary to antibiotic therapy [31–35]. In our previous work, we demonstrated the high activity of EOs against *E. coli* for coriander (*Coriandrum sativum* L.), peppermint (*Mentha piperita* L.), and juniper (*Juniperus communis* L.) [36].

#### *4.3.1. Materials and methods*

We are interested in evaluating of the efficiency of some EOs against carbapenem-resistant *Acinetobacter baumannii* and *E. coli* ATCC 25922. *A. baumannii* is a ubiquitous nonfermenter species, found in soil, water, and clinical units, and *E. coli* is a constant presence of the normal microbiocenosis of humans and warm-blood animals. Of hundreds of natural products commercially available, without prescription, only 21 volatile extracts (**Table 1**) were tested undiluted by two methods—diffusimetric method and aromatogram—described elsewhere [36]. Diffusimetric sensibility testing demonstrates the antibacterial activity by charging 5 mm diameter sterile paper disk with 2 or 5 μl of EOs. The aromatogram method is illustrated in **Figure 3**. Each experiment was performed three times at intervals of 2–3 days. The results are presented as mean and standard deviation (SD).

| No | EO | Species | Family | Producer | Administration |
|---|---|---|---|---|---|
| 1 | Thyme | *Thymus vulgaris* | Lamiaceae | Fares | Internal use, aromatherapy, massage |
| 2 | Clove | *Eugenia cayophyllata* | Myrtaceae | Fares | Internal use, aromatherapy, massage |
| 3 | Eucalyptus | *Eucalyptus globulus* | Myrtaceae | Fares | Internal use, aromatherapy, massage |
| 4 | Juniper | *Juniperus communis* | Cupressaceae | Fares | Internal use, aromatherapy, massage |
| 5 | Lavander | *Lavandula angustifolia* | Lamiaceae | Fares | Internal use, aromatherapy, massage |
| 6 | Mint | *Mentha piperita* | Labiatae | Fares | Internal use, aromatherapy, massage |
| 7 | Pine | *Pinus silvestris* | Pinaceae | Fares | Internal use, aromatherapy, massage |
| 8 | Rosemary | *Rosmarinus officinalis* | Lamiaceae | Fares | Internal use, aromatherapy, massage |
| 9 | Tea tree | *Melaleuca alternifolia* | Myrtaceae | Fares | Internal use, aromatherapy, massage |
| 10 | Oregano | *Origanum vulgare* | Lamiaceae | Steaua Divina | Internal use, aromatherapy, massage |
| 11 | Negril | *Nigella sativa* | Ranunculaceae | Steaua Divina | Internal use, aromatherapy, massage |
| 12 | Lemon | *Citrus limonum* | Rutaceae | Steaua Divina | Internal use, aromatherapy, massage |
| 13 | Fennel | *Foeniculi fructus* | Apiaceae | Hofigal | Internal use |
| 14 | Sage | *Salvia officinalis* | Lamiaceae | Solaris | Aromatherapy, massage |

| No | EO | Species | Family | Producer | Administration |
|---|---|---|---|---|---|
| 15 | Sandalwood | *Santal amyris* | Rutaceae | Herbavit | Aromatherapy, massage |
| 16 | Seeds of apricots | *Prunus armeniaca* | Rosaceae | Herbavit | Internal use |
| 17 | Incense | *Boswellia serrata* | Burseraceae | Bionovativ | Internal use |
| 18 | Inhalant | *Pinus sylvestis, Salvia officinalis, Chamommilla recutita, Lavandula angustifolia* extracts, *Propolis cera,* Eucalyptus oil | | Tisofit | Inhalations |
| 19 | Grapefruit | *Citrus paradisi* | Rutaceae | Solaris | Aromatherapy, massage |
| 20 | Orange | *Citrus sinensis* | Rutaceae | Solaris | Aromatherapy, massage |
| 21 | Rosewood | *Aniba rosaeodora* | Lauraceae | Solaris | Aromatherapy, massage |

**Table 1.** The characteristics of the essential oils.

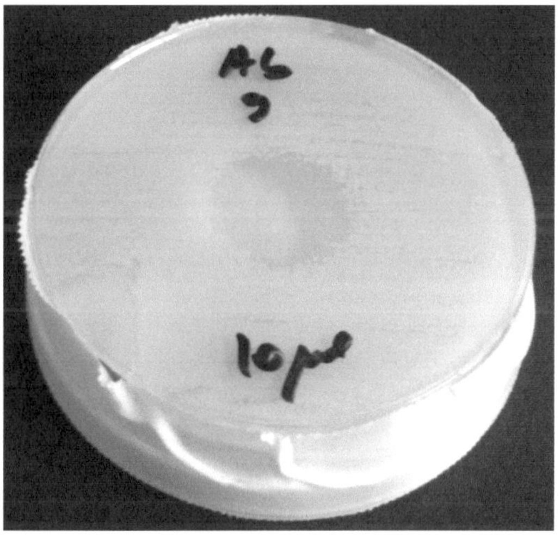


**Figure 3.** Aromatogram. In the middle of a sterile paper disk, with diameter of a Petri dish lid, 10 μl of essential oil was deposed. After sealing the assembly, the volatile effect was tested.

### *4.3.2. Results*

#### *4.3.2.1. Diffusimetric method*

**Figures 4–7** showing EOs inhibitory activity, demonstrate antibacterial activity for the two Gram-negative species tested. Before we comment on the implication of these results, it is worth considering the obvious antibacterial effect of some EOs. In particular, it is worth mentioning that we obtain more precise results—the smallest SDs—when 5 μl EOs are tested.

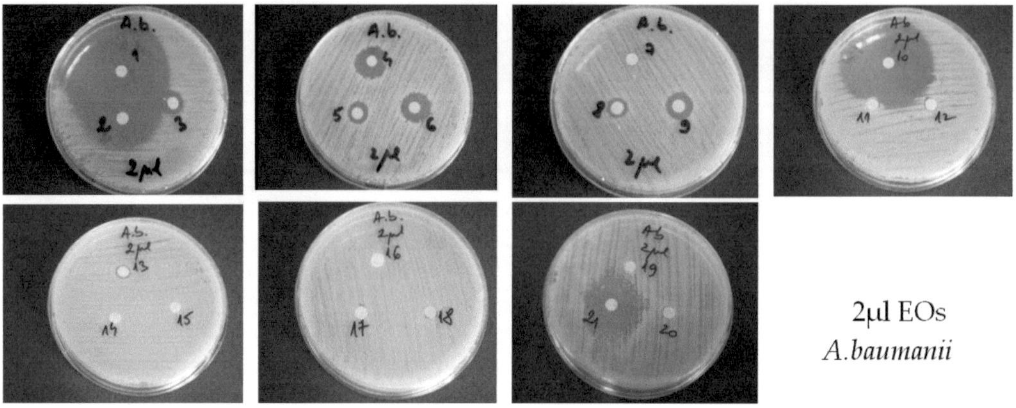


**Figure 4.** Diffusimetric method carbapenem-resistant *A. baumanii* tested by 2 µl EOs (see **Table 1** for the coresponding numbers).

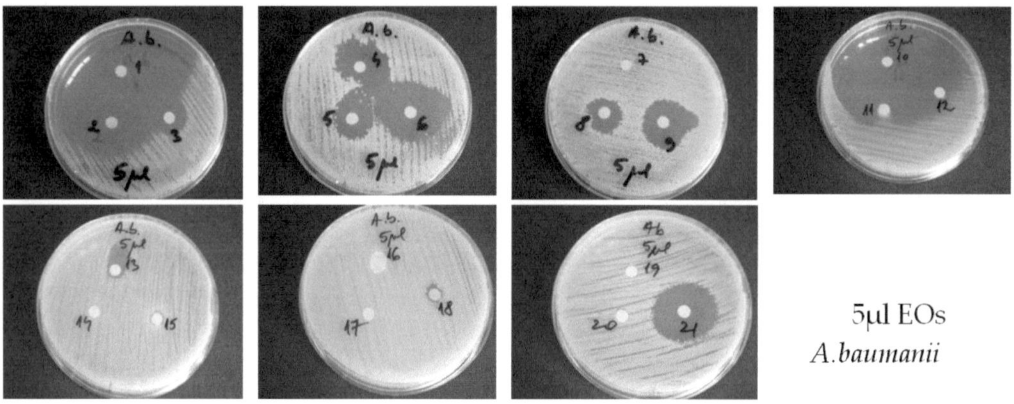


**Figure 5.** Diffusimetric method carbapenem-resistant *A. baumanii* tested by 5 µl EOs (see **Table 1** for the coresponding numbers).

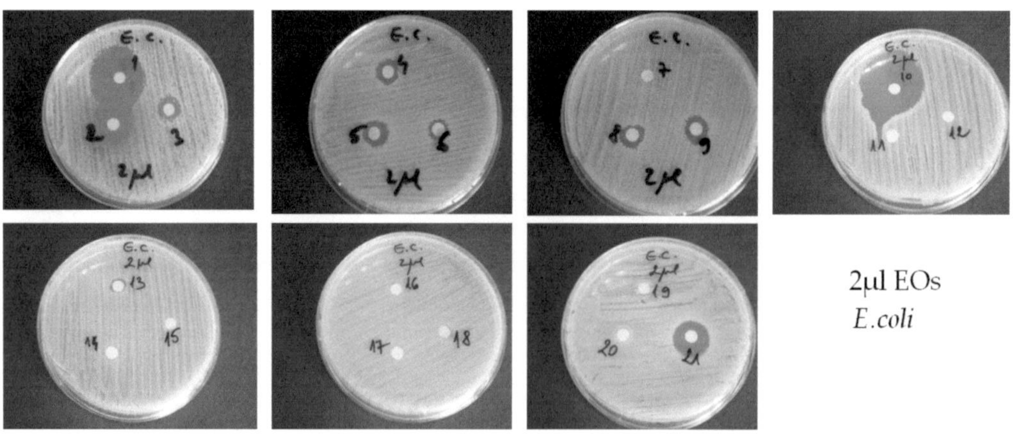


**Figure 6.** Diffusimetric method *E. coli* ATCC 25922 tested by 2 µl EOs (see **Table 1** for the coresponding numbers).

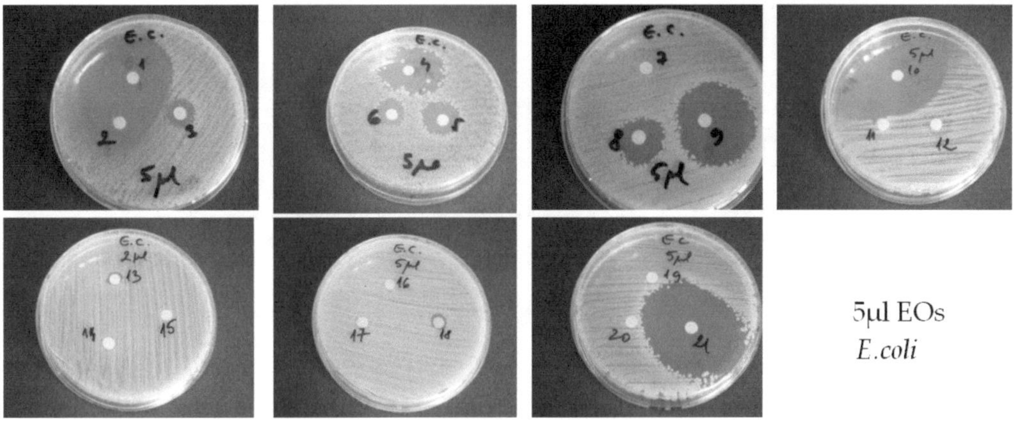


**Figure 7.** Diffusimetric method *E. coli* ATCC 25922 tested by 5 µl EOs (see **Table 1** for the coresponding numbers).

*Thymus vulgaris, Eugenia cayophyllata, Origanum vulgare,* and *Aniba rosaeodora* oils not only are by far the most effective but also obviously inhibit *A. baumannii* more efficiently than *E. coli.* Alternatively, *Melaleuca alternifolia* is slightly more effective against *E. coli* when diffusimetric method was used. Diffusimetric method also permits observing other important details. Although only clear inhibition zone was measured, *E. cayophyllata* shows residual growing, which is not measured and demonstrates a very good inhibitory activity. Also, it demonstrates an agonist effect in combination with *T. vulgaris*. Contrary, *O. vulgare* and *Nigella sativa* show an antagonistic effect.

#### *4.3.2.2. Aromatogram*

Aromatogram method (**Figures 8** and **9**) reveals more interesting evidence of usefulness of volatile effects of at least seven essential oils: *T. vulgaris, E. caryophyllata, O. vulgare, A. rosaeodora, Lavandula angustifolia, Mentha piperita,* and *M. alternifolia.* Surprisingly, some EOs, like mint, proved to be more effective when volatile effect is tested. The susceptibility testing was repeated after several weeks, but the results are inconsistent, mostly for mint, which showed no inhibitory effect after several weeks after opening the bottle. For other EOs (thyme, clove, eucalyptus, oregano, and rosewood) the antibacterial effect was not changed in time. Anyway, using single-use vials may be an option.

Synthetic results are listed in **Table 2**. At first glance, we noticed a remarkable antibacterial activity for *T. vulgaris, E. caryophyllata, O. vulgare,* and *A. rosaeodora*. Three other EOs could be considered as being efficient (*M. alternifolia, Lavandula angustifolia,* and *M. piperita*), but ten of them proved to have no antibacterial effect at any concentration tested. *Eucalyptus globulus* and *J. communis* could be considered for topical use, but not for their volatile properties. Four EOs (*E. globulus, Lavandula angustifolia, M. piperita,* and *Rosmarinus officinalis*) show multiple resistant colonies inside inhibition zone when *E. coli* was tested by aromatogram. Therefore, we consider them without antibacterial activity when volatile effect is considered.

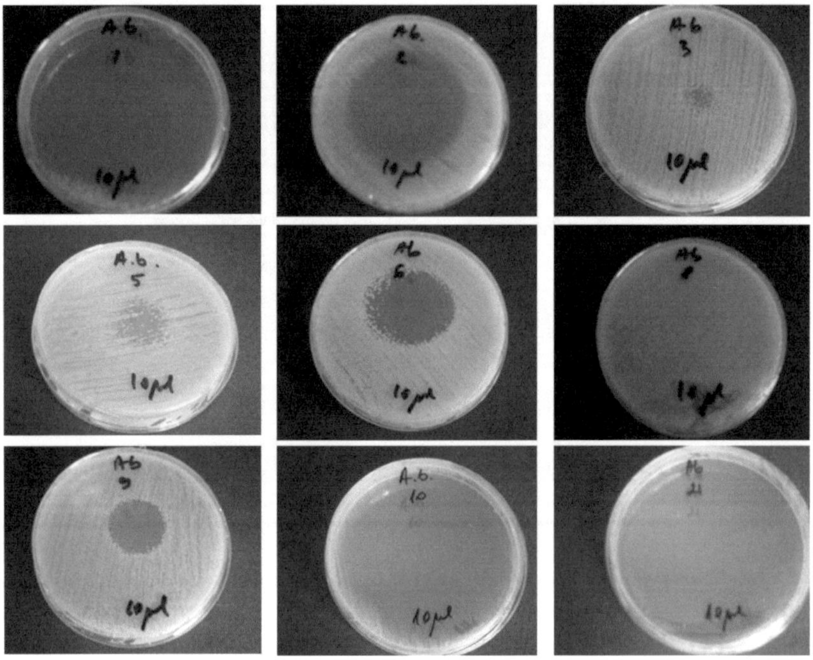


**Figure 8.** Aromatogram carbapenem-resistant *A. baumanii* tested by 10 µl EOs (see **Table 1** for the coresponding numbers).

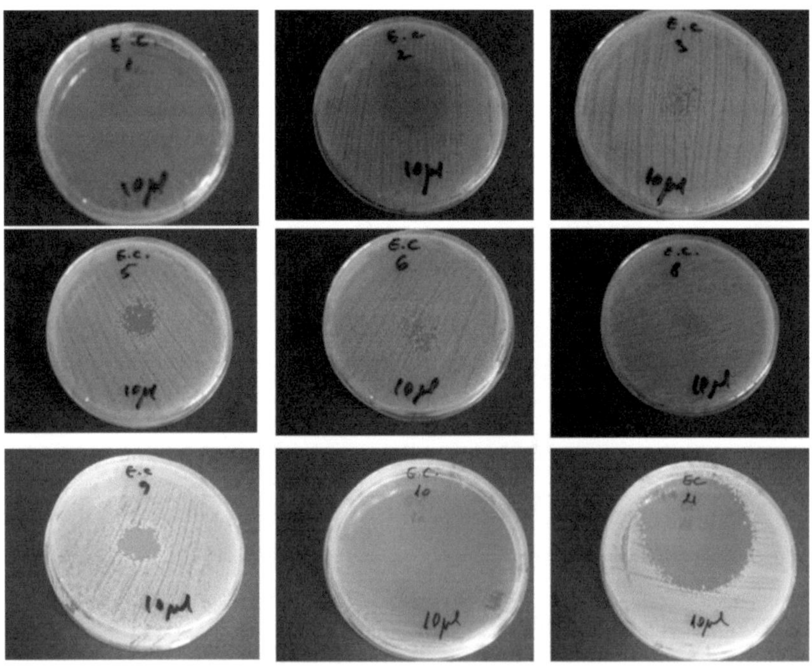


**Figure 9.** *E. coli* ATCC 25922 tested by 10 µl EOs (see **Table 1** for the coresponding numbers).

| EOs | | Carbapenem-resistant *A. baumannii* | | | *E. coli* ATCC 25922 | | |
|---|---|---|---|---|---|---|---|
| | | 2 μl | 5 μl | 10 μl | 2 μl | 5 μl | 10 μl |
| | | Mean (SD) | Mean (SD) | Mean (SD) | Mean (SD) | Mean (SD) | Mean (SD) |
| 1 | Thyme | 38.33 mm (10.41) | 66.67 mm (5.77) | 70.00 mm (5.00) | 28.00 mm (3.61) | 65.00 mm (8.66) | **75.00 mm** (5.00) |
| 2 | Clove | 21.67 mm (6.51) | 32.33 mm (2.52) | 46.67 mm (2.89) | 19.00 mm (5.29) | 29.33 mm (2.31) | **33.33 mm** (7.64) |
| 3 | Eucalyptus | 9.67 mm (2.52) | 16.00 mm (3.61) | NI | 8.00 mm (1.73) | 16.00 mm (3.46) | NI mrc |
| 4 | Juniper | 16.33 mm (2.52) | 23.00 mm (1.73) | NI | 14.67 mm (4.62) | 27.33 mm (2.52) | NI |
| 5 | Lavander | 10.33 mm (0.58) | 14.67 mm (2.52) | 19.67 mm (5.51) | 11.67 mm (0.58) | 20.33 mm (3.51) | NI mcr |
| 6 | Mint | 13.67 mm (2.31) | 20.67 mm (6.51) | 39.00 mm (6.56) | 7.00 mm (0.00) | 15.00 mm (1.00) | NI mcr |
| 7 | Pine | NI | NI | NI | NI | NI | NI |
| 8 | Rosemary | 12.33 mm (±4.62) | 16.33 mm (±1.53) | NI | 10.33 mm (±3.51) | 18.67 mm (±1.53) | NI mcr |
| 9 | Tea tree | 15.67 mm (8.14) | 24.67 mm (3.51) | 26.33 mm (4.16) | 18.33 mm (7.64) | 23.33 mm (2.89) | 11.00 mm (6.56) |
| 10 | Oregano | 46.00 mm (±2.00) | 70.00 mm (0.00) | 77.67 mm (2.52) | 29.67 mm (0.58) | 40.33 mm (1.53) | 76.00 mm (1.73) |
| 11 | Negril | NI | NI | NI | NI | NI | NI |
| 12 | Lemon | NI | NI | NI | NI | NI | NI |
| 13 | Fennel | 6.00 mm (0.00) | 6.33 mm (0.58) | NI | 6.00 mm (0.00) | NI | NI |
| 14 | Sage | NI | NI | NI | NI | NI | NI |
| 15 | Sandalwood | NI | NI | NI | NI | NI | NI |
| 16 | Seeds of apricots | NI | NI | NI | NI | NI | NI |
| 17 | Incense | NI | NI | NI | NI | NI | NI |
| 18 | Inhalant | NI | NI | NI | NI | NI | NI |
| 19 | Grapefruit | NI | NI | NI | NI | NI | NI |
| 20 | Orange | NI | NI | NI | NI | NI | NI |
| 21 | Rosewood | 16.00 mm (1.00) | 32.33 mm (11.59) | 80.00 mm (0.00) | 14.67 mm (0.58) | 30.33 mm (9.50) | 50.00 mm (2.00) |

NI—no inhibition; mrc—multiple resistant colonies.

**Table 2.** The inhibition of carbapenem-resistant *A. baumannii* and *E. coli* ATCC 25922 by 21 EOs. The results are reported as the mean (SD—standard deviation) of three independent experiments.

### 4.4. Discussion

In this study, commercial undiluted EOs were tested. There are some differences on viscosity, dispersion, vaporization, and other physical properties that, no doubt, influence the antibacterial activity. Although no proof can be given, the presence of antibiotic-resistance genes does not influence the efficiency of EOs. Therefore, an intuitive feeling turned our attention to the utility of these products in prevention or, why not, treatment of antibiotic-resistant Gram-negative bacillary respiratory infections. Although there are precise methods for identifying the chemicals with antibacterial activity, these are not important for our purpose. Note that here we are speaking of a screening of some commercial EOs that anyone can buy without medical prescription. Some authors demonstrate discrepancy of antimicrobial activity of EOs from different herbal varieties [37–40]. Of course, as we observed in our study, accurate description of physicochemical properties are needed [41], but for clinical purpose, the overall activity of EOs is relevant. In our opinion, a plant product should be considered as a distinct entity, and we can be certain that each component is synergistic to each other in a manner that exceeds the individual action of separated molecules. As we are speaking of living things, plant properties greatly depends on geographic area of collection, weather influence, manufacturing protocols, preservation conditions, species variety, and so on. Because natural plant products are considered safe, diverse possible applications were investigated: in agriculture for preventing crop diseases, monitoring soil characteristics [42, 43], or as industrial preservation solutions [44].

## 5. Environmental source of carbapenem-resistant strains

### 5.1. General considerations

Extensive studies are devoted to the ecotoxicity of industrial compounds or of pharmaceutical wastes [45]. Even though existing tools permit measurement of the concentration of any chemical in a certain geographic area, it is almost impossible to accurately estimate the influence of external factors that, no doubt, interfere with the spread or chemical transformation of any substance—like antibiotics. When biology occurs, the problems become more complicated. Nowadays, a different approach in follow-up to the intricate relationships of abundant microorganisms from a specific environment is needed. Antibiotics, like any other chemicals, do not differ in the way of spreading, accumulation, and changing certain environmental characteristics. It is not an exaggeration to state that multidrug-resistant microorganisms from hospital facilities are the nightmare of health practitioners. Analyzing bacterial species one by one provides certain information, but the big picture contains much more. Before starting to accumulate new data, there are huge unexplored resources, like public databases. Our concern was related to the magnitude of change on environmental microbiome by medical activities, especially the use of carbapenems. We extensively searched carbapenemases, or similar beta-lactamases, in protein databases available, and we compared their similitudes depending on their isolation source. The goal of searching similitudes between carbapenemase of clinical samples and their counterpart of environmental origin was to assess the influence of medical activities in changing soil and water microbiota.

### 5.2. Data collection and methods

Herein, we have focused on comparison of the carbapenemases, from different sources, deposited in public databases—NCBI/National Center for Biotechnology Information (https://www.ncbi.nlm.nih.gov/protein). The preliminary results were briefly presented in the First Conference of the Romanian Association of Laboratory Medicine [46]. Carbapenemase sampling was carried out to cover all beta-lactamase classes. In summary, 40 FASTA carbapenemase sequences were collected, and then a pairwise sequence alignment (EMBOSS Needle Program) and multiple sequence alignment (Clustal Omega tool) were performed [47–49]. The default settings were used. **Table 3** lists the characteristics of the sequences used for further comparisons. Sequences for Classes A, B, and D belonging to Archaea and bacteria were selected. Alignment sequence based on protein crystal structure was not possible due to lack of crystal structures available for beta-lactamases isolated from environmental samples.

### 5.3. Results and discussion

The major limit of the present study is the scarcity of carbapenemases of environmental source deposited in the public databases. Most of environmental beta-lactamases found belong to Classes B and D. The archaeal beta-lactamases found are metallo-hydrolase, and metal ions probably contribute to enzymes stability in extreme environmental conditions. Searching was extended to Eukaryota domain of life, but any sequences were included in the present study. Only two beta-lactamases-like of eukaryotic origin were retrieved—*Homo sapiens* (NP_057111) and *Caenorhabditis elegans* (NP_497107). Even they show MBL-folding, their similarity with other class B carbapenemases are very low, being more close to one hypothetical protein from *Sulfolobus acidocaldarius* (WP_01538554)—20.5% identity with NP_057111; 23.2% with NP_497107, respectively.

On the other hand, environmental Classes A, B, and D carbapenem-hydrolyzing enzymes are very similar with carbapenemases of clinical sources. Some carbapenemases, such as IMI-2, IMI-3, NDM-1, or OXA-48, are the same regardless their origin as observed by sequences pairwise comparison [50, 51]. For further statistical analysis, identity percent was recovered. Student's *t*-test assuming unequal sample variance was performed. The limit of this approach is due to the differences in the sequences length. The Needle program calculates identity, similarity, and score according to number of residues. Anyway, observing the data from **Table 4**, we noticed that environmental serine beta-lactamases are more similar with their clinical enterobacterial counterparts than with nonfermenters carbapenemases. The most striking differences are observed for subgroups IMI-3 of uncultured bacteria (ALJ52278) isolated from river sediment in China and OXA-48-like of uncultured bacteria (AJF40233) isolated from river sediment in Portugal. For ALJ52278 (IMI-3) beta-lactamase, 73.03% identity mean (CI 95 ± 25.33) with Class A carbapenemases of clinical *Enterobacteria* was noticed. More, sequences pairwise comparison reveals 93.50% identity with subgroups IMI-2 (*Enterobacter asburidae* WP_032491237), IMI-2 (*E. coli* AEU10762), and IMI-14 (*Enterobacter hormaechei*

| Class | Source | Organism (accession number) isolation source | Beta-lactamase | Residues |
|---|---|---|---|---|
| **Archaea** | | | | |
| MBL-fold | ES | *Sulfolobus acidocaldarius* (WP_011278945) | MBL fold metallo-hydrolase | 305 |
| | | *Sulfolobus acidocaldarius* (WP_015385554) | Hypothetical protein | 298 |
| | | *Hadesarchaea* archaeon (KUO42968) | MBL fold metallo-hydrolase | 395 |
| | | *Archaeoglobus fulgidus* (WP_010877604) | MBL fold metallo-hydrolase | 293 |
| | | *Vulcanisaeta distributa* (WP_013336995) | MBL fold metallo-hydrolase | 306 |
| **Bacteria** | | | | |
| A | ES | *Enterobacter asburiae* (AIL29239)/water | IMI-2 | 192 |
| | | uncultured bacterium (ALJ52278)/river sediment, Haithe River, China | IMI-3 | 280 |
| | E | *Escherichia coli* (WP_015059046) | GES-20 | 287 |
| | | *Serratia fonticola* (4EV4) | SFC-1 E166A mutant | 283 |
| | | *Serratia marcescens* (1DY6) | SME-1 | 267 |
| | | *Enterobacter asburiae* (WP_032491237) | IMI-2 | 292 |
| | | *Escherichia coli* (AEU10762) | IMI-2 | 292 |
| | | *Enterobacter hormaechei* (APY16311) | IMI-14 | 292 |
| | N | *Pseudomonas aeruginosa* (WP_021018677) | KPC | 293 |
| | | *Pseudomonas aeruginosa* (4GNU) | GES-5 | 287 |
| | | *Acinetobacter baumannii* (3TSG) | GES-14 | 287 |
| B | ES | *Serratia* sp. Sr_CGKV333_2014 (ALL98459)/ poultry flock soil, India | NDM_FIM-like_MBL-B1 | 270 |
| | | *Acinetobacter junii* (YP_009062718)/livestock farms, China | NDM-1 (plasmid) | 270 |
| | | *Acinetobacter calcoaceticus* (YP_009060354)/ livestock farms, China | NDM-1 (plasmid) | 270 |
| | E | *Klebsiella pneumoniae* (4UWS) | VIM-26 | 266 |
| | | *Klebsiella pneumoniae* (5A87) | VIM-5 | 248 |
| | | *Klebsiella pneumoniae* (3SPU) | NMD-1 | 265 |
| | N | *Pseudomonas aeruginosa* (4NQ2) | VIM-2 | 261 |
| | | *Pseudomonas aeruginosa* (AAR15341) | SPM-1 | 276 |
| | | *Pseudomonas aeruginosa* (ALU10771) | NMD-1 | 270 |
| | | *Pseudomonas aeruginosa* (AGH20684) | IMP-15 | 246 |
| | | *Aeromonas hydrophila* (1X8I) | CphA complex with Biapenem | 227 |

| Class | Source | Organism (accession number) isolation source | Beta-lactamase | Residues |
|---|---|---|---|---|
| D | ES | *Escherichia coli* (AJA05008)/*Halimione portulacoides*, Portugal | OXA-48 like | 215 |
| | | *Citrobacter freundii* (AJA05009)/*Halimione portulacoides*, Portugal | OXA-48 like | 190 |
| | | *Pantoea eucalypti* (AJA05006)/*Halimione portulacoides*, Portugal | OXA-181 | 173 |
| | | Uncultured bacterium (AJF40233)/river water, Portugal | OXA-48-like | 248 |
| | E | *Klebsiella pneumoniae* (5FAT) | Oxa-48 complex with Fpi-1602 | 243 |
| | | *Klebsiella pneumoniae* (4WMC) | Oxa-48 complex with Avibactam | 242 |
| | | *Escherichia coli* (3QNC) | OXA-10 | 244 |
| | | *Klebsiella pneumoniae* (AGC60012) | OXA-244 | 265 |
| | N | *Pseudomonas aeruginosa* (AAQ76282) | OXA-50 | 262 |
| | | *Acinetobacter baumannii* (ADB28891) | OXA-160 | 275 |
| | | *Acinetobacter baumannii* (4WM9) | OXA-24 | 245 |
| | | *Acinetobacter radioresistens* (ACE63186) | OXA-23 | 273 |
| | | *Acinetobacter baylyi* (ACH99101.1) | OXA-72 | 275 |

**Table 3.** The main characteristics of beta-lactamase sequences.

APY16311) (data not shown). The Class D carbapenemase AJF40233 (OXA-48-like) displays 80.35% identity mean (CI 95 ± 34.61) with its clinical *Enterobacteria* counterparts. Sequences pairwise comparison shows 91.00% identity with OXA-48-like (*Klebsiella pneumoniae* 5FAT and *K. pneumoniae* 4WMC) and 91.70% identity with OXA-244 (*K. pneumoniae* AGC60012) (data not shown). In contrast, for Class B carbapenemases, there are no notable differences when comparing environmental carbapenemases with those of clinical *Enterobacteria* or non-fermenters of Gram-negative bacilli origin. Particularly, all three NDM-1 carbapenemases of environmental sources included in the present study (**Table 3**) are identical with the carbapenemases isolated from *K. pneumoniae* (3SPU), *Enterobacteria*, or from the nonfermenter *Pseudomonas aeruginosa* (ALU10771). This is the most obvious illustration of long-term consequences of antibiotics use in livestock farms. Contrary, as it is shown in **Table 4**, Archaeal metallo-hydrolases show low similarities with other Class B carbapenemases.

Multiple sequence alignment of Classes A and D carbapenemases demonstrate that the active-site residues are very well conserved. Class B carbapenems, which mediate resistance to all beta-lactamases except aztreonam, are particularly interesting; they are found in bacteria, Archaea, and similar proteins, even in eukaryotes. Further, multiple sequence alignment (**Figure 10**)

| Environmental samples | *Enterobacteria* | Nonfermenters | *P*-value |
|---|---|---|---|
| | Identity% Mean (CI 95) | Identity% Mean (CI 95) | |
| **Class B** | | | |
| Bacteria | | | |
| *Serratia* sp. (ALL98459) | 51.07 (±70.37) | 40.30 (±42.34) | 0.65 |
| *A.junii* (YP_009062718) | 51.07 (±70.37) | 40.30 (±42.34) | 0.65 |
| *A. calcoaceticus* (YP_009060354) | 51.07 (±70.37) | 40.30 (±42.34) | 0.65 |
| Archaea | | | |
| *S. acidocaldarius* (WP_011278945) | 15.47 (±0.75) | 15.56 (±3.04) | 0.93 |
| *S. acidocaldarius* (WP_015385554) | 14.93 (±1.11) | 14.48 (±2.88) | 0.69 |
| *H. archaeon* (KUO42968) | 11.00 (±5.81) | 13.18 (±2.57) | 0.25 |
| *A. fulgidus* (WP_010877604) | 15.27 (±2.67) | 15.38 (±1.59) | 0.89 |
| *V. distributa* (WP_013336995) | 16.50 (±1.51) | 16.60 (±2.21) | 0.91 |
| **Class A** | | | |
| *E. asburiae* (AIL29239) | 54.87 (±17.00) | 31.40 (±18.06) | 0.02 |
| Uncultured (ALJ52278) | 73.03 (±26.33) | 40.20 (±26.23) | 0.03 |
| **Class D** | | | |
| *E. coli* (AJA05008) | 69.85 (±29.32) | 28.54 (±2.37) | 0.02 |
| *C. freundii* (AJA05009.1) | 67.78 (±25.43) | 27.94 (±2.63) | 0.01 |
| *Peucalypti* (AJA05006) | 60.93 (±21.63) | 25.58 (±2.28) | 0.01 |
| Uncultured (AJF40233) | 80.35 (±34.61) | 32.26 (±3.02) | 0.02 |

CI 95—Confidence Intervals 95%.

**Table 4.** Pairwise comparison of beta-lactamase sequences of environmental sources with *Enterobacteria* and non-fermenters carbapenemases.

highlights the notable differences between Archaea and bacteria. Residues involved in $Zn^{2+}$ ions are very well conserved with the exception of Cys221, which is replaced by Asp in Archaea. However, nearby Cys residues were noticed. Since their crystal structures are not solved, we can just assume their involvement in metal ion binding.

The observation that Archaea contain different beta-lactamases demonstrates that human behavior has not profoundly altered natural environment. Or some microorganism communities have regulatory mechanisms so flexible that rapidly adapt at new environmental factors. For example, *Acinetobacter* is no longer considered just a free-living organism found in soil, water, and skin of human and warm-blooded animals, but an important multidrug-resistant pathogen.

```
                                    201                                                        260
Hypothetical protein S.acidocaldarius CVKY--GENLFCGDHILPNVTPNVSLHAPYDDP-------LGR------------YLDSL
Hydrolase Hadersarchaea archaeon      FTYFEEEKVLFPCDFFGAHYAGP-EN--FDDEMGELLIHEAKRYYAEIMMPFKPPVSRAL
Hydrolase A.fulgidus                  YIYIPQKKVVFCGDLLFAKPCTPLAV--G--GS-------VRG------------SVNAL
Hydrolase S.acidocaldarius            FIYFPDEKVVFTGDLLFSPPCTPFAL--M--GY-------LQG------------YIKTL
Hydrolase V.distributa                YIYIPDSRVVFAGDLLFAEPCTPFVL--F--GS-------VSG------------SIEAL
CphA A.hydrophila                     FVYFPDEQVLYGGCILK----EKLGN--LSFAD-------VKA------------YPQTL
NDM Serratia sp. (ES)                 TVGIDGTDIAFGGCLIKDSKAKSLGN--LGDAD-------TEH------------YAASA
NDM-1 A.junii (ES)                    TVGIDGTDIAFGGCLIKDSKAKSLGN--LGDAD-------TEH------------YAASA
NDM-1 A.calcoaceticus (ES)            TVGIDGTDIAFGGCLIKDSKAKSLGN--LGDAD-------TEH------------YAASA
NDM-1 P.aeruginosa                    TVGIDGTDIAFGGCLIKDSKAKSLGN--LGDAD-------TEH------------YAASA
NDM-1 K.pneumoniae                    TVGIDGTDIAFGGCLIKDSKAKSLGN--LGDAD-------TEH------------YAASA
VIM-2 P.aeruginosa                    VVYVPSASVLYGGCAIYELSRTSAGN--VADAD-------LAE------------WPTSI
VIM-26 K.pneumoniae                   VVYVPSANVLYGGXAVLELSSTSAGN--VADAD-------LAE------------WPTSV
VIM-5 K.pneumoniae                    VVYVPSANVLYGGCAVLALSRTSAGN--VADAD-------LAE------------WPTSV
SPM-1 P.aeruginosa                    VVYFPKKKLLFGGCMIK---PKELGY--LGDAN-------VKA------------WPDSA
IMP-15 P.aeruginosa                   VVWLPENRVLFGGCFVK---PYGLGN--LGDAN-------LEA------------WPKSA
                                                :    .                                          :
```

**Figure 10.** Multiple sequence alignment of Class B beta-lactamase. The cysteine residues involved in the second $Zn^{2+}$ binding, highly conserved in bacteria, are written in white on black background; the residues noticed in Archaea are highlighted - the aspartic acid are underlined and the cysteine are written on grey background.

## 6. Final remarks

Carbapenems remain a valid option for the treatment of ESBL *Enterobacteriaceae* pneumonia. Prolonged treatments with beta-lactamine associated with other co-morbidities of the patients, rapidly changed the phenotypic pattern of resistance.

Essential oils have, no doubt, beneficial effects, but some providers excessively claim many possible effects—from antibacterial activity to neurological benefits—not always consistent with reality. Moreover, nowadays, there exists all sort of mixtures, and we can only hope that the ingredients are chosen following logical connections between their activities. Herein, these problems were not debated, but it is not a trivial question about the validity of all plant extracts. Just notice that the only mixture tested (an inhalant) proved no antibacterial activity, at least against *A. baumannii* and *E. coli* strains. On the other hand, tyme-clove association proved to be beneficial in Gram-negative bacilli respiratory infections. The oregano EO has an excellent antibacterial activity, but its effect is antagonized by negril EO. Other plant extracts could be added for their anti-inflammatory effect or just for changing the scent [52].

One important question arises from here—what else, apart from widely using of antibiotics, could influence the persistence of antibiotic genes in hospital facilities? Industrial wastes could remain for a long period of time in the environment, notably in groundwater [8]. Carbapenemases from hospital sources are, no doubt, the major factor in the evolution of these enzymes, hospital residues being, definitely, a source of wastewater pollution. Further, the carbapenemases produced by natural environmental bacteria and Archaea significantly contribute to selection of new mutations. Soil bacterial species greatly influences our life; therefore, a genome-scale metabolic network [53] has proved to be a valid approach to evaluate the complex dynamics of soil bacterial species, mostly in geographic areas near huge hospitals with many departments. Also, innate resistance to antibiotics has raised over time a growing interest for a rational design of new antibacterial compounds [54].

## 7. Conclusion

Carbapenem-resistant Gram-negative bacilli are one of the leading causes of nosocomial pneumonia. They are particularly involved in the outbreaks in ICUs. These strains are very often multidrug resistant, putting additional pressure on physicians and clinical microbiologists. Bacteriological diagnosis provides essential evidence for carbapenem-resistant Gram-negative bacillary pneumonia. From the very beginning, the Gram smear from respiratory specimens shows to be indispensable for an accurate diagnosis. Preventing respiratory infections in ICUs is a challenging issue; antibiotic prescription for any kind of acute respiratory tract infection does not benefit the patients. Besides, carbapenem-resistant bacilli already exist not only in clinical units but also alter environmental microbiota. It is time for a different approach in dealing with the antibiotic-resistance issues. An endless struggle with microorganisms does not work; these tiny creatures have incredible resources to deal with any new chemotherapeutic agent. We do not have the slightest idea of the long-term impact of widespread antibiotic use on environmental microorganisms. Careful analysis of existing data, like the evidence deposited in public databases, and reconsidering the antibacterial efficiency of natural products, such as EOs, could help at dealing with multidrug-resistant organisms.

## Acknowledgments

I gratefully acknowledge the financial support received from the Fares Bio Vital Laboratories, Orăştie, România for covering part of the cost to publish in open access.

## Conflicts of Interest

The author declare no conflict of interest. The funder had no role in the design of the study, in the collection, analyses, or interpretation of data, in the writing of the manuscript, and in the decision to publish the results.

## Author details

Mihaela Ileana Ionescu

Address all correspondence to: mionescu@umfcluj.ro

Microbiology Department, "Iuliu Hatieganu" University of Medicine and Pharmacy, Cluj-Napoca, Romania

## References

[1] Sutherasan Y, Peñuelas O, Muriel A, Vargas M, Frutos-Vivar F, Brunetti I, et al. Management and outcome of mechanically ventilated patients after cardiac arrest. Critical Care. 2015;**19**:215. DOI: 10.1186/s13054-015-0922-9

[2] Suwantarat N, Carroll KC. Epidemiology and molecular characterization of multi-drug-resistant gram-negative bacteria in Southeast Asia. Antimicrobila Resistance and Infection Control. 2016;**5**:15. DOI: 10.1186/s13756-016-0115-6

[3] Le NK, Hf W, Vu PD, Khu DTK, Le HT, Hoang BTN, et al. High prevalence of hospital-acquired infections caused by gram-negative carbapenem resistant strains in Vietnamese pediatric ICUs: A multi-centre point prevalence survey. Medicine (Baltimore). 2016;**95**:e4099. DOI: 10.1097/MD.0000000000004099

[4] Tamma PD, Han JH, Rock C, Harris AD, Lautenbach E, Hsu AJ, et al. Carbapenem therapy is associated with improved survival compared with piperacillin-tazobactam for patients with extended-spectrum β-lactamase bacteremia. Clinical Infectious Diseases. 2015;**60**:1319-1325. DOI: 10.1093/cid/civ003

[5] Shapira S, Pleban S, Kazanov D, Tirosh P, Arber N. Terpinen-4-ol: A novel and promising therapeutic agent for human gastrointestinal cancers. PLoS One. 2016;**11**:e0156540. DOI: 10.1371/journal.pone.0156540

[6] Arweiler NB, Donos N, Netuschil L, Reich E, Sculean A. Clinical and antibacterial effect of tea tree oil—A pilot study. Clinical Oral Investigation. 2000;**4**:70-73

[7] Biak-Bielinska A, Kumirska J, Stepnowski P. What do we know about the chronic and mixture toxicity of the residues of sulfonamides in the environment? Organic Pollutants—Monitoring Risk and Treatment. InTech, Croatia; 2013. DOI: 10.5772/53732

[8] Ory J, Bricheux G, Togola A, Bonnet JL, Donnadieu-Bernard F, Nakusi L, et al. Ciprofloxacin residue and antibiotic-resistant biofilm bacteria in hospital effluent. Environmental Pollution. 2016;**214**:635-645. DOI: 10.1016/j.envpol.2016.04.033

[9] Munsch-Alatossava P, Ikonen V, Alatossava T, Gauchi J-P. Trends of antibiotic resistance (AR) in mesophilic and psychrotrophic bacterial populations during cold storage of raw milk, produced by organic and conventional farming systems. Antibiotic Resistance Bacteria—A Continuous Challenge New Millennium, InTech, Croatia; 2012. DOI: 10.5772/29994

[10] Woese CR. There must be a prokaryote somewhere: Microbiology's search for itself. Microbiological Reviews. 1994;**58**:1-9. DOI: 10146-0749/94/$04.00+0

[11] Silva TP, Gamalier JP, Melo RCN. TEM as an important tool to study aquatic microorganisms and their relationships with ecological processes. Modern Electron Microscopy in Physical and Life Sciences. InTech, Croatia; 2016. DOI: 10.5772/61804

[12] Abed RMM, Al-Kharusi S, Prigent S, Headley T. Diversity, distribution and hydrocarbon biodegradation capabilities of microbial communities in oil-contaminated cyanobacterial mats from a constructed wetland. PLoS One. 2014;**9**:e114570. DOI: 10.1371/journal.pone.0114570

[13] Ritchey S, Gandhapudi S, Coyne M. Stability of antibiotic resistance patterns in agricultural pastures: Lessons from Kentucky, USA. Antibiotic Resistance Bacteria—A Continuous Challenge in the New Millennium. InTech, Croatia; 2012. DOI: 10.5772/31258

[14] Brandão MA da R, Lopes ATS, Neta MT da S, de Oliveira RBF, Rezende RP, Albuquerque GR, et al. Microbiological quality and prevalence of β-lactam antibiotic resistance genes in oysters (*Crassostrea rhizophorae*). Journal of Food Protection. 2017;**80**:488-496. DOI: 10.4315/0362-028X.JFP-16-098

[15] Bush K, Jacoby Ga, Medeiros Aa. A functional classification scheme for β-lactamases and its correlation with molecular structure. Antimicrobial Agents and Chemotherapy. 1995;**39**:1211-1233. DOI: 10.1128/AAC.39.6.1211

[16] Hall BG, Barlow M. Structure-based phylogenies of the serine β-lactamases. Journal of Molecular Evolution. 2003;**57**:255-260. DOI: 10.1007/s00239-003-2473-y

[17] Antunes NT, Lamoureaux TL, Toth M, Stewart NK, Frase H, Vakulenko SB. Class D β-lactamases: Are they all carbapenemases? Antimicrobial Agents of Chemotherapy. 2014;**58**:2119-2125. DOI: 10.1128/AAC.02522-13

[18] Bush K, Jacoby GA. Updated functional classification of beta-lactamases. Antimicrobila Agents of Chemotherapy. 2010;**54**:969-976. DOI: 10.1128/AAC.01009-09

[19] Bush K. Proliferation and significance of clinically relevant β-lactamases. Annals of New York Academy of Sciences. 2013;**1277**:84-90. DOI: 10.1111/nyas.12023

[20] Bajaj H, Scorciapino Ma, Moynié L, Page MGP, Naismith JH, Ceccarelli M, et al. Molecular basis of filtering carbapenems by porins from β-lactam-resistant clinical strains of *Escherichia coli*. Journal of Biological Chemistry. 2016;**291**:2837-2847. DOI: 10.1074/jbc.M115.690156

[21] Walther-Rasmussen J, Høiby N. Class A Carbapenemases. Journal of Antimicrobial Chemotherapy. 2007;**60**:470-482. DOI: 10.1093/jac/dkm226

[22] Walsh TR, Toleman MA, Poirel L, Nordmann P. Metallo-lactamases: the Quiet before the Storm? Clinical Microbiology Reviews. 2005;**18**:306-325. DOI: 10.1128/CMR.18.2.306-325.2005

[23] Queenan AM, Bush K. Carbapenemases: The versatile beta-lactamases. Clinical Microbiology Reviews. 2007;**20**:440-458, table of contents. DOI: 10.1128/CMR.00001-07

[24] Wang B, Sun D. Detection of NDM-1 carbapenemase-producing *Acinetobacter calcoaceticus* and *Acinetobacter junii* in environmental samples from livestock farms. Journal of Antimicrobial Chemotheray. 2015;**70**:611-613. DOI: 10.1093/jac/dku405

[25] Mandell LA, Wunderink RG, Anzueto A, Bartlett JG, Campbell GD, Dean NC, et al. Infectious diseases Society of America/American Thoracic Society consensus guidelines on the management of community-acquired pneumonia in adults. Clinical Infectious Diseases. 2007;**44**:S27-S72. DOI: 10.1086/511159

[26] Masterton RG, Galloway A, French G, Street M, Armstrong J, Brown E, et al. Guidelines for the management of hospital-acquired pneumonia in the UK: Report of the Working Party on Hospital-Acquired Pneumonia of the British Society for Antimicrobial Chemotherapy. Journal of Antimicrobial Chemotherapy. 2008;**62**:5-34. DOI: 10.1093/jac/dkn162

[27] Bartlett JG, Dowell SF, Mandell LA, File TM, Musher DM, Fine MJ. Practice guidelines for the management of community-acquired pneumonia in adults. Clinical Infectious Diseases. 2000;**31**:347-382. DOI: 10.1086/313954

[28] Tuon FF, Graf ME, Merlini A, Rocha JL, Stallbaum S, Arend LN, et al. Risk factors for mortality in patients with ventilator-associated pneumonia caused by carbapenem-resistant *Enterobacteriaceae*. Brazilian Journal of Infectious Diseases. 2017;**21**:1-6. DOI: 10.1016/j.bjid.2016.09.008

[29] Rouby J-J, Bouhemad B, Monsel A, Brisson H, Arbelot C, Lu Q. Aerosolized antibiotics for ventilator-associated pneumonia. Anesthesiology. 2012;**117**:1364-1380. DOI: 10.1097/ALN.0b013e3182755d7a

[30] Kim UJ, Kim HK, An JH, Cho SK, Park K-H, Jang H-C. Update on the epidemiology, treatment, and outcomes of carbapenem-resistant *Acinetobacter* infections. Chonnam Medical Journal. 2014;**50**:37-44. DOI: 10.4068/cmj.2014.50.2.37

[31] Lahmar A, Bedoui A, Mokdad-Bzeouich I, Dhaouifi Z, Kalboussi Z, Cheraif I, et al. Reversal of resistance in bacteria underlies synergistic effect of essential oils with conventional antibiotics. Microbial Pathogens. 2017;**106**:50-59. DOI: 10.1016/j.micpath.2016.10.018.

[32] Arslan M. Effects of intra-row spacing on herbage yield, essential oil content and composition of *Micromeria fruticosa*. Farmacia. 2012;**60**:925-931

[33] Ashraf A, Fatma I, Tamer F, Wedad A. Antimicrobial activity of some essential oils against *S. aureus* and *Candida albicans* with mastitic relevance. Behna Veterinary Medical Journal. 2015;**28**:281-288

[34] Herman AAP, Herman AAP, Domagalska BW, Młynarczyk A, Przemysław A, Beata H @bullet, et al. Essential oils and herbal extracts as antimicrobial agents in cosmetic emulsion. Indian Journal of Microbiology. 2013;**53**:232-237. DOI: 10.1007/s12088-012-0329-0

[35] Rojas J, Buitrago A. Essential oils and their products as antimicrobial agents: Progress and prospects. Therapeutic Medicinal Plants From Lab to Mark. 2015;**253**

[36] Şerban ES, Ionescu M, Matinca D, Maier CS, Bojiţă MT. Screening of the antibacterial and antifungal activity of eight volatile essential oils. Farmacia. 2011;**59**:440-446

[37] Adaszyńska M, Swarcewicz M, Dzięcioł M, Dobrowolska a. Comparison of chemical composition and antibacterial activity of lavender varieties from Poland. Natural Products Research. 2013;**27**:1497-1501. DOI: 10.1080/14786419.2012.724408

[38] Jianu C, Pop G, Gruia AT, Horhat FG. Chemical composition and antimicrobial activity of essential oils of lavender (*Lavandula angustifolia*) and lavandin (Lavandula x intermedia) grown in Western Romania. International Journal of Agricultural Biology. 2013;**15**:772-776

[39] Kasture A, Patel S, Chauhan J, Krishnamurthy R, Iriti M, Taralkar S V. In vitro antimicrobial effect of essential oil from leaf and rhizome of various accessions of *Acorus calamus* Linn. and its phytochemical screening. European Journal of Medicinal Plants. 2015;**9**. DOI: 10.9734/EJMP/2015/17318

[40] Salwa HA, Maqtari MA Al, Alhamzy EH, Alghalibi Saeed M, Ali NAA. Antimicrobial activity of *Lavandulla pubescens* essential oil from two places in Yemen. Journal of Advanced Biology. 2014;**4**:446-454

[41] Skwirzyńska MA, Swarcewicz M, Dobrowolska A. The potential of use lavender from vegetable waste as effective antibacterial and sedative agents. Medicinal Chemistry (Los Angeles). 2014;**4**. DOI: 10.4172/2161-0444.1000222

[42] Hugues K, Kouassi S, Bajji M, Jijakli H. Author's personal copy the control of postharvest blue and green molds of citrus in relation with essential oil–wax formulations, adherence and viscosity. Postharvest Biology and Technology. 2012;**73**:122-128

[43] Mazhar R, Ilyas N, Saeed M, Bibi F, Batool N. Biocontrol and Salinity Tolerance Potential of *Azospirillum lipoferum* and its Inoculation Effect in Wheat Crop. International Journal of Agriculture and Biology. 2016;**18**:494-500. ISSN Online n.d.:1560-8530. DOI: 10.17957/IJAB/15.0115

[44] Manikandan A, Saxena S, Sri Nidhi N, Sivakumar A. Antioxidant and antibacterial studies on essential oils used as alternatives for chemical preservatives. Journal of Natural Product and Plant Resources. 2015;**5**:9-14

[45] Wright GD. The antibiotic resistome: The nexus of chemical and genetic diversity. Natural Reviews of Microbiology. 2007;**5**:175-186. DOI: 10.1038/nrmicro1614

[46] Ionescu MI, Deac LM, Corneanu ER. The presence of environmental carbapenemases—an indicator for industrial pollution? 1st Conf. Rom. Assoc. Lab. Med. with Int. Particip, vol. 24, Romanian Journal of Laboratory Medicine; 2016. p. 118

[47] Rice P, Longden I, Bleasby A. EMBOSS: The European molecular biology open software suite. Trends in Genetics. 2000;**16**:276-277. DOI: 10.1016/S0168-9525(00)02024-2

[48] McWilliam H, Li W, Uludag M, Squizzato S, Park YM, Buso N, et al. Analysis tool web services from the EMBL-EBI. Nucleic Acids Research. 2013;**41**:W597-W600. DOI: 10.1093/nar/gkt376

[49] Li W, Cowley A, Uludag M, Gur T, McWilliam H, Squizzato S, et al. The EMBL-EBI bioinformatics web and programmatic tools framework. Nucleic Acids Research. 2015;**43**:W580-W584. DOI: 10.1093/nar/gkv279

[50] Dang B, Mao D, Luo Y. Complete nucleotide sequence of pGA45, a 140,698-bp IncFIIY plasmid encoding blaIMI-3-mediated carbapenem resistance, from river sediment. Frontiers in Microbiology. 2016;**7**:188. DOI: 10.3389/fmicb.2016.00188

[51] Wang B, Sun D. Detection of NDM-1 carbapenemase-producing *Acinetobacter calcoaceticus* and *Acinetobacter junii* in environmental samples from livestock farms. Journal of Antimicrobial Chemotherapy. 2015;**70**:611-613. DOI: 10.1093/jac/dku405

[52] Zehra S, Saeed A, Fatima S. Antioxidant and antibacterial studies of *Phoenix dactylifera* and its varieties. International Journal of Applied Microbiology and Biotechnology Research. 2015;**3**:81-88

[53] Mei J, Xu N, Ye C, Liu L, Wu J. Reconstruction and analysis of a genome-scale metabolic network of *Corynebacterium glutamicum* S9114. Gene. 2016;**575**:615-622. DOI: 10.1016/j.gene.2015.09.038

[54] Esthela I, Jess L, Guerra G, Ayala Snchez NE. Bioactive compounds from bacteria associated to marine algae. Biotechnology—Molecular Studies and Novel. Applications for Improved Quality of Human Life, InTech, Croatia; 2012. DOI: 10.5772/27842

Chapter 4

# Multidrug-Resistant Gram-Negative Pneumonia and Infection in Intensive Care Unit

Mauricio Rodriguez and Salim R. Surani

Additional information is available at the end of the chapter

http://dx.doi.org/10.5772/intechopen.69377

**Abstract**

Multidrug-resistant (MDR) pneumonia can be problematic and challenging to treat in an era of increasing resistance and limited treatment armamentarium. Multidrug-resistant pathogens are associated with increased morbidity and mortality, thus early empiric appropriate antibiotics are critical for survival. Many factors play a role in the selection, optimization, and duration of therapy that should be made on an individual basis. New technologies such as "rapid diagnostics" may provide the clinician with early phenotypic or genotypic result, thus improving early appropriate therapy. The increasing antibiotic resistance is a global threat to patients worldwide and is an economic burden. In the United States, drug-resistant bacteria cause approximately 2 million cases of illnesses and contribute to 23,000 deaths each year. The inappropriate use of antibiotics has contributed to the healthcare burden that ranges from $27 to $42 billion annually. As a result, several governmental agencies have placed forth regulatory mandates to enforce antimicrobial stewardship programs in acute care hospitals. Education will be vital across all healthcare disciplines to ultimately ensure optimal prescribing and reduce the emergence of resistance.

**Keywords:** multidrug-resistant infections, intensive care unit, pneumonia, healthcare-associated infections, critically ill patients, antibiotic stewardship

## 1. Introduction

In this chapter, we will focus on the critically ill patients with Gram-negative **pneumonia**, the prevalence of multidrug resistance, factors associated with patients developing these resistance infections. Surveillance, infection control, and early detection by means of utilizing rapid diagnostics and other methodologies are important for early prevention of disease. The reader will be able to understand how and why the administration of early appropriate empiric antibiotics is

INTECH
open science | open minds

© 2017 The Author(s). Licensee InTech. This chapter is distributed under the terms of the Creative Commons Attribution License (http://creativecommons.org/licenses/by/3.0), which permits unrestricted use, distribution, and reproduction in any medium, provided the original work is properly cited.

key for survival in the critically ill. We will emphasize on the importance of robust antimicrobial stewardship programs, which are in accordance with Centers for Disease Control and Prevention (CDC) core elements. New regulatory mandates from the Joint Commission (TJC) on antimicrobial stewardship programs will require hospitals to be compliant for accreditation. Finally, we will end the chapter with an outlook on future antibiotics in Phase III development to aid in the combat against multidrug-resistant (MDR) organisms.

## 2. Global resistance and global economic impact

The preantibiotic era is a reality for many parts around the world, especially among the developed countries, driven in part by antibiotic overuse and misuse. Increasing antibiotic resistance is a global threat to patients worldwide and an economic burden. According to the U.S. Centers for Disease Control and Prevention (CDC), each year in the United States, drug-resistant bacteria cause approximately 2 million cases of illnesses and contribute to 23,000 deaths. A key driver has been the inappropriate use of antibiotics, which as an avoidable cost and burden to healthcare dollars, ranges from $27 billion to 42 billion annually [1, 2]. The Infectious Diseases Society of America (IDSA) white paper entitled "Bad Bugs, No Drugs" commented on the declining research investments in antimicrobial development, as did an update on this article from clinical infectious disease (CID) in 2009 [3]. These papers identified certain Gram-negative bacteria that are particularly problematic pathogens, which tend to "escape" the activity of many antibiotics. These problematic pathogens are known as, the "ESKAPE" pathogens, which include: *Enterococcus faecium, Staphylococcus aureus, Klebsiella pneumoniae, Acinetobacter baumannii, Pseudomonas aeruginosa, Enterobacter species* and can *Clostridium difficile* is also include to the list. In addition to the "ESKAPE" pathogens, the prevalence of *C. difficile* infection (CDI) has risen dramatically in just the last 2 decades. Since 2001, surveillance data has shown a dramatic increase. The number of CDI cases (any diagnosis) per 10,000 hospital discharges increased from 25.0 to 40.0, a 60% increase. However, over the next 4 years (2001–2005), a 92% increase was observed (from 40.0 to 76.9) [3–5]. The CDC has placed these resistant pathogens into three categories: urgent, serious, and concerning threat levels. Several recent efforts have attempted to raise awareness and focus attention on antibiotic overuse in healthcare including: the World Health Organization, the CDC, and White House. The White House issued executive order 13,676: combating antibiotic-resistant bacteria, which is a roadmap to guide the nation that was issued by President Obama on September 18, 2014. This executive order will implement the *National Action Plan for Combating Antibiotic-Resistant Bacteria*, a plan that intends to have major reductions in the occurrence of urgent and serious threating pathogens, including methicillin-resistant *S. aureus* (MRSA), carbapenem-resistant *Enterobacteriaceae* (CRE), and *C. difficile* [6]. Recent studies have demonstrated that critically ill patients colonized with multidrug-resistant pathogens also have a high prevalence of being infected with that particular organism. In such, antimicrobial resistance (AMR) as an independent risk factor also increases morbidity and mortality [7, 8].

## 3. Prevalence of MDROs and risk factors in the critically ill

The CDC in 2013 published *Antibiotic Resistance Threats in the United States*. Regarding the level of concern, CDC has, for the first time, prioritized bacteria in this report into one of three categories: urgent, serious, and concerning (**Table 1**).

The CDC has placed carbapenem-resistant *Enterobacteriaceae* (CRE) as an urgent threat level. CRE confers resistance to last-line antibiotics such as carbapenems, by producing a β-lactamase enzyme called KPC (*K. pneumoniae* carbapenemase-producing). The CDC reports their laboratories have confirmed CRE in 44 states within healthcare facilities across the United States. CRE causes more than 9000 healthcare-associated infections (HAI) annually, among these the two most common types are carbapenem-resistant *Klebsiella* and carbapenem-resistant *E. coli*. The percentages of the United States CRE healthcare-associated infections for *Klebsiella* spp. and carbapenem-resistant *Escherichia coli* are 11 and 2%, respectively. These serious infections contribute to roughly 600 deaths each year [5].

| |
|---|
| **Urgent threats** |
| *Clostridium difficile* |
| Carbapenem-resistant *Enterobacteriaceae* (CRE) |
| Drug-resistant *Neisseria gonorrhoeae* |
| **Serious threats** |
| Multidrug-resistant *Acinetobacter** |
| Drug-resistant *Campylobacter* |
| Fluconazole-resistant *Candida* (a fungus) |
| Extended spectrum β-lactamase producing *Enterobacteriaceae* (ESBLs)* |
| Vancomycin-resistant *Enterococcus* (VRE) |
| Multidrug-resistant *Pseudomonas aeruginosa** |
| Drug-resistant nontyphoidal *Salmonella* |
| Drug-resistant *Salmonella* Typhi |
| Drug-resistant *Shigella* |
| Methicillin-resistant *Staphylococcus aureus* (MRSA)* |
| Drug-resistant *Streptococcus pneumoniae** |
| Drug-resistant tuberculosis* |
| **Concerning threats** |
| Vancomycin-resistant *Staphylococcus aureus* (VRSA) |
| Erythromycin-resistant Group A *Streptococcus* |
| Clindamycin-resistant Group B *Streptococcus* |

*Notes*: *MDROs associated with pneumonia. Reproduced from CDC. Antibiotic resistance threats in the United States, 2013 [5].

**Table 1.** CDC antibiotic resistance threats in the United States, 2013.

The first case of *K. pneumoniae* carbapenemase-producing CRE was reported in North Carolina in 2001. Since then, cases have been reported in almost every state. Carbapenemase-producing CRE carries antimicrobial resistance genes on mobile plasmids that can move between organisms, thus potentially facilitating a wider and more rapid spread. A clone known as *K. pneumoniae* sequence type 258 was responsible for this global dissemination, particularly in the United States. Knowing the genotype level aids in tracking the epidemiology worldwide [9]. Guh et al. conducted a 2-year surveillance period, which included 599 incident CRE cases that were reported across 7 Emerging Infections Program (EIP) sites (Georgia, Minnesota, Oregon, Colorado, Maryland, New Mexico, and New York). They concluded that the overall crude incidence CRE was 2.93 per 100,000 populations [10]. The overall CRE incidence may be underreported as many hospital laboratories may not preform confirmatory testing [11].

CRE is encountered in patients with extensive healthcare exposure. Patients can be hospitalized in an acute short stay hospital, residents of LTCFs (long-term care facilities), LTACHs (long-term acute care hospitals), or outpatients with recent healthcare exposure. These patients also frequently have multiple comorbidities, poor functional status, recent intravenous antibiotic exposure (within 90 days), and indwelling devices (urinary catheter, mechanical ventilation, indwelling lines). Patients that recover from their acute hospitalization are frequently discharged to LTCFs or LTACHs, thus contributing to a viscous cycle [10, 12]. LTACHs play an important role in the regional epidemiology of CRE. In a recent study, 30% of LTACH residents were colonized with *K. pneumoniae* carbapenemase-producing CRE. This represented a ninefold higher prevalence in LTACHs compared to intensive care unit (ICU) patients in acute short-stay hospitals in the same area. Various efforts to reduce the burden of CRE in LTACHs have had only a slight impact [13].

Common sites of infection include respiratory, bloodstream, -wounds, and urinary tract. Urine is the most common site for infection and colonization. Outcomes associated with CRE infections are poor with high mortality rates as high as 50% in some studies. Outcomes vary by the site of infection with blood stream infections carrying the highest mortality and urinary tract infection the lowest [10, 13].

According to the CDC, *Acinetobacter* in the United States causes approximately 12,000 healthcare-associated infections annually. Approximately 7000 of these infections are considered to be multidrug-resistant *Acinetobacter* at a staggering 63%, meaning at least three different classes of antibiotics no longer cures these infections, which contributes to 500 deaths per year. The CDC 2013 publication does not estimate long-term care hospitals or long-term care facilities in the prevalence statistics [10]. Others [14] have estimated that there may be as many as approximately 46,000 cases of *Acinetobacter*-related infections per year in the U.S. and approximately 1 million cases per year globally. In the United States, a 2006–2007 report of 463 hospitals participating in the National Healthcare Safety Network (NHSN) indicated that infections due to *Acinetobacter baumannii* accounted for 3% of all healthcare-associated infections (HAI). Focusing on the ICU, approximately 7% of all HAIs were associated with critically ill patients on mechanical ventilation in the United States, which were caused by *Acinetobacter* [11].

A further concern is that the prevalence of resistance among *Acinetobacter* infections is increasing. Between 2000 and 2009, the percentage of imipenem-resistant *A. baumannii* increased from ~5% to an approaching 40%, an increase that has been observed across most of U.S. states [15]. *Acinetobacter* is uniquely able to survive in hospital environments and to develop resistance to antibiotics. When combined these attributes result in both a high potential for endemicity and epidemicity, resulting in both hospital outbreaks and persistent colonization [16]. Studies have indicated that key sources of *Acinetobacter* transmission within hospital units include the following: hands of hospital personnel, contamination of environmental surfaces and medical equipment, environmental shedding by colonized patients, procedures that result in a spray of contaminated fluids, and airborne particles are believed to play a role in transmission [17].

In critically ill patients, *A. baumannii* can invade through breaches in skin integrity or airway protection. This pathogen is associated with high mortality [18]. Debilitated patients in ICUs are especially prone to *Acinetobacter* infections [15]. High-risk patients include:

a) Severe underlying illness or comorbidities such as diabetes mellitus and chronic lung disease.

b) Circumstances of hospitalization, such as length of stay, high workload, and admission to units in the acute care center with high a density of infected.

c) Infection or colonization of specific sites, respiratory, urinary, gastrointestinal tracts, burns, or surgical wounds.

d) Exposure to prolonged antimicrobial therapy with broad-spectrum antibiotics, which include carbapenems, fluoroquinolones, aminoglycosides, third generation cephalosporins.

e) Administration of blood product transfusions, enteral feeding and contaminated parenteral solutions.

Common sites of infection include respiratory, bloodstream, skin and soft tissue and urine. Mortality associated with *A. baumannii* infections ranges from 7.8 to 23% in general hospital patients and from 10 to 43% in ICU patients. Bacteremia has the highest mortality, and in hematopoietic stem cell transplantation (HSCT) recipients, mortality rates associated with *Acinetobacter* bacteremia may reach up to 70% [19].

Extended spectrum β-lactamase (ESBLs) producing *Enterobacteriaceae* produce a hydrolytic β-lactamase enzyme that confers resistance to various penicillins, which also include extended spectrum cephalosporins. Given the resistance, clinicians' remaining treatment option is a carbapenem antibiotic. Carbapenems are last-line antibiotics, and their use in ESBL infections has also contributing to additional resistance [20, 21]. In the United States, the CDC reports an estimated 140,000 healthcare-associated *Enterobacteriaceae* infections occur each year. The CDC also reports that approximately 26,000 of these infections are caused by ESBL-containing *Enterobacteriaceae* bloodstream infections, which contribute to 1700 deaths. The total excess hospital charges per episode of ESBL-bacteraemia are roughly $40,000 per occurrence. ESBL-producing *Klebsiella* spp. and ESBL-producing *E. coli* are the most common and percentage resistant to extended spectrum cephalosporins are 23 and 14%, respectively [5].

Sequence type 131 (ST131) is a pathogenic clone of *E. coli* and it also frequently expresses a hydrolytic β-lactamase enzyme called CTX-M-type and has rapidly disseminated worldwide. *E. coli* expressing CTX-M-type enzymes containing ESBLs have been increasingly seen in the community [12, 22–26]. Residency of a long-term care facility has been recognized as a prominent risk factor for acquisition of ESBL infections in the community. Various studies have also identified ESBL bacteremia as an independent risk factor from exposure to fluoroquinolones, first-generation cephalosporins, and finally, a previously known colonization history with an ESBL [25, 27]. Patients are 57% more likely to die from bloodstream infections associated with ESBL-producing *Enterobacteriaceae* than those with bloodstream infections caused by a non ESBL-producing strain [26].

In a study by Ha et al. [28], they concluded that significant risk factors associated with ESBL-producing *E. coli* bacteremia were prior treatment with fluoroquinolones and cephalosporins, as previous studies have also demonstrated. Moreover, recent surgery, liver disease, and immunosuppressant use were also deemed as significant risk factors. The study resulted in an overall 30-day mortality rate of 14.9%. As described previously, the mortality rate was higher in patients with ESBL-producing *E. coli* than in those without ESBL bacteremia (22.1 vs. 12.2%; $P = 0.02$). A multivariate analysis in this study demonstrated an independent risk factor for mortality (odds ratio = 3.01, 95% confidence interval 1.45–6.28; $P = 0.003$) for ESBL bacteremia [26, 28].

*P. aeruginosa* is a common cause of healthcare-associated infections including pneumonia, bloodstream infections, urinary tract infections, and surgical site infections. *P. aeruginosa* can easily adapt to the environment it inhabits, this ability can lead to colonization, and ultimately invade the human host defenses and cause serious infections. According to the CDC, approximately 7.1% of all healthcare-associated infections in the United States are caused by *P. aeruginosa*. This organism was the second most common cause of pneumonia in the hospital setting, and the third most common cause of Gram-negative bloodstream infections [5]. Kollef et al. recently conducted a global prospective epidemiological study on the prevalence of *P. aeruginosa* causing Ventilator-associated pneumonia (VAP). They concluded that global incidence was 4.1%, and did not differ among countries significantly [29].

In 2013, the CDC's National Healthcare Safety Network (NSHN) reported that 8% of all healthcare-associated infections are caused by *P. aeruginosa*. Among these 8% reported to the NSHN, approximately 13% were considered severe healthcare-associated infections caused by MDR *P. aeruginosa*. By definition, MDR is resistance to at least three different antibiotics classes (mainly antipseudomonal penicillins, aminoglycosides, cephalosporins, and carbapenems). Each year, approximately 51,000 healthcare-associated *P. aeruginosa* infections occur in the United States (according to the CDC). Of these infections, more than 13% are classified as multidrug-resistant (MDR) *P. aeruginosa* and contribute roughly to 400 deaths per year [5].

The true prevalence of multidrug-resistant *P. aeruginosa* is not well established, mainly because there are considerable different definitions used in the literature. Upon reviewing many studies, they tend to report on both MDR and "pan-drug resistant" *P. aeruginosa* infections. In 2011, a new standardized definition was proposed, which classified *Pseudomonas* as MDR, XDR, or pan drug-resistant (PDR) bacteria. MDR as described above is resistant to at least one antibiotic in three or more classes. Extensively drug-resistant (XDR), resistance to all FDA-approved, systemically active agents except for those known to be substantially more toxic than or inferior in efficacy to alternative agents when used to treat susceptible organisms [30]. Finally, PDR, defined, is resistant to all commercially available antibiotics in all classes. MDR *P. aeruginosa* should not be synonymous with carbapenem resistance, as multiple mechanisms of can contribute to resistance. Risk factors for multidrug-resistant (MDR) infections include the following: length of hospital stay, prior use of IV antibiotics, history of *P. aeruginosa* infection, or colonization within the previous year, bedridden in the intensive care unit, mechanical ventilation, history of chronic obstructive pulmonary disease, and malignant disease. Nseir et al. concluded that a new patient admission into a previously occupied ICU room with a patient that had either MDR *P. aeruginosa* or *A. baumannii* was at an independent risk factor for acquisition of those pathogenic organisms. Many studies have examined multidrug-resistant infections as an independent risk factor for mortality, especially when combined with inappropriate antimicrobial therapy [31, 32].

## 4. Infection control

Environmental reservoirs may be unrecognized as the culprit for outbreaks or ongoing sporadic transmission. Recent studies suggest that the risk of acquiring multidrug-resistant pathogens such as *Acinetobacter* spp., *Pseudomonas* spp., vancomycin-resistant Enterococcus (VRE), MRSA, or *C. difficile* is increased if a new patient admission is placed in a room previously occupied by a colonized or infected patient with one of the above pathogens [33–38]. "Terminal cleans" have been utilized for multidrug-resistant Gram-negative organisms and may be integrated with infection control measures, along with surveillance to limit the horizontal transmission of multidrug-resistant organisms.

Environmental survival times of infectious pathogens [39]:

a) MRSA survival time ranges from 7 days to >7 months

b) *Acinetobacter* survival time ranges from 3 days to >5 months

c) *C. difficile* survival is >5 months

d) *Vancomycin-resistant Enterococcus* ranges from 5 days to >4 months

e) *E. coli* from 2 h to 16 months

f) *Klebsiella* from 2 h to >30 months.

Environmental surfaces are routinely disinfected in hospitals based on infection control policies and procedures. Several factors dictate the type and frequency for these cleanings such as surface characteristics, intensity of people traffic, clinical risk, and patient turnover. Following a patient discharge that was known to be colonized or infected with a multidrug-resistant pathogen, a terminal or deep cleaning may be performed. The cleaning regimen is usually tailored with a disinfectant and strength of choice for that particular pathogen. This process usually includes initial removal of all detachable objects from the room, such as bedding and curtains. The terminal clean also includes wiping down any ventilation components on the ceiling or lighting. Finally, all other surfaces and sites are cleaned downward toward the floor level, and all equipment and items that were removed from the room are wiped over with disinfectant before returning to the room. Automated technologies have been recently introduced and may offer enhanced decontamination. Although these technologies are automated they do not replace routine daily cleaning [39].

In the following study, terminal cleaning, combined with standard infection control polices resulted in 70–40% reduction in patients colonized with MDR *Enterobacteriaceae*. These results were attributed to the overall combined intervention. Universal decolonization has been conducted in many ICUs; particularly, after the results of a landmark trial called REDUCE MRSA [33]. Huang et al. concluded that routine ICU practice and universal decolonization was more effective than targeted decolonization or screening [40]. The universal decolonization was effective at reducing rates of MRSA and bloodstream infection from any pathogen. In the treatment group, the number needed to treat (to prevent one) bloodstream infection was per 99 patients. Other technologies have been explored such automated decontamination devices which include peroxide and UV light. As mentioned earlier, these automated technologies could possibly offer some improvement, but they should not replace routine daily cleaning. Common pitfalls for these techniques include additional training of staff, management and personnel oversight, logistical complexities, and costs of equipment. Future studies are warranted to evaluate overall costs versus benefits [39].

The Affordable Care Act in 2015 mandated that the hospital-acquired condition (HAC) reduction program reduce hospital payments by 1% for hospitals performing at the lowest ranked 25% with regard to hospital-acquired conditions. These conditions include Catheter Associated Urinary Tract Infections (CAUTI) and Central Line Associated Bloodstream Infections (CLABSI). As of 2017, CMS has also added both CDI and MRSA to the program. Given that hospitals are now accountable for these conditions, it is imperative that they have robust infection control policies and procedures and have also successfully implemented antimicrobial stewardship programs as defined by the Joint Commission Medication Management (MM) Standard MM.09.01.01 [41–43].

## 5. Surveillance

Surveillance systems allow the evaluation of the local and regional healthcare associated infections (HAI) and antimicrobial resistance (AMR) patters. Surveillance systems contribute to the early detection of HAI and new patterns of AMR, including identifying new clusters or outbreaks. Surveillance is a key component on a local, regional, national, and even on a global scale (WHO) for determining these patterns [44]. Knowing and identifying resistance patterns can help provide guidance to practitioners by means of antibiograms. Antibiograms give the clinician the most appropriate empiric antibiotic information choice while awaiting further confirmation by either phenotypic or genotypic means. The CDC will soon require hospitals to report their antimicrobial use and resistance patterns into the National Healthcare Safety Network (NSHN). This tracking system is the nation's most widely used for healthcare-associated infection. This process will enable the CDC to benchmark hospitals and assess antimicrobial use by measuring the Standardized Antimicrobial Administration Ratio (SAAR). The measurement is a ratio of observed-to-expected (O-to-E). Ratio values greater than 0, and a value of 1.0 suggests equivalency between the observed and predicted antimicrobial use. Values above 1.0 may indicate statistically significant excessive antimicrobial use [44]. In addition to the CDC, many hospital regulatory agencies such as the Joint Commission and CMS will be enforcing this element as part of complying with antimicrobial stewardship program mandates [42, 43].

## 6. Mechanisms of resistance

Microorganisms are tenacious at survival, they have been on the Earth for billions of years, and their sole existence is based on their ability to adapt to the environment. This ability for survival despite the introduction of antibiotics is best described antimicrobial resistance. The mechanisms of antimicrobial resistance are as follows: (a) enzymatic degradation of antibiotics via hydrolytic enzymes, (b) alteration of bacterial proteins or target sites, and (c) changes in membrane permeability to antibiotics either by penetration or by expulsion of the actual antibiotic from within the bacteria. Antibiotic resistance can be either plasmid or chromosomal mediated. One of the most important mechanisms of resistance to beta-lactams is enzymatic hydrolysis of the ring structure resulting in inactivity [45]. The chromosomal β-lactamases expression can either be depressed or induced or by the exposure to β-lactam antibiotics. Overcoming resistance to β-lactam antibiotics includes the coadministration of inhibitors to protect the ring structure, and the development of new antibiotics that are stable against enzymatic degradation. By adding a β-lactamase inhibitor to a β-lactam antibiotic, this allows the β-lactam to avoid enzymatic hydrolysis and perform its bactericidal effects. The following are examples of resistance [45]:

a) Efflux pumps (especially overexpression), which pump the drug out of the cell.

b) Changes in porin protein channels in outer membrane (decreased number or channel charge alteration), which decreases drug uptake.

c) Circumvent metabolic pathways.

d) Enzymatic hydrolysis, i.e., beta-lactamases in Enterobacteriaceae, and nonfermentative Gram-negatives (Acinetobacter).

e) Change in binding affinity of antibiotic for target, i.e., penicillin-binding proteins, DNA topoisomerases, and ribosomal targets.

Bacterial resistance to β-lactam antibiotics as mentioned earlier is mediated via β-lactamases; this mode is the primary mechanism of resistance. Ambler molecular classification is used to classify β-lactamases and is based on the amino acid sequence and divides the class into four

(A, B, C, and D). A, C, and D enzymes utilize serine for β-lactam hydrolysis and class B metalloenzymes require zinc bivalent metal ion, usually $Zn^{2+}$ ions for substrate hydrolysis [46–48].

Example enzymes are as follows:

a) Class A enzymes TEM, SHV, ESBL, CTX-M, KPC, PC1, SME, IMI/NMC, GES/IBC.

b) Class B enzymes MP, VIM, SIM, GIM, SPM, NDM-1.

c) Class C enzymes AmpC, CMY.

d) Class D OXA superfamily (OXA-23, OXA-40 in US outbreaks).

Multidrug efflux mechanisms in bacteria contribute significantly to intrinsic and acquired resistance to many antibiotics. Whole genome sequencing has confirmed the broad distribution of these systems in Gram-negative as well as in Gram-positive bacteria. Multidrug efflux systems have given rise to high-level resistance to Gram-negatives, particularly when multiple mechanisms or resistances are simultaneously produced by a single isolate. The efflux system is mediated by transport proteins, which confer resistance antimicrobial agents. The tripartite efflux system in Gram-negative bacteria is necessary to expel the antibiotic to the outer medium. The system consists of (a) protein localized in the cytoplasmic membrane, (b) protein located in the periplasmatic space, and (c) a third protein located in the outer membrane. These active transport proteins are grouped in families, which are based on their amino acid sequences and mechanisms. The most identified and studied multidrug efflux systems among Gram-negative bacteria are *P. aeruginosa* and *E. coli* [49].

## 7. Early detection

The surviving sepsis guidelines now recommend IV antibiotics to be started within 1 h of sepsis recognition and should include combination therapy (at least two classes of antibiotics to cover a known or suspected pathogen) for patients with septic shock. Combination therapy should not routinely be used for patients without shock. Many studies have demonstrated improved survival in early appropriate administration of antibiotics at the first presence of septic shock [50]. Kumar et al. concluded for each hour of delay of appropriate antimicrobials resulted in a mean increase in mortality by 7.6%, with a range 3.6–9.9% [51]. Ferrer et al. published the results of a large population, which concluded that a delay in first antibiotic administration was associated with increased in-hospital mortality in patients with severe sepsis and septic shock [45]. It was also noted that there was a linear risk increase in mortality for every hour delay in antibiotic administration. Another study by Vazquez-Guillamet concluded that improved targeting in multidrug-resistant bacteria would have the greatest impact on reducing overall mortality. In their study, they calculated the number of patients needed to treat and found for every four patients treated with appropriate antimicrobial therapy in severe sepsis and septic shock, it prevents one patient death [52]. The appropriateness of early empiric antibiotics is driven by local hospital-resistance patterns. At times, selection of the most appropriate empiric antimicrobial regimen may be difficult for the clinician based, appropriate history, comorbidities, risk factors for resistant pathogens, and the complexity of patient transitions of care. Clinicians for decades have depended on phenotypic testing that detects the activity of enzymes (i.e., hydrolysis of antibiotics such as beta-lactams *in vitro*) to provide definitive guidance on antimicrobial therapy. These tests provide the clinician pathogen identity with sensitivity, which may have a turn-around time of up to 72 h. As mentioned above, timing of appropriate antimicrobial therapy is key for patient survival in the critically ill, especially with septic shock. New technological advancements in both phenotypic and genotypic testing (molecular tests that detect the resistance mechanisms of a specific gene) commonly known as "rapid diagnostics" will be able to provide detailed information within several hours versus current standards (48–72 h) [53–56].

See **Tables 2** and **3**.

Procalcitonin (PCT) is an inflammatory biomarker that is an acute phase reactant that reflects host response to bacterial infections. PCT synthesis is up regulated in the presence of bacterial toxins and certain bacterial pro-inflammatory mediators such as TNF$\alpha$ (tumor necrosis factor alpha), interleukin (IL)-1b, IL-6. PCT is neutral to cytokines that are normally released for viral

| **Rapid nonnucleic acid–based tests and other phenotypic tests (MHT/CIM)** | | | |
|---|---|---|---|
| **Manufacturer/product name** | **Methodology** | **Detection results** | **Turnaround time** |
| BioMérieux<br>Rapidec Carba -NP | Detects pH shifts by phenol red indicator that occurs when imipenem is hydrolyzed | Detects (w/o distinction) all three types of carbapenemases:<br>Class A: KPC<br>Class B: NDM/VIM/IMP<br>Class D: OXA | <2 h (after positive culture growth, ~24–48 h) |
| BioMerieux<br>MALDI-TOF MS<br>VItek—MS<br>(matrix-assisted laser desorption ionization time of flight mass spectrometry) | Detects change in native carbapenem mass | Provides bacterial (or fungal) identification at the species, genus, or group level (detects carbapenemase activity) | 2–4 h |
| Modified Hodge test (MHT) | CLSI suggested phenotypic confirmatory test.<br>Enhanced growth = (+) for carbapenemase production<br>No enhanced growth = (-) for carbapenemase production | Only confirms the presence of carbapenemases (does not identify specific carbapenemase (i.e., KPC vs. NDM) | 18–24 h (after positive culture growth, ~24–48 h) |
| Carbapenemase Inactivation method (CIM) | Phenotypic confirmatory test | Only confirms the presence of carbapenemases (does not identify specific carbapenemase (i.e., KPC vs. NDM) | If results required within same day can be read after 6 h, but prefer reading results after 12–24 h (after positive culture growth, ~24–48 h) |

**Table 2.** Rapid diagnostic testing methodologies.

| Rapid nucleic acid–based tests (molecular test) | | | | | |
|---|---|---|---|---|---|
| **Manufacturer/ product name** | **Methodology** | **Specimen type** | **Organisms identified** | **Resistance mechanisms identified** | **Turnaround time** |
| BioFire Diagnostics LLC/ Film Array® Blood Culture Identification Panel (BCID) | Multiplex PCR (detects 23 bacterial species, four resistance mechanisms and *Candida* spp.) | Blood Other FDA Cleared Panels: Respiratory, GI, Meningitis | Gram-positives: *Staph/Strep/ Enterococcus/ Listeria* Gram-negatives: *Enterobacteriaceae, Pseudomonas aeruginosa*, and *Acinetobacter* species. Fungus: *Candida spp.* | *mecA* *vanA/vanB* $bla_{KPC}$ | 1 h (after blood culture positivity, ~8–24 h) |
| Nanosphere/ Verigene® | Microarray (detects 15 different Gram-positive targets and 14 different Gram-negative targets (including nine resistance mechanisms) | Blood Other FDA Cleared Panels: Respiratory, GI | Gram-positives: *Staph/Strep/ Enterococcus/ Listeria* Gram-negatives: *Enterobacteriaceae, Pseudomonas aeruginosa*, and *Acinetobacter* species | *mecA* *vanA/vanB* IMP/KPC/NDM OXA/VIM/ CTX-M ESBLs | 2.5 h (after blood culture positivity, ~8–24 h) |
| Cepheid GeneXpert Carba R | "On demand" PCR | Rectal swabs | Gram-negative: *Enterobacteriaceae, Pseudomonas aeruginosa*, and *Acinetobacter* species | IMP/KPC/NDM/ OXA*/VIM *(Includes OXA-48, OXA-181, OXA-232) | 48 min (can test directly from clinical specimen) |

**Table 3.** Rapid diagnostic testing methodologies.

infections such as interferon-γ. PCT concentrations are undetectable (less than 0.05 ng/mL). However, PCT is immediately released within 2–4 h upon exposure to bacterial toxins. The plasma half-life of PCT is approximately 24 h. Concentrations in the literature have varied for infected patients; however, as higher max concentrations of PCT are released during infection, this tends to correlate with a higher incidence of mortality. In the critically ill baseline PCT levels should be obtained with signs and symptoms of infection as a means of trending. A low PCT level or an ample decrease from baseline along with clinical review during the course of therapy should be interpreted to discontinue antimicrobial therapy. This methodology is part of an antimicrobial stewardship program, which reduces unnecessary antibiotics and also decreases duration. PCT has been proven to effective and safe in various critically ill patients. Many published studies have evaluated the utility of a PCT-guided strategy for determining the appropriate time to discontinue and/or de-escalate antibiotics in patients with varying severity of illnesses with documented infections. These studies have resulted in decreased unnecessary use of antibiotics [50].

## 8. Treatment

As described earlier, prompt administration with appropriate empiric broad-spectrum antibiotics within 1 h of recognizing sepsis or septic shock has shown to improve survival. The surviving sepsis guidelines recommend initial selection of antimicrobial therapy to broad or "shot gun" approach. This approach ensures that the likely pathogen will be covered. If not, survival may decrease as much as fivefold for septic shock if the initial empiric regimen fails to cover the offending pathogen [50]. The choice of empiric antimicrobial therapy depends on factors related to clinical status, the patient's history, and local epidemiologic factors (see below). Due to the high mortality associated with inappropriate initial therapy, empiric treatment choices should be broad initially, with constant evaluation to de-escalate the regimen once cultures and results have been determined. The guidelines also address several factors in determining the appropriate antimicrobial regimens:

a) The site of infection, pathogen profile, and antimicrobial pharmacokinetics and pharmacodynamics (PK/PD) as it relates to penetration at the site.

b) Prevalence of pathogens in the community, hospital, and specific hospital locations, i.e., critical care unit by means of surveillance is an important determinant.

c) The resistance patterns of prevalent pathogens in the form of antibiograms or surveillance programs.

d) Status of the patient, i.e., immunocompromised patients such as HIV infection, splenectomy, neutropenia, congenital defects of immunoglobulin, complement, or leukocyte dysfunction.

e) Age and patient comorbidities, the presence of invasive devices that compromise the host defenses [50].

Since majority of the patients with severe sepsis do have some form of immunocompromised status, the broad-spectrum antibiotics should be initiated [50]. Clinicians should assess these statuses of β-lactam and carbapenem resistance in their local communities. Physicians should also consider adding another Gram-negative coverage to cover *Pseudomonas* or *Acinetobacter* infections [57]. It holds true for covering for MRSA infections in patients with suspicion or risk factors for those infections. In patients who are immunocompromised with immunosuppressive medications, neutropenia, liver or renal failure, on total parenteral nutrition the coverage for the candida infection needs to be considered [58].

Dosing patients with severe sepsis and septic shock should be centered on pharmacokinetics/pharmacodynamics (PK/PD) and drug properties as per the recommendation of surviving sepsis committee [50]. In most instances, the inability to achieve a therapeutic response can be attributed to the failure of optimizing PK/PD, i.e., failure of target attainment by means of reduced initial dosing or inadequate achievable troughs with subsequent dosing [59]. For optimum dosing for fluoroquinolones and aminoglycoside, it requires to optimize the peak plasma level. For aminoglycoside, it can be achieved by 5–7 mg/kg daily gentamicin dose or equivalent. For fluoroquinolones, one should consider dosing for ciprofloxacin at 600 mg, every 12 hourly and for levofloxacin at 750 mg Q 24 hourly [60–62].

For vancomycin, trough levels of 15–20 mg/L have been advocated. In addition, drugs with a low volume of distribution such as vancomycin and colistin, a higher loading dose is suggested [63–65]. For the β-lactams, it is the time when the plasma concentration of the drug should be above the pathogen minimum inhibitory concentration (MIC) level. It is suggested to have the T > MIC (time above the minimum inhibitory concentration) of 60% and greater to have good efficacy, but among patients with sepsis a level of T > MIC of 100% may be needed. This is achieved by prolonging the infusion either as an extended or continuous infusion [50, 66].

In regard to the duration of antimicrobial therapy, per surviving sepsis guidelines, the duration of 7–10 days is adequate for most serious infections associated with sepsis and septic shock. In the 2016, management of adults with hospital-acquired and ventilator-associated pneumonia, 7 days are appropriate for those patients that respond to therapy early on and show clinical improvement (see below). Longer courses can be appropriate for patients who are slow responders or immunocompromised patients, and patients with MDR organisms, some fungal, or viral infections or MRSA [50]. Patients with endocarditis, osteomyelitis and larger abscesses may also require longer duration of therapy [50].

Multidrug-resistant pathogens are associated with increased morbidity and mortality and are certainly challenging to treat. We have described the surviving sepsis guidelines and recently published the 2016 Management of Adults With Hospital-acquired and Ventilator-associated Pneumonia: Clinical Practice Guidelines by the Infectious Diseases Society of America. These guidelines make recommendations for the diagnosis and treatment of Hospital-acquired pneumonia (HAP) and Ventilator-associated pneumonia (VAP) and are evidence-based derived from systematic literature reviews (**Table 4**).

Detailed pathogen recommendation is beyond the scope of this chapter, but we included an extensive review on Minocin IV. Minocin IV has an FDA approved indication for *Acinetobacte*r *spp*. and not referenced in the guidelines above, but it has been used with success against *Acinetobacte*r, including MDR and XDR strains. MINOCIN® (minocycline) [67] IV has been reformulated, the new formulation contains magnesium sulfate heptahydrate and can be infused in as low as 100 mL to as high as 1000 mL over 60 min. It has a new pH of 4.5–6.0 when diluted.

Resistance to β-lactams has resulted in the resurrection of shelf toxic agents, i.e., the polymyxins. Tigecycline and sulbactam are not FDA approved for treatment of infections due to *Acinetobacter*. A recent meta-analysis evaluating the use of tigecycline against *Acinetobacter* infections disfavor its use due to an associated higher in-hospital mortality (OR = 1.57, 95% CI 1.04–2.35; $P = 0.03$) [68].

Tetracyclines, as a class, have shown consistent *in vitro* activity against *Acinetobacte*r [20, 21]. Increasing levels of multidrug resistance with *Acinetobacter* have led clinicians to reevaluate certain tetracyclines with good *in vitro* activity. Studies of minocycline in *Acinetobacter* infections have shown clinical success ranging from 67 to 88% [21, 69–73]. Minocycline has approved breakpoints for *Acinetobacter* set forth by the Clinical and Laboratory Standards Institute (CLSI) [54]. These breakpoints are shown in **Table 5**.

| A. Gram-positive antibiotics with MRSA activity | B. Gram-negative antibiotics with antipseudomonal activity: β-lactam–based agents | C. Gram-negative antibiotics with antipseudomonal activity: non–β-lactam–based agents |
|---|---|---|
| Glycopeptides<br>Vancomycin 15 mg/kg IV q8-12h<br>(Consider a loading dose of 25–30 mg/kg × 1 for severe illness) | Antipseudomonal penicillins<br>Piperacillin-tazobactam 4.5 g IV q6h | Fluoroquinolones<br>Ciprofloxacin 400 mg IV q8h<br>Levofloxacin 750 mg IV q24h |
| OR | OR | OR |
| Oxazolidinones<br>Linezolid 600 mg IV q12h | Cephalosporins<br>Cefepime 2 g IV q8h<br>Ceftazidime 2 g IV q8h | Aminoglycosides<br>Amikacin 15–20 mg/kg IV q24h<br>Gentamicin 5–7 mg/kg IV q24h<br>Tobramycin 5–7 mg/kg IV q24h |
| | OR | OR |
| | Carbapenems<br>Imipenem 500 mg IV q6hd<br>Meropenem 1 g IV q8h | Polymyxins<br>Colistin 5 mg/kg IV × 1 (loading dose) followed by 2.5 mg × (1.5 × CrCl + 30) IV q12h (maintenance dose)<br>Polymyxin B 2.5–3.0 mg/kg/d divided in 2 daily IV doses |
| | OR | |
| | Monobactams<br>Aztreonam 2 g IV q8h | |

Notes: Please refer to these guidelines for the compete table, HAP recommendations and detailed pathogen recommendations that can be found at: https://www.thoracic.org/statements/resources/tb-opi/hap-vap-guidelines-2016.pdf

**Table 4.** Summary of recommendations for suggested empiric treatment options for clinically suspected ventilator-associated pneumonia.

| MIC (μg/mL) | Interpretation |
|---|---|
| ≤4.0 | Susceptible (S) |
| 8.0 | Intermediate (I) |
| ≥16.0 | Resistant (R) |

**Table 5.** Clinical and Laboratory Standards Institute MIC and disk breakpoints available for minocycline and *Acinetobacter spp*.

CLSI recommends separate *Acinetobacter* susceptibility results for minocycline since surrogate testing with other tetracyclines will underestimate susceptibility. Several retrospective studies have documented that lower mortality rates seen with combination therapy are used against MDR *A. baumannii* infections.

Minocycline IV has been used in combination therapy to achieve synergistic activity and to maximize antimicrobial activity in severely ill patients, or to prevent emergence of resistance [74]. Minocycline and colistin combinations demonstrated bactericidal and synergistic activity against imipenem-resistant *A. baumannii* and MDR *A. baumannii* clinical isolates [75]. Combinations of minocycline plus meropenem and minocycline plus colistin were found to be synergistic *in vitro* against XDR *A. baumannii*. The package insert (PI) has an initial dose of 200 mg, with subsequent doses of 100 mg administered over 60 min every 12 h. Minocycline is very lipophilic compared to other tetracyclines. It has a very unique pharmacokinetic/pharmacodynamic profile (PK/PD) [67]:

a) Peak concentrations following 200-mg load (mean) = 4.18 μg/mL (range, 2.52–6.63 μg/mL).

b) Trough concentration of (1.4–1.8 μg/mL) with 100-mg dosing every 12 h.

c) These achievable peak and trough serum concentrations with standard human doses of minocycline intravenous exceed the mutant prevention concentration of 1 μg/mL, which has been reported with *Acinetobacter*.

d) Half-life of 15–23 h.

e) The mean concentration of minocycline in lung parenchyma has been reported to be 378% of that in plasma.

f) Urinary excretion 11%.

g) Renal dysfunction does not appear to alter the maximum serum concentrations of mino cycline.

h) Bactericidal activity in combination with carbapenems or colistin against *A. baumannii*.

## 9. Importance of antimicrobial stewardship programs, outcomes, and new regulatory mandate from the Joint Commission (7 CDC elements)

According to the World Health Organization (WHO), "Antimicrobial resistance threatens the effective prevention and treatment of an ever-increasing range of infections caused by bacteria, parasites, viruses, and fungi." The Centers for Disease Control and Prevention (CDC) has identified that 20–50% of all antibiotics prescribed in the U.S. acute care hospitals are either inappropriate or unnecessary. The CDC has also stated that "Antibiotics are among the most commonly prescribed medications in nursing homes. Up to 70% of long-term care facilities' residents receive an antibiotic every year [76]."

White House held the antibiotic stewardship program in June, 2015, in which the Joint Commission participated along with more than 150 major healthcare organizations and other relevant organizations for helping to implement changes over the next 5 years to decrease the rate of emergence of antibiotic-resistant bacteria, to help detect the resistant strains, help preserve the efficacy of existing antibiotics, and also more importantly regulate to prevent the spread of resistant infections [76].

The Joint Commission has also developed the antimicrobial stewardship standard for hospitals, critical access hospitals, nursing care centers, ambulatory care organizations, and

Official Publication of Joint Commission Requirements New Antimicrobial Stewardship Standard Applicable to Hospitals and Critical Access Hospitals Effective January 1, 2017 Medication Management (MM) Standard MM.09.01.01 The critical access hospital has an antimicrobial stewardship program based on current scientific literature.

**1.** Leaders establish antimicrobial stewardship as an organizational priority. (*See also* LD.01.03.01, EP 5)
**Note:** *Examples of leadership commitment to an antimicrobial stewardship program are as follows:*

- Accountability documents
- Budget plans
- Infection prevention plans
- Performance improvement plans
- Strategic plans
- Using the electronic health record to collect antimicrobial stewardship data

**2.** The critical access hospital educates staff and licensed independent practitioners involved in antimicrobial ordering, dispensing, administration, and monitoring about antimicrobial resistance and antimicrobial stewardship practices. Education occurs upon hire or granting of initial privileges and periodically thereafter, based on organizational need

**3.** The critical access hospital educates patients, and their families as needed, regarding the appropriate use of antimicrobial medications, including antibiotics. (For more information on patient education, refer to Standard PC.02.03.01)
**Note:** *An example of an educational tool that can be used for patients and families includes the Centers for Disease Control and Prevention's Get Smart document, "Viruses or Bacteria—What's got you sick? At https://www.cdc.gov/antibiotic-use/community/pdfs/Viruses-or-Bacteria-Factsheet-Eng.pdf*

**4.** The critical access hospital has an antimicrobial stewardship
multidisciplinary team that includes the following members, when available in the setting:

- Infectious disease physician
- Infection preventionist(s)
- Pharmacist(s)
- Practitioner

**Note 1:** *Part-time or consultant staff are acceptable as members of the antimicrobial stewardship multidisciplinary team*
**Note 2:** *Telehealth staffs are acceptable as members of the antimicrobial stewardship multidisciplinary team*

**5. The critical access hospital's antimicrobial stewardship program includes the following CDC core elements:**

- Leadership commitment: Dedicating necessary human, financial, and information technology resources.
- Accountability: Appointing a single leader responsible for program outcomes. Experience with successful programs shows that a physician leader is effective.
- Drug expertise: Appointing a single pharmacist leader responsible for working to improve antibiotic use.
- Action: Implementing recommended actions, such as systemic evaluation of on-going treatment need, after a set period of initial treatment (for example, "antibiotic time out" after 48 h).
- Tracking: Monitoring the antimicrobial stewardship program, which may include information on antibiotic prescribing and resistance patterns.
- Reporting: Regularly reporting information on the antimicrobial stewardship program, which may include information on antibiotic use and resistance, to doctors, nurses, and relevant staff.
- Education: Educating practitioners, staff, and patients on the antimicrobial program, which may include information about resistance and optimal prescribing. (*See also* IC.02.01.01, EP 1 and NPSG.07.03.01, EP 5)

**Note:** *These core elements were cited from the Centers for Disease Control and Prevention's Core Elements of Hospital Antibiotic Stewardship Programs (https://www.cdc.gov/antibiotic-use/healthcare/pdfs/core-elements.pdf)*

| | |
|---|---|
| **6**. The critical access hospital's antimicrobial stewardship program uses organization-approved multidisciplinary protocols (for example, policies and procedures).<br>**Note:** *Examples of protocols are as follows:*<br>• *Antibiotic Formulary Restrictions*<br>• *Assessment of Appropriateness of Antibiotics for Community-Acquired Pneumonia*<br>• *Assessment of Appropriateness of Antibiotics for Skin and Soft Tissue Infections*<br>• *Assessment of Appropriateness of Antibiotics for Urinary Tract Infections*<br>• *Care of the Patient with Clostridium difficile (c. -diff)*<br>• *Guidelines for Antimicrobial Use in Adults*<br>• *Guidelines for Antimicrobial Use in Pediatrics*<br>• *Plan for Parenteral to Oral Antibiotic Conversion*<br>• *Preauthorization Requirements for Specific Antimicrobials*<br>• *Use of Prophylactic Antibiotics* | **7**. The critical access hospital collects, analyzes, and reports data on its antimicrobial stewardship program<br>**Note:** *Examples of topics to collect and analyze data on may include evaluation of the antimicrobial stewardship program, antimicrobial prescribing patterns, and antimicrobial resistance patterns* |
| **8**. The critical access hospital takes action on improvement opportunities identified in its antimicrobial stewardship program. (*See also* MM.08.01.01, EP 6) | |
| Adopted from https://www.jointcommission.org/assets/1/6/New_Antimicrobial_Stewardship_Standard.pdf. | |

**Table 6.** The New Joint Commission antimicrobial stewardship standard: MM.09.01.01.

office-based surgery practices in standard with the following governmental and professional organizations: Centers for Medicare & Medicaid Services (CMS), the CDC, and the Society for Healthcare Epidemiology of America (SHEA) (**Table 6**).

## 10. Future pipeline in phase III development

There has been emergence and increase of MDR pathogens. Efforts have been made toward adequate treatment, daily de-escalation regimen as well as antibiotic stewardship programs. The pipeline for the new drugs is still sparse. **Table 7** illustrates the antibiotics that are in the phase 3 trials. Only very few have an expected activity against the CDC urgent threat potential (**Table 7**).

## 11. Conclusion

Antimicrobial resistance has risen at threating levels within the past few decades and has contributed to an economic burden on healthcare expenditures. Several governmental agencies including the WHO, CDC, and the White House are focused on combating antimicrobial resistance at various steps. Acquisition of multidrug-resistant organisms in patients has established an

http://dx.doi.org/10.5772/intechopen.69377

| Drug name | Development phase | Company | Drug class | Expected activity against resistant Gram-negative ESKAPE pathogens? | Expected activity against a CDC urgent threat pathogen?4 |
|---|---|---|---|---|---|
| Zabofloxacin | Phase 3 | Dong Wha Pharmaceutical Co. Ltd | Fluoroquinolone | No | No |
| S-649266 | Phase 3 | Shionogi Inc. | Cephalosporin | Yes | Yes |
| Omadacycline | Phase 3 | Paratek Pharmaceuticals Inc. | Tetracycline | Yes | Possible |
| Lefamulin (BC-3781) | Phase 3 | Nabriva Therapeutics AG | Pleuromutilin | No | No<br>No |
| Imipenem/ cilastatin+relebactam (MK-7655) | Phase 3 | Merck & Co. Inc. | Carbapenem+novel beta-lactamase inhibitor | Yes | Yes |
| Iclaprim | Phase 3 | Motif Bio PLC | Dihydrofolate reductase (DHFR) inhibitor | No | No |
| Cadazolid | Phase 3 | Actelion Pharmaceuticals Ltd. | Quinolonyl- oxazolidinone | No | Yes |
| Taksta (fusidic acid) | Phase 3 | Cempra Inc. | Fusidane | No | No |
| Carbavance (vaborbactam+ meropenem) | Phase 3 | Rempex Pharmaceuticals Inc. (wholly owned subsidiary of the Medicines Co.) | Meropenem+novel boronic beta-lactamase inhibitor | Yes | Yes |
| Baxdela (delafloxacin) | Phase 3 | Melinta Therapeutics Inc. | Fluoroquinolone | Possible | Possible |
| Eravacycline | Phase 3 | Tetraphase Pharmaceuticals Inc. | Tetracycline | Yes | Yes |
| Plazomicin | Phase 3 | Achaogen Inc. | Aminoglycoside | Yes | Yes |
| Solithromycin | Phase 3 | Cempra Inc. | Macrolide (fluoroketolide) | No | Yes |

*Source*: Adopted with permission from: http://www.pewtrusts.org/~/media/assets/2016/05/antibiotics-currently-in-clinical-development.pdf. Full table for drugs in phase 1 and phase 2 is available from this site.

**Table 7.** New antibiotics currently in clinical development.

independent risk factor for mortality. Clinical expertise, risk stratification, surveillance, infection control, and the use of rapid diagnostics may be key to early identification of resistant pathogens; furthermore, appropriate antimicrobial selection and dose optimization via PK/PD are critical in improving outcomes and survival. Various studies have demonstrated the correlation between survival and appropriate early initial antibiotics. Antimicrobial stewardship programs have been shown to reduce antimicrobial resistance and are now considered a regulatory mandate. CMS and TJC have developed guidance for accreditation as it relates to demonstrating an effective antimicrobial stewardship program, including developing publicly reportable measures.

In recent years, we have seen high-level resistance to last-line agents such as carbapenems. Inappropriate usage and a reduced antimicrobial pipeline have driven this crisis. Several companies are dedicated to the research and development of new antimicrobials for our armamentarium in combating multidrug-resistant organisms and preventing a preantibiotic era. Education will be vital across all healthcare disciplines, including to patients, as this will ultimately ensure optimal prescribing.

## Conflict of Interest

Salim Surani has no conflict of interest to disclose. Mauricio Rodriguez is an employee of Medicine Company. No conflict persists pertaining to this chapter.

## Author details

Mauricio Rodriguez[1] and Salim R. Surani[2,3*]

*Address all correspondence to: srsurani@hotmail.com

1 Global Health Sciences-Infectious Disease Care, The Medicines Company, TX, USA

2 Texas A&M University, TX, USA

3 University of North Texas, TX, USA

## References

[1] Ventola CL. The antibiotic resistance crisis: Part 1: Causes and threats. P & T: A Peer-Reviewed Journal for Formulary Management. 2015;**40**(4):277-283 [PMID: 25859123 PMCID: 4378521]

[2] Ventola CL. The antibiotic resistancecrisis: Part 2: Management strategies and new agents. P & T: A Peer-Reviewed Journal for Formulary Management. 2015;**40**(5):344-352 [PMID: 25987823 PMCID: 4422635]

[3] Boucher HW, Talbot GH, Bradley JS, Edwards JE, Gilbert D, Rice LB, Scheld M, Spellberg B, Bartlett J. Bad bugs, no drugs: No ESKAPE! An update from the Infectious Diseases Society of America. Clinical Infectious Diseases: An Official Publication of the Infectious Diseases Society of America. 2009;**48**(1):1-12 [PMID: 19035777 DOI: 10.1086/595011]

[4] Talbot GH, Bradley J, Edwards Jr JE, Gilbert D, Scheld M, Bartlett JG, Antimicrobial availability task force of the infectious diseases society of A. Bad bugs need drugs: An update on the development pipeline from the Antimicrobial availability task force of the infectious diseases society of America. Clinical Infectious Diseases: An Official Publication of the Infectious Diseases Society of America. 2006;**42**(5):657-668 [PMID: 16447111 DOI: 10.1086/499819]

[5] Antibiotics Resistance Threat in the US. US Department of Health & Human Services; Centers for Disease Control and Prevention [Internet]. 2013. Available from: http://www.cdc.gov/drugresistance/pdf/ar-threats-2013-508.pdf [Accessed: March 16, 2017]

[6] President Advisory Council on Combating Antibiotic-resistant Bacteria. HHS. Gov. 2015. Available from: http://www.hhs.gov/ash/advisory.committees/paccarb/$ [Accessed: March 16, 2017]

[7] Detsis M, Karanika S, Mylonakis E. ICU acquisition rate, risk factors, and clinical significance of digestive tract colonization with extended-spectrum beta-lactamase-producing enterobacteriaceae: A systematic review and meta-analysis. Critical Care Medicine. 2017;**45**(4):705-714. [PMID: 28157141 DOI: 10.1097/CCM.0000000000002253]

[8] Vardakas KZ, Rafailidis PI, Konstantelias AA, Falagas ME. Predictors of mortality in patients with infections due to multi-drug resistant Gram negative bacteria: The study, the patient, the bug or the drug? The Journal of Infection. 2013;**66**(5):401-414 [PMID: 23142195 DOI: 10.1016/j.jinf.2012.10.028]

[9] Munoz-Price LS, Poirel L, Bonomo RA, Schwaber MJ, Daikos GL, Cormican M, Cornaglia G, Garau J, Gniadkowski M, Hayden MK, Kumarasamy K, Livermore DM, Maya JJ, Nordmann P, Patel JB, Paterson DL, Pitout J, Villegas MV, Wang H, Woodford N, Quinn JP. Clinical epidemiology of the global expansion of *Klebsiella pneumoniae* carbapenemases. The Lancet Infectious Diseases. 2013;**13**(9):785-796 [PMID: 23969216 PMCID: 4673667 DOI: 10.1016/S1473-3099(13)70190-7]

[10] Guh AY, Bulens SN, Mu Y, Jacob JT, Reno J, Scott J, Wilson LE, Vaeth E, Lynfield R, Shaw KM, Vagnone PM, Bamberg WM, Janelle SJ, Dumyati G, Concannon C, Beldavs Z, Cunningham M, Cassidy PM, Phipps EC, Kenslow N, Travis T, Lonsway D, Rasheed JK, Limbago BM, Kallen AJ. Epidemiology of carbapenem-resistant enterobacteriaceae in 7 US communities, 2012-2013. Journal of the American Medical Association. 2015;**314**(14):1479-1487 [PMID: 26436831 DOI: 10.1001/jama.2015.12480]

[11] Spellberg B, Rex JH. The value of single-pathogen antibacterial agents. Nature Reviews Drug Discovery. 2013;**12**(12):963 [PMID: 24232373 PMCID: 4012226 DOI: 10.1038/nrd3957-c1]

[12] van Duin D, Perez F, Rudin SD, Cober E, Hanrahan J, Ziegler J, Webber R, Fox J, Mason P, Richter SS, Cline M, Hall GS, Kaye KS, Jacobs MR, Kalayjian RC, Salata RA, Segre JA, Conlan S, Evans S, Fowler Jr VG, Bonomo RA. Surveillance of carbapenem-resistant *Klebsiella pneumoniae*: Tracking molecular epidemiology and outcomes through a regional network. Antimicrobial Agents and Chemotherapy. 2014;**58**(7):4035-4041 [PMID: 24798270 PMCID: 4068524 DOI: 10.1128/AAC.02636-14]

[13] Lin MY, Lyles-Banks RD, Lolans K, Hines DW, Spear JB, Petrak R, Trick WE, Weinstein RA, Hayden MK, Centers for Disease C, Prevention Epicenters P. The importance of long-term acute care hospitals in the regional epidemiology of *Klebsiella pneumoniae* carbapenemase-producing enterobacteriaceae. Clinical Infectious Diseases: An Official Publication of the Infectious Diseases Society of America. 2013;**57**(9):1246-1252 [PMID: 23946222 DOI: 10.1093/cid/cit500]

[14] Kim UJ, Kim HK, An JH, Cho SK, Park KH, Jang HC. Update on the epidemiology, treatment, and outcomes of carbapenem-resistant acinetobacter infections. Chonnam Medical Journal. 2014;**50**(2):37-44 [PMID: 25229014 PMCID: 4161759 DOI: 10.4068/cmj.2014.50.2.37]

[15] Munoz-Price LS, Weinstein RA. Acinetobacter infection. The New England Journal of Medicine. 2008;**358**(12):1271-1281 [PMID: 18354105 DOI: 10.1056/NEJMra070741]

[16] Cerqueira GM, Peleg AY. Insights into *Acinetobacter baumannii* pathogenicity. IUBMB Life. 2011;**63**(12):1055-1060 [PMID: 21989983 DOI: 10.1002/iub.533]

[17] Bennett JE, Raphael D, Blaser MJ. Mandell, Douglas and Bennett's Principles and Practices of Infectious Disease. 8th ed. Philadelphia: Saunders; 2014

[18] Al-Anazi KA, Abdalhamid B, Alshibani Z, Awad K, Alzayed A, Hassan H, Alsayiegh M. *Acinetobacter baumannii* septicemia in a recipient of an allogeneic hematopoietic stem cell transplantation. Case Reports in Transplantation. 2012;**2012**:646195 [PMID: 23259136 PMCID: 3504248 DOI: 10.1155/2012/646195]

[19] Al-Anazi KA, Al-Jasser AM. Infections caused by *Acinetobacter baumannii* in recipients of hematopoietic stem cell transplantation. Frontiers in Oncology. 2014;**4**:186 [PMID: 25072028 PMCID: 4095644 DOI: 10.3389/fonc.2014.00186]

[20] Castanheira M, Mendes RE, Jones RN. Update on *Acinetobacter* species: Mechanisms of antimicrobial resistance and contemporary in vitro activity of minocycline and other treatment options. Clinical Infectious Diseases: An Official Publication of the Infectious Diseases Society of America. 2014;**59(**Suppl 6):S367–S373 [PMID: 25371512 DOI: 10.1093/cid/ciu706]

[21] Denys GA, Renzi PB, Koch KM, Wissel CM. Three-way comparison of BBL CHROMagar MRSA II, MRSASelect, and spectra MRSA for detection of methicillin-resistant *Staphylococcus aureus* isolates in nasal surveillance cultures. Journal of Clinical Microbiology. 2013;**51**(1):202-205 [PMID: 23135930 PMCID: 3536262 DOI: 10.1128/JCM.02022-12]

[22] Doi Y, Park YS, Rivera JI, Adams-Haduch JM, Hingwe A, Sordillo EM, Lewis 2nd JS, Howard WJ, Johnson LE, Polsky B, Jorgensen JH, Richter SS, Shutt KA, Paterson DL.

Community-associated extended-spectrum beta-lactamase-producing *Escherichia coli* infection in the United States. Clinical Infectious Diseases: An Official Publication of the Infectious Diseases Society of America. 2013;**56**(5):641-648 [PMID: 23150211 PMCID: 3563390 DOI: 10.1093/cid/cis942]

[23] Ben-Ami R, Schwaber MJ, Navon-Venezia S, Schwartz D, Giladi M, Chmelnitsky I, Leavitt A, Carmeli Y. Influx of extended-spectrum beta-lactamase-producing enterobacteriaceae into the hospital. Clinical Infectious Diseases: An Official Publication of the Infectious Diseases Society of America. 2006;**42**(7):925-934 [PMID: 16511754 DOI: 10.1086/500936]

[24] Ben-Ami R, Rodriguez-Bano J, Arslan H, Pitout JD, Quentin C, Calbo ES, Azap OK, Arpin C, Pascual A, Livermore DM, Garau J, Carmeli Y. A multinational survey of risk factors for infection with extended-spectrum beta-lactamase-producing enterobacteriaceae in nonhospitalized patients. Clinical Infectious Diseases: An Official Publication of the Infectious Diseases Society of America. 2009;**49**(5):682-690 [PMID: 19622043 DOI: 10.1086/604713]

[25] Denisuik AJ, Lagace-Wiens PR, Pitout JD, Mulvey MR, Simner PJ, Tailor F, Karlowsky JA, Hoban DJ, Adam HJ, Zhanel GG, Canadian Antimicrobial Resistance A. Molecular epidemiology of extended-spectrum beta-lactamase-, AmpC beta-lactamase- and carbapenemase-producing *Escherichia coli* and *Klebsiella pneumoniae* isolated from Canadian hospitals over a 5 year period: CANWARD 2007-11. The Journal of Antimicrobial Chemotherapy. 2013;**68**(Suppl 1):i57–i65 [PMID: 23587779 DOI: 10.1093/jac/dkt027]

[26] Harris PN. Clinical management of infections caused by Enterobactericeae that express extended-spectrum Beta-lactamase and AmpC enzymes. Seminars in Respiratory and Critical Care Medicine. 2015;**36**(1):56-73

[27] Stuart RL, Kotsanas D, Webb B, Vandergraaf S, Gillespie EE, Hogg GG, Korman TM. Prevalence of antimicrobial-resistant organisms in residential aged care facilities. The Medical Journal of Australia. 2011;**195**(9):530-533 [PMID: 22060088]

[28] Ha YE, Kang CI, Cha MK, Park SY, Wi YM, Chung DR, Peck KR, Lee NY, Song JH. Epidemiology and clinical outcomes of bloodstream infections caused by extended-spectrum beta-lactamase-producing *Escherichia coli* in patients with cancer. International Journal of Antimicrobial Agents. 2013;**42**(5):403-409 [PMID: 24071027 DOI: 10.1016/j.ijantimicag.2013.07.018]

[29] Kollef MH, Chastre J, Fagon JY, Francois B, Niederman MS, Rello J, Torres A, Vincent JL, Wunderink RG, Go KW, Rehm C. Global prospective epidemiologic and surveillance study of ventilator-associated pneumonia due to *Pseudomonas aeruginosa*. Critical Care Medicine. 2014;**42**(10):2178-2187 [PMID: 25054674 DOI: 10.1097/CCM.0000000000000510]

[30] Magiorakos AP, Srinivasan A, Carey RB, Carmeli Y, Falagas ME, Giske CG, Harbarth S, Hindler JF, Kahlmeter G, Olsson-Liljequist B, Paterson DL, Rice LB, Stelling J, Struelens MJ, Vatopoulos A, Weber JT, Monnet DL. Multidrug-resistant, extensively drug-resistant and pan drug-resistant bacteria: An international expert proposal for interim standard definitions for acquired resistance. Clinical Microbiology and Infection: The Official

Publication of the European Society of Clinical Microbiology and Infectious Diseases. 2012;**18**(3):268-281 [PMID: 21793988 DOI: 10.1111/j.1469-0691.2011.03570.x]

[31] Hirsch EB, Tam VH. Impact of multidrug-resistant *Pseudomonas aeruginosa* infection on patient outcomes. Expert Review of Pharmacoeconomics & Outcomes Research. 2010;**10**(4):441-451 [PMID: 20715920 PMCID: 3071543 DOI: 10.1586/erp.10.49]

[32] McCarthy K. Pseudomonas aeruginosa: Evolution of antimicrobial resistance and implications for therapy. Seminars in Respiratory and Critical Care Medicine. 2015;**36**(1):44-55 [PMID: 25643270 DOI: 10.1055/s-0034-1396907]

[33] Huang SS, Datta R, Platt R. Risk of acquiring antibiotic-resistant bacteria from prior room occupants. Archives of Internal Medicine. 2006;**166**(18):1945-1951 [PMID: 17030826 DOI: 10.1001/archinte.166.18.1945]

[34] Drees M, Snydman DR, Schmid CH, Barefoot L, Hansjosten K, Vue PM, Cronin M, Nasraway SA, Golan Y. Prior environmental contamination increases the risk of acquisition of vancomycin-resistant enterococci. Clinical Infectious Diseases: An Official Publication of the Infectious Diseases Society of America. 2008;**46**(5):678-685 [PMID: 18230044 DOI: 10.1086/527394]

[35] Wilks M, Wilson A, Warwick S, Price E, Kennedy D, Ely A, Millar MR. Control of an outbreak of multidrug-resistant Acinetobacter baumannii-calcoaceticus colonization and infection in an intensive care unit (ICU) without closing the ICU or placing patients in isolation. Infection Control and Hospital Epidemiology. 2006;**27**(7):654-658 [PMID: 16807837 DOI: 10.1086/507011]

[36] Nseir S, Blazejewski C, Lubret R, Wallet F, Courcol R, Durocher A. Risk of acquiring multidrug-resistant Gram-negative bacilli from prior room occupants in the intensive care unit. Clinical Microbiology and Infection: The Official Publication of the European Society of Clinical Microbiology and Infectious Diseases. 2011;**17**(8):1201-1208 [PMID: 21054665 DOI: 10.1111/j.1469-0691.2010.03420.x]

[37] Shaughnessy MK, Micielli RL, DePestel DD, Arndt J, Strachan CL, Welch KB, Chenoweth CE. Evaluation of hospital room assignment and acquisition of *Clostridium difficile* infection. Infection Control and Hospital Epidemiology. 2011;**32**(3):201-206 [PMID: 21460503 DOI: 10.1086/658669]

[38] Dancer SJ, Carling PC. All that glistens may be neither gold nor clean. The Journal of Hospital Infection. 2010;**76**(2):177-178 [PMID: 20691502 DOI: 10.1016/j.jhin.2010.06.008]

[39] Dancer SJ. Controlling hospital-acquired infection: Focus on the role of the environment and new technologies for decontamination. Clinical Microbiology Reviews. 2014;**27**(4):665-690 [PMID: 25278571 PMCID: 4187643 DOI: 10.1128/CMR.00020-14]

[40] Huang SS, Septimus E, Kleinman K, Moody J, Hickok J, Avery TR, Lankiewicz J, Gombosev A, Terpstra L, Hartford F, Hayden MK, Jernigan JA, Weinstein RA, Fraser VJ, Haffenreffer K, Cui E, Kaganov RE, Lolans K, Perlin JB, Platt R, Program

CDCPE, Network AD, Healthcare-Associated Infections P. Targeted versus universal decolonization to prevent ICU infection. The New England Journal of Medicine. 2013;**368**(24):2255-2265 [PMID: 23718152 DOI: 10.1056/NEJMoa1207290]

[41] Patient Safety 2015. National Quality Forum, 2015. 2015. Available from: http://www.qualityforum.org/qps/2720 [Accessed: July 3, 2017]

[42] Commission TJ. New Antimicrobial Stewardship Standard. 2016. Available from: http://www.jointcommission.org/assets/1/6/hap-cah_antimicrobial_prepub.pdf [Accessed: July 3, 2017]

[43] Forum NQ. National Quality Partners Playbook: Antibiotic Stewardship in Acute Care. National Quality Forum. 2016. Available from: http://www.qualityforum.org/nqp/antibiotic_stewardship_playbook.aspx [Accessed: July 2, 2017]

[44] Storr J, Twyman A, Zingg W, Damani N, Kilpatrick C, Reilly J, Price L, Egger M, Grayson ML, Kelley E, Allegranzi B, Group WHOGD. Core components for effective infection prevention and control programmes: New WHO evidence-based recommendations. Antimicrobial resistance and Infection Control. 2017;**6**:6 [PMID: 28078082 PMCID: 5223492 DOI: 10.1186/s13756-016-0149-9]

[45] Ferrer R, Martin-Loeches I, Phillips G, Osborn TM, Townsend S, Dellinger RP, Artigas A, Schorr C, Levy MM. Empiric antibiotic treatment reduces mortality in severe sepsis and septic shock from the first hour: Results from a guideline-based performance improvement program. Critical Care Medicine. 2014;**42**(8):1749-1755 [PMID: 24717459 DOI: 10.1097/CCM.0000000000000330]

[46] Tenover FC. Mechanisms of antimicrobial resistance in bacteria. The American Journal of Medicine. 2006;**119**(6 Suppl 1):S3-S10; discussion S62-70 [PMID: 16735149 DOI: 10.1016/j.amjmed.2006.03.011]

[47] Jacoby GA, Munoz-Price LS. The new beta-lactamases. The New England Journal of Medicine. 2005;**352**(4):380-391 [PMID: 15673804 DOI: 10.1056/NEJMra041359]

[48] Bush K, Jacoby GA. Updated functional classification of beta-lactamases. Antimicrobial Agents and Chemotherapy. 2010;**54**(3):969-976 [PMID: 19995920 PMCID: 2825993 DOI: 10.1128/AAC.01009-09]

[49] Li XZ, Ma D, Livermore DM, Nikaido H. Role of efflux pump(s) in intrinsic resistance of *Pseudomonas aeruginosa*: Active efflux as a contributing factor to beta-lactam resistance. Antimicrobial Agents and Chemotherapy. 1994;**38**(8):1742-1752 [PMID: 7986004 PMCID: 284631]

[50] Rhodes, A., Evans, L.E., Alhazzani, W., Levy, M.M., Antonelli, M., Ferrer, R., Kumar, A., Sevransky, J.E., Sprung, C.L., Nunnally, M.E. and Rochwerg, B. Surviving sepsis campaign: international guidelines for management of sepsis and septic shock: 2016. Intensive care medicine. 2017;**43**(3):304-377. [DOI: 10.1007/s00134-017-4683-6]

[51] Kumar A, Ellis P, Arabi Y, Roberts D, Light B, Parrillo JE, Dodek P, Wood G, Kumar A, Simon D, Peters C, Ahsan M, Chateau D, Cooperative Antimicrobial Therapy of Septic Shock Database Research G. Initiation of inappropriate antimicrobial therapy results in a fivefold reduction of survival in human septic shock. Chest. 2009;**136**(5):1237-1248 [PMID: 19696123 DOI: 10.1378/chest.09-0087]

[52] Vazquez-Guillamet C, Scolari M, Zilberberg MD, Shorr AF, Micek ST, Kollef M. Using the number needed to treat to assess appropriate antimicrobial therapy as a determinant of outcome in severe sepsis and septic shock. Critical Care Medicine. 2014;**42**(11):2342-2349 [PMID: 25072764 DOI: 10.1097/CCM.0000000000000516]

[53] Lutgring JD, Limbago BM. The problem of carbapenemase-producing-carbapenem-resistant-enterobacteriaceae detection. Journal of Clinical Microbiology. 2016;**54**(3):529-534 [PMID: 26739152 PMCID: 4767976 DOI: 10.1128/JCM.02771-15]

[54] CLSI Performance Standards for Natimicrobial Susceptibility Testing (note: document pages 56, 63, 67, 122-35). Clinical Laboratory Standard Institute; 2016 [Internet]. Available from: http://shop.clsi.org/site/sample_pdf/M100s26_sample.pdf [Accessed: July 2, 2017]

[55] Laboratory Detection and Reporting of Carbepenem-resistant Enterobacteriaceae (CRE): Specifically, slides 37-54. CLSI Outreach Working Group (ORWG) [Internet]. 2016. Available from: http://clsi.org/wp-content/uploads/sites/14/2013/11/orwg-cre-laboratory-role-5.30.16.pdf [Accessed: July 2, 2016]

[56] Banerjee R, Humphries R. Clinical and laboratory considerations for the rapid detection of carbapenem-resistant Enterobacteriaceae. Virulence. 2016;**0**(0)1-13 [PMID:27168451 DOI:10.1080/21505594.2016.1185577]

[57] Micek ST, Welch EC, Khan J, Pervez M, Doherty JA, Reichley RM, Kollef MH. Empiric combination antibiotic therapy is associated with improved outcome against sepsis due to Gram-negative bacteria: A retrospective analysis. Antimicrobial Agents and Chemotherapy. 2010;**54**(5):1742-1748 [PMID: 20160050 PMCID: 2863648 DOI: 10.1128/AAC.01365-09]

[58] Pittet D, Monod M, Suter PM, Frenk E, Auckenthaler R. Candida colonization and subsequent infections in critically ill surgical patients. Annals of Surgery. 1994;**220**(6):751-758 [PMID: 7986142 PMCID: 1234477]

[59] Moore RD, Smith CR, Lietman PS. The association of aminoglycoside plasma levels with mortality in patients with gram-negative bacteremia. The Journal of Infectious Diseases. 1984;**149**(3):443-448 [PMID: 6715900]

[60] van Zanten AR, Polderman KH, van Geijlswijk IM, van der Meer GY, Schouten MA, Girbes AR. Ciprofloxacin pharmacokinetics in critically ill patients: A prospective cohort study. Journal of Critical Care. 2008;**23**(3):422-430 [PMID: 18725050 DOI: 10.1016/j.jcrc.2007.11.011]

[61] Barza M, Ioannidis JP, Cappelleri JC, Lau J. Single or multiple daily doses of aminoglycosides: A meta-analysis. British Medical Journal (Clinical Research ed). 1996;**312**(7027):338-345 [PMID: 8611830 PMCID: 2350289]

[62] Hatala R, Dinh T, Cook DJ. Once-daily aminoglycoside dosing in immunocompetent adults: A meta-analysis. Annals of Internal Medicine. 1996;**124**(8):717-725 [PMID: 8633831]

[63] Rybak MJ, Lomaestro BM, Rotschafer JC, Moellering RC, Craig WA, Billeter M, Dalovisio JR, Levine DP. Vancomycin therapeutic guidelines: A summary of consensus recommendations from the infectious diseases Society of America, the American Society of Health-System Pharmacists, and the Society of Infectious Diseases Pharmacists. Clinical Infectious Diseases: An Official Publication of the Infectious Diseases Society of America. 2009;**49**(3):325-327 [PMID: 19569969 DOI: 10.1086/600877]

[64] Steinmetz T, Eliakim-Raz N, Goldberg E, Leibovici L, Yahav D. Association of vancomycin serum concentrations with efficacy in patients with MRSA infections: A systematic review and meta-analysis. Clinical Microbiology and Infection: The Official Publication of the European Society of Clinical Microbiology and Infectious Diseases. 2015;**21**(7):665-673 [PMID: 25887712 DOI: 10.1016/j.cmi.2015.04.003]

[65] Mohamed AF, Karaiskos I, Plachouras D, Karvanen M, Pontikis K, Jansson B, Papadomichelakis E, Antoniadou A, Giamarellou H, Armaganidis A, Cars O, Friberg LE. Application of a loading dose of colistin methanesulfonate in critically ill patients: Population pharmacokinetics, protein binding, and prediction of bacterial kill. Antimicrobial Agents and Chemotherapy. 2012;**56**(8):4241-4249 [PMID: 22615285 PMCID: 3421626 DOI: 10.1128/AAC.06426-11]

[66] McKinnon PS, Paladino JA, Schentag JJ. Evaluation of area under the inhibitory curve (AUIC) and time above the minimum inhibitory concentration (T>MIC) as predictors of outcome for cefepime and ceftazidime in serious bacterial infections. International Journal of Antimicrobial Agents. 2008;**31**(4):345-351 [PMID: 18313273 DOI: 10.1016/j.ijantimicag.2007.12.009]

[67] Minocin (minocycline) for injection. Available from: www.minociniv.com [Accessed: March 15, 2017]

[68] Ni W, Han Y, Zhao J, Wei C, Cui J, Wang R, Liu Y. Tigecycline treatment experience against multidrug-resistant *Acinetobacter baumannii* infections: A systematic review and meta-analysis. International Journal of Antimicrobial Agents. 2016;**47**(2):107-116 [PMID: 26742726 DOI: 10.1016/j.ijantimicag.2015.11.011]

[69] Chan JD, Graves JA, Dellit TH. Antimicrobial treatment and clinical outcomes of carbapenem-resistant *Acinetobacter baumannii* ventilator-associated pneumonia. Journal of Intensive Care Medicine. 2010;**25**(6):343-348 [PMID: 20837632 DOI: 10.1177/0885066610377975]

[70] Goff DA, Bauer KA, Mangino JE. Bad bugs need old drugs: A stewardship program's evaluation of minocycline for multidrug-resistant Acinetobacter baumannii infections. Clinical Infectious Diseases: An Official Publication of the Infectious Diseases Society of America. 2014;**59(**Suppl 6):S381–S387 [PMID: 25371514 DOI: 10.1093/cid/ciu593]

[71] Bishburg E, Bishburg K. Minocycline—An old drug for a new century: Emphasis on methicillin-resistant *Staphylococcus aureus* (MRSA) and *Acinetobacter baumannii*. International Journal of Antimicrobial Agents. 2009;**34**(5):395-401 [PMID: 19665876 DOI: 10.1016/j.ijantimicag.2009.06.021]

[72] Wood GC, Hanes SD, Boucher BA, Croce MA, Fabian TC. Tetracyclines for treating multidrug-resistant *Acinetobacter baumannii* ventilator-associated pneumonia. Intensive Care Medicine. 2003;**29**(11):2072-2076 [PMID: 14556048 DOI: 10.1007/s00134-003-1811-2]

[73] Jankowski CA. A stewardship approach to combating multidrug-resistant *Acinetobacter baumannii* infections with minocycline. Infectious Disease in Clinical Practice. 2012;**20**:184-187

[74] Karageorgopoulos DE, Falagas ME. Current control and treatment of multidrug-resistant *Acinetobacter baumannii* infections. The Lancet Infectious Diseases. 2008;**8**(12):751-762 [PMID: 19022191 DOI: 10.1016/S1473-3099(08)70279-2]

[75] Tan TY, Ng LS, Tan E, Huang G. In vitro effect of minocycline and colistin combinations on imipenem-resistant *Acinetobacter baumannii* clinical isolates. The Journal of Antimicrobial Chemotherapy. 2007;**60**(2):421-423 [PMID: 17540671 DOI: 10.1093/jac/dkm178]

[76] Prevention CfDCa. Core Elements of Hospital Antibiotic Stewardship Program [Internet]. 2016. Available from: http://www.cdc.gov/getsmart/healthcare/implementation/core-elements.html [Accessed: July 20, 2016]

Chapter 5

# Microbiology of Ventilator-Associated Pneumonia

Valério Monteiro-Neto, Lídio G. Lima-Neto,
Afonso G. Abreu and Cinara Regina A. V. Monteiro

Additional information is available at the end of the chapter

http://dx.doi.org/10.5772/intechopen.69430

**Abstract**

Ventilator-associated pneumonia (VAP) is a pulmonary infection that appears after 2 days of endotracheal intubation and when invasive mechanical ventilation is used. VAP is considered the most common nosocomial infection in the intensive care unit (ICU) and presents high morbidity and mortality rates, principally when caused by multi-resistant bacteria. Several risk factors are associated with VAP, including the microbiota, advanced age, immunocompromising conditions, pulmonary illness, length of mechanical ventilation, the aspiration technique, tracheostomy, supine positioning, enteral feeding, previous antibiotic exposure, among other endogenous and exogenous factors. The main pathogens are *Staphylococcus aureus*, *Pseudomonas aeruginosa*, *Acinetobacter baumannii*, and Enterobacteriaceae members, which are considered potentially multidrug-resistant pathogens. Conventional microbiology methods continue to be used for laboratory diagnosis. However, it is necessary to validate rapid and accurate laboratory methods, such as molecular assays that detect multiple gene sequences of a wide range of bacterial species and resistance markers. Therefore, the objective of this chapter is to review and update several aspects related to VAP, including risk factors, etiology, laboratory diagnosis, bacterial virulence and VAP severity, and antibiotic susceptibility.

**Keywords:** ventilator-associated pneumonia, respiratory infections, nosocomial infections, microbiology

## 1. Introduction

Pneumonia is a serious public health problem associated with high morbidity and mortality rates that leads to a significant increase in healthcare costs. It results from an infectious process of the lower airways through aspiration or inhalation of pathogenic microorganisms. It can be acquired in the community or in the hospital environment, after 48 h of admission [1].

INTECH
open science | open minds

© 2017 The Author(s). Licensee InTech. This chapter is distributed under the terms of the Creative Commons Attribution License (http://creativecommons.org/licenses/by/3.0), which permits unrestricted use, distribution, and reproduction in any medium, provided the original work is properly cited. (cc) BY

Hospital-acquired infections usually have a high mortality rate (approx. 20%) when compared to the community acquisition (10%), this rate increases even more when it is associated with mechanical ventilation [2].

According to the guidelines of the American Thoracic Society, hospital pneumonia is divided into ventilator-associated pneumonia (VAP), which develops after 48–72 h of endotracheal intubation and the one that occurs in nonhospitalized patients, but that have constant contact with health services [3]. VAP is the infection of the pulmonary parenchyma with onset after 48–72 h of endotracheal intubation. Early-onset VAP occurs during the first 4 days of mechanical ventilation, whereas late-onset VAP occurs on 5 or more days of mechanical ventilation [4–7]. VAP corresponds to 70–80% of cases of hospital-acquired pneumonia in intensive care units [1].

VAP is characterized by the presence of new or progressive pulmonary infiltrates, systemic alterations such as fever and leukocyte alterations, altered sputum, and diagnosis of an infectious agent [8]. Mortality due to VAP is high, principally because of the association with multidrug-resistance (MDR) bacteria [9]. In pediatrics and neonatology, the frequency of VAP is 3–19%, with a mortality rate ranging from 10 to 20% of patients [10].

Many microorganisms can be involved in VAP. In this chapter, data on microbiology of VAP are reviewed, including risk factors, etiology, virulence features of main pathogens contributing to VAP severity, antimicrobial susceptibility, and laboratory diagnosis.

## 2. Risk factors for VAP

The use of mechanical ventilation is a significant risk factor for hospital-acquired pneumonia associated with aspiration, lowering of consciousness level, excessive management and patient transport, and chronic lung disease. The risk of VAP increases by 3% in the first 5 days of ventilation, 2% in 5–10 days, and 1% in 10 days of ventilation [11].

Although other routes may lead to VAP, such as hematogenous spread, inhalation of contaminated air, and also by extension of an infection of the pleural space, the main entry of pathogens into the lower respiratory tract occurs by aspiration of secretions containing microorganisms (from oropharynx or reflux of the stomach). Pathogens that cause VAP may be part of the upper airway microbiota or are acquired exogenously after hospital admission [8].

**Figure 1** shows the different risk factors that are associated with VAP. Among risk factors inherent to the host (endogenous), it was observed that patients with advanced age, immunosuppressed individuals or pulmonary diseases have an increased risk for the development of VAP [4, 12, 13]. In a multicenter cohort study that analyzed the frequency of VAP among middle-aged, elderly, and very elderly patients, it was concluded that the highest frequency of VAP was in elderly patients (16.6%), associated to increased mortality among the elderly and very elderly (51%) when compared to middle-aged patients (35%) [4].

Long-term mechanical ventilation in patients with acute respiratory distress syndrome (ARDS) increases the risk of VAP [5]. Evaluation of the association between ARDS and VAP found that 55% of patients with ARDS developed nosocomial infection compared to 28%

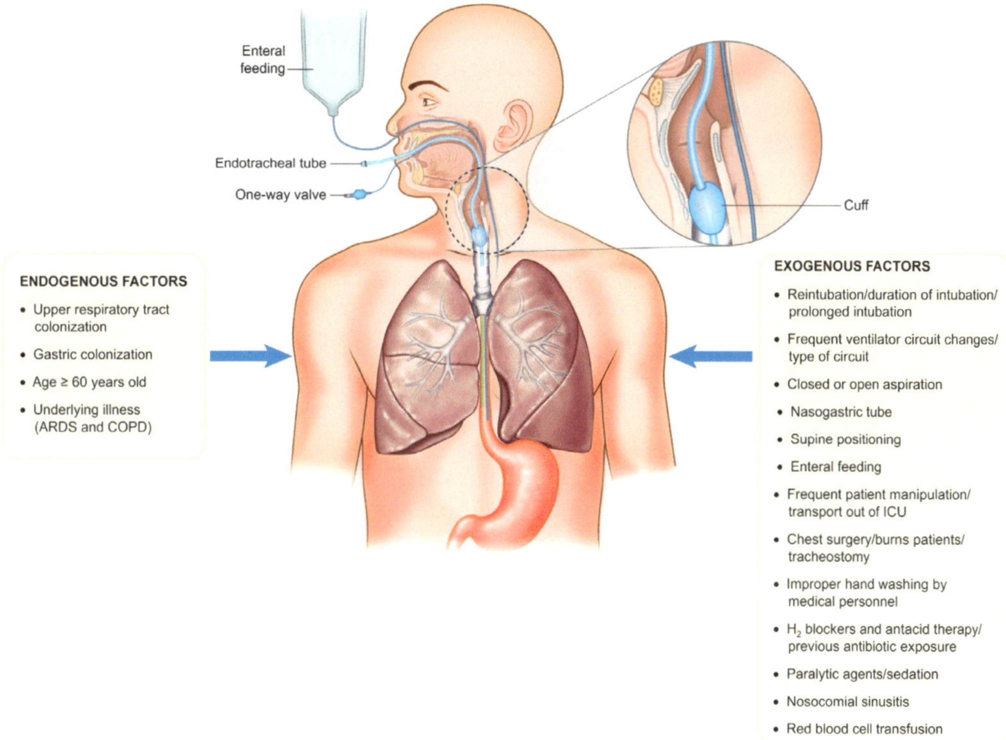


**Figure 1.** Main endogenous and exogenous risk factors for VAP.

without the syndrome [14]. Cigarette smoking, inhibition of mucociliary function, and reduction of cough reflex due to obstruction of airflow make chronic obstructive pulmonary disease (COPD) patients more susceptible to ventilation-associated infections [5].

The exogenous risk factors are due to the interventions undergone by the patient in intensive care units (ICUs) (**Figure 1**). Mechanical ventilation equipment is a primary source of infection, in which respiratory circuit condensations can be sources of microorganisms [8]. The endotracheal tube, as well as other invasive devices, promotes bacterial colonization of the trachea. Bacteria may have access to the lower respiratory tract through a partial blockage around the cuff or through the lumen of the endotracheal tube.

Prolonged intubation may promote the formation of a layer of microorganisms adhered to the inner surface of the endotracheal tube. This formation, known as biofilm, represents an important virulence mechanism and contributes to pathogen persistence as well as therapeutic failures, since microorganisms in the biofilm state are more resistant to host defenses and also metabolically less active, therefore, are more resistant to antibiotics [8, 15]. To inhibit the biofilm formation on the surface of polymeric medical devices, many studies have focused on the development of new biomaterials with modifications that alter the biophysical interactions of the cell surface or impede biofilm growth. A wide range of new coatings with antimicrobials, cationic antimicrobial peptides, or metal nanoparticles (e.g., copper, gold, iron, magnesium, silver, titanium, or zinc) have been applied to medical devices such as endotracheal tubes [16, 17]. Other approach consists in the use of polymers that exhibit antimicrobial activity by themselves, with positively charged active groups (biguanide, cyclic *N*-halamine, quaternary ammonium, pyridinium or phosphonium salts, and polyionenes) or other polymers, such as synthetic poly(phenylene ethynylenes), polynorbornenes, and polymethacrylates that display similar antimicrobial activities of human peptides [17]. Both types of devices display advantages and disadvantages, but in the near future one expects to have nontoxic and biocompatible products available, which display broad-spectrum antibiofilm activities for the prevention of biofilm formation on endotracheal tubes [18].

The aspiration technique of endotracheal secretions also plays an important role as a risk factor for the establishment of VAP. The open method where a sterile aspiration probe is introduced has disadvantages such as loss of oxygenation, since the patient is temporarily disconnected from the ventilator and the system is opened with exposure of the patient, and the maximum duration of use of each circuit is not known [5].

Tracheostomy is an indicated procedure after 2 weeks of translaryngeal intubation of critically ill patients. Apparently, early tracheostomy may be associated with a lower incidence of pneumonia when compared to the late procedure or nonprocedure [19]. Frequent reintubations are also associated with VAP because of the risk of aspiration of gastric contents through the use of the nasogastric tube, subglottic dysfunction, and lowering of the level of consciousness [5].

The VAP prevention guidelines recommend the placement of the patient in the bed between 30 and 45° semi-reclined [20]. The supine position to which the patient is subjected may lead to lesions such as atelectasis in the dorsal lung region, barotrauma in the ventral lung region [5]. Experiments performed on rats proved the advantage of lateral decubitus in improving gas exchange, reducing gastroesophageal reflux, and avoiding pulmonary infection by gastric aspiration due to gravity [21]. Recently, the semi-decubitus position (30–60°) was shown to reduce the risk of VAP compared to supine positioning (0–10°) [20].

Nasal feeding by nasogastric tube increases gastric secretions and pH, leading to colonization by Gram-negative bacilli. Aspiration of this gastric content increases the risk of VAP. The use of sedative medications used in therapeutic procedures can cause prolonged relaxation of the muscles, increasing the risk of aspiration [5].

In addition, in the neonatal intensive care unit (NICU), some risk factors are associated with characteristics peculiar to this age group, including: length of stay in the NICU, enteral and parenteral feeding, blood transfusion, low birth weight, prematurity, and bronchopulmonary dysplasia [10, 13].

## 3. Etiology of VAP

VAP is usually caused by bacteria, whereas fungi and viruses are rarely involved [3, 6]. Generally, early-onset VAP is caused by pathogens more susceptible to antibiotics, including *Streptococcus pneumoniae, Haemophilus influenzae,* and methicillin-susceptible *Staphylococcus aureus*. On the other hand, late-onset VAP is usually caused by antibiotic-resistant bacteria, such as *Pseudomonas aeruginosa, Acinetobacter* spp., methicillin-resistant *S. aureus* (MRSA), and extended-spectrum β-lactamase producing Enterobacteriaceae, such as *Klebsiella pneumoniae, Escherichia coli, Enterobacter* spp., among others [5–7]. However, some studies have reported that both susceptible and antibiotic-resistant microorganisms can have similar frequencies in early and late-onset VAP [22, 23].

In many cases, VAP can be caused by more than one pathogen (polymicrobial infection). This fact can be ignored sometimes when isolates are reported only as a percentage of the total number of isolates. In a recent study, performed in medical and surgical ICUs of a hospital in Spain, of 147 VAP patients, 32 (21%) had more than one pathogen associated. Interestingly, the clinical outcomes were not influenced by the polymicrobial etiology, when appropriate antibiotic therapy was administered [24].

The etiology of VAP varies in different countries and even between ICUs of the same city, distinct patients groups (like the ARDS patients, immunocompromised, and so on), or settings of the same hospital [25]. However, among Gram-negative bacteria, a high frequency is generally reported for *P. aeruginosa, Acinetobacter* spp., and Enterobacteriaceae members. Among Gram-positive isolates, *S. aureus* and *Streptococcus* spp. are considered as important pathogens [3, 5, 14, 25–27]. **Table 1** shows a list of the most frequently and also some uncommon microorganisms detected in VAP patients.

| Microorganisms | Frequency (%) |
|---|---|
| (1) Gram-positive bacteria | |
| *Staphylococcus aureus* | 20–32 |
| *Streptococcus* spp. | 2–8 |
| Coagulase-negative staphylococci | 1–2 |
| (2) Gram-negative bacteria | |
| *Pseudomonas aeruginosa* | 20–28 |
| *Acinetobacter* spp. | 4–13 |
| *Klebsiella pneumoniae* | 8–12 |
| *Escherichia coli* | 4–10 |
| *Haemophilus influenzae* | 4–8 |
| *Enterobacter* spp. | 6–7 |
| *Serratia* spp. | 2–4 |
| *Neisseria* spp. | 2–3 |
| *Stenotrophomonas maltophilia* | 2–3 |
| (3) Other bacteria | <1 each |
| Anaerobes | |
| *Corynebacterium* spp. | |

| Microorganisms | Frequency (%) |
|---|---|
| *Enterococcus* spp. | |
| *Moraxella* spp. | |
| (4) Viruses | <1 each |
| *Influenza* virus | |
| *Herpes simplex* virus | |
| *Cytomegalovirus* | |
| (5) Fungi | <1 each |
| *Aspergillus* spp. | |
| *Candida* spp. | |
| *Pneumocystis carinii* | |

**Table 1.** Frequency of etiologic agents of VAP.

## 4. Virulence of major pathogens and VAP severity

Clinical outcomes of VAP depend on a variety of factors, which are inherent to the patient, the hospital assistance, and also the microorganism, including host immune system status, underlying diseases associated, appropriate antibiotic therapy, accurate and rapid clinical and laboratory diagnosis, antimicrobial susceptibility, and virulence of the pathogen. Antimicrobial susceptibility is discussed in Section 5. Here, we present significance of major virulence factors associated with VAP severity of four selected pathogens: *Acinetobacter baumannii*, *K. pneumoniae*, *P. aeruginosa*, and *S. aureus*.

### 4.1. *Acinetobacter baumannii*

There are more than 20 *Acinetobacter* species, with *A. baumannii* being the most commonly isolated in clinical settings, in which it represents important emerging nosocomial pathogen. *A. baumannii* is a Gram-negative bacterium, strictly aerobic, nonfermentative coccobacillus, nonmotile, nonpigmented, and catalase-positive. It is ubiquitous in nature and has been recovered from soil, water, and animals and found as part of the normal skin, throat, and rectal flora of human. Although a frequent colonizer, *A. baumannii* can be the cause of severe and sometimes lethal infections, frequently of nosocomial origin, principally VAP. A survey in U.S. hospitals showed that the majority of the isolates (57.6%) were from the respiratory tract, and *Acinetobacter* species ranked fifth as the causative organism of VAP (6.6%) [28–30].

In recent years, it has been designated a "red alert" human pathogen and has caused considerable concern in the medical community. This pathogen can adhere to surfaces, and it specifically targets moist tissues such as mucous membranes or skin that has been exposed due to accident or injury, and can cause a wide variety of infections. Most of the cases involve the respiratory tract, but bacteremia, meningitis, and wound infection may also occur. A recent systematic review and meta-analysis showed that some invasive procedures frequently used in the ICU increase the risk of *A. baumannii* bacteremia: mechanical ventilation, central venous or urinary catheterization, and nasogastric tube use [31, 32].

The virulence of *A. baumannii* can be attributed to several factors: capacity to form biofilms; its ability to adhere, to colonize, and invade human epithelial cells; its antibiotic resistance mechanisms; and its ability to acquire foreign genetic material to promote its own survival under antibiotic and host selection pressures. Approximately 30% of *Acinetobacter* strains also produce an exopolysaccharide, which is a major virulence factor protecting bacteria from host defenses [28, 31].

### 4.2. *Klebsiella pneumoniae*

*K. pneumoniae* is generally considered an opportunistic pathogen that affects mainly immunocompromised individuals. It can be found normally in the intestine, oral cavity, and skin, as well as in hospital settings and medical devices [33]. *K. pneumoniae* is able to form biofilms in catheters and endotracheal tubes, which represent major sources of infection in patients with invasive devices [34].

Infections by *K. pneumoniae* that involves biofilm formation tend to be persistent or chronic, since the biofilm protects the pathogen of the host immune response and also of the antibiotic action [35]. An additional risk factor for chronic infections caused by nosocomial strains includes resistance to multiple antibiotics, making difficult for the choice of suitable antibiotics for the treatment [36].

*K. pneumoniae* has about 78 capsular serotypes (or K antigens) [37]. Some of them present an increase in the production of the capsule and present very viscous colonies, which are called hypermucoviscous. Such isolates have also been considered to be hypervirulent because capsule is the most important virulence factor of *K. pneumoniae* [38].

A practical way to check if an isolate is hypermucoviscous is by using the string test. If there is the formation of a viscous chain greater than 5 mm after touching bacterial growth on agar and try to stretch it with a platinum loop. The degree of mucoviscosity correlates with the establishment of invasive infections. Hypervirulent *K. pneumoniae* is highly invasive and can affect previously healthy persons, causing fatal infections, including severe pneumonia among them [38]. The bacterium with the phenotype of hypermucoviscosity is capable of spreading from one organ to other organs (metastatic spread) [39].

The capsule consists of polysaccharides and is generally constituted by repeating units of three to six sugars [38]. The main functions assigned to it include: (1) protection of *K. pneumoniae* against opsonization and phagocytosis [40]; (2) interference with dendritic cells (DCs) maturation and, consequently, in the production of pro-Th1 cytokines mediated by DCs [41]; (3) anti-inflammatory effect by the inhibition of IL-8 expression [42–44]; and (4) reduction of the amount of antimicrobial peptides reaching the bacterial surface, thus, promoting resistance to them [45].

In addition to capsule, iron acquisition is a virulence property that also contributes to the persistence of the microorganism in the patient body and, consequently, to VAP, since iron is essential for bacterial growth. Pathogenic members of the Enterobacteriaceae family usually display a variety of iron uptake systems, of which at least 12 have been described in *K. pneumoniae.* Isolates associated with pulmonary infections also produce yersiniabactin and salmochelin, which are not sequestered by the host protein lipocalin 2 of the innate immune defense [46, 47]. Additionally, hypervirulent *K. pneumoniae* produces a higher amount and more active siderophore molecules than classical *K. pneumoniae*, which increases its pathogenic potential [48].

### 4.3. *Pseudomonas aeruginosa*

VAP caused by *P. aeruginosa* has been associated with higher case fatality rates than that by other bacteria. This pathogen is a noninvasivefermenting Gram-negative, aerobic, rod-shaped polar-flagella, with unipolar motility. *P. aeruginosa* is considered emerging as an important nosocomial pathogen worldwide and is responsible for an extensive spectrum of infections in humans associated with significant morbidity and mortality. It is an opportunistic pathogen that is normally found in plants, soils, and in a variety of aquatic environments. The adaptability and high antibiotic resistance allow it to survive in a wide range of other natural and artificial settings, including surfaces in medical facilities. In addition, *P. aeruginosa* is recognized for its ability to form biofilms and directly increase the VAP-induced lung injury. In the United States, *P. aeruginosa* is among the most common hospital pathogens and is the second most common pathogen isolated from patients with VAP and has been associated with prolonged hospitalization, increased cost, and mortality [49–52].

Cell surface virulence factors of *P. aeruginosa* play an important role in colonization of the lower respiratory tract. These factors include *flagellum*, *pili* or fimbriae, lipopolysaccharide (LPS), as well as type III secretion system (T3SS), which is a major determinant of virulence. The T3SS expression is frequently associated with acute invasive infections and has been linked to increased mortality in infected patients, and it is shared among many pathogenic Gram-negative bacteria as a means of injecting toxins directly into host cells [49, 53].

Additionally, several proteases are produced by *P. aeruginosa*. These proteases have established roles in distinct infectious process, such as hydrolysis of immunoglobulin, fibrin, fibrinogen, and also disruption of epithelial tight junctions. Main *P. aeruginosa* proteases include pyocyanin, which induces damage to the respiratory tract, such as epithelial necrosis and reduced ciliary movement; pyoverdin, its main secreted siderophore; protease IV, a serine protease responsible to degradation of complement proteins, fibrinogen, immunoglobulin G, and plasminogen; elastase and metalloproteinases that degrade elastin, collagen types III and IV, surfactant, immunoglobulins, complement factors, and cytokines; and exotoxin A, one of the most potent toxins with cytopathic activity, among others, such as *quorum-sensing*, a very sophisticated gene regulatory mechanism that allows bacteria to coordinate activity through the production of small diffusible molecules. These functions include the formation of biofilms, motility, secretion of virulent factors, and exopolysaccharide production [49, 54].

### 4.4. *Staphylococcus aureus*

*S. aureus* strains produce several virulence factors that contribute to the pathogenesis and severity of lower respiratory infections. Some of them can hinder host defenses, such as protein

http://dx.doi.org/10.5772/intechopen.69430

A, coagulase, leukocidin, and γ-toxin [55]. Protein A is an important virulence factor in the pathogenesis of experimental staphylococcal pneumonia in mice [56]. Moreover, protein A mediates: (1) invasion across airway epithelial cells through activation of RhoA GTPase signaling and proteolytic activity; (2) binding to tumor necrosis factor receptor 1 (TNFR1) on lung epithelial cells, and (3) activation of a specific intracellular signaling causing the recruitment of neutrophils. These activities increase inflammation of the airway epithelium and, thus, contribute to tissue damage [57].

Cysteine proteases, in particular staphopain A (ScpA), cleave the pulmonary surfactant protein-A (SP-A), a major surfactant component with immune functions that is important during *S. aureus* infections [55]. Additionally, *S. aureus* releases enzymes with significant roles as virulence factors, including proteases, nucleases, lipases, hyaluronidase, and staphylokinase that facilitate the invasion of the infected tissue [58].

Interestingly, *S. aureus* display a great ability to subvert innate and adaptive immune responses to favor its replication [59]. In some situations, such as in immunocompromising conditions, there is a higher susceptibility to acquire *S. aureus* infection, mainly by hospitalized patients. In this context, *S. aureus* and especially the epidemic methicillin-resistant *S. aureus* strains cause severe necrotizing pneumonia by producing Panton-Valentine leukocidin (PVL) that has been reported to cause rapidly progressive necrosis of the lung tissue in young immunocompetent patients. The severity of disease, survival, and clinical outcome of VAP patients can also be associated with the presence of the Panton-Valentine leukocidin genes in MRSA [60]. The role of PVL in the pathogenesis of MRSA infection is not clear, but recently, it was demonstrated that the PVL have strong affinity for host extracellular matrix proteins being, therefore, implicated as a *S. aureus* adherence molecule. Moreover, PVL as a cytotoxin targets human polymorphonuclear neutrophils, and monocytes or macrophages, or both, leading to their apoptosis or necrosis as result of the Bax-independent apoptosis occurring by means of a novel pathway that presumably involved PVL-mediated pore formation in the mitochondria membranes.

## 5. Antimicrobial susceptibility and management of patients

Choosing an initial antibiotic for suspected VAP is a difficult task. A scheme of empiric antibiotic therapy must take into account that *S. aureus, P. aeruginosa, Acinetobacter* spp., and Enterobacteriaceae members together represent more than 80% of VAP cases worldwide and several strains are defined as MDR pathogens [26]. To provide suitable antibiotic exposure regarding the possibility of infection by MDR pathogens, the empiric therapy should contain multiple agents with broader spectrum of activity [25].

However, antibiotic choices should be based on local prevalence and the antimicrobial susceptibility profile of the usual pathogens, since data from guidelines or other hospitals can be ineffective [61]. For empiric MRSA coverage, vancomycin or linezolid are strongly recommended. On the other hand, if it is indicated as MSSA coverage, the following antibiotics should be used: piperacillin-tazobactam, cefepime, levofloxacin, imipenem, or meropenem. Suspected etiology for MRSA or MSSA should be based on the presence of risk factors [61].

It has been reported that more than 50% of MRSA are also resistant to macrolides, lincosamides, fluoroquinolones, and aminoglycosides. This high level of resistance not only impedes successful therapy but also allows the microorganism to persist in the hospital, expanding its reservoir. So, vancomycin is the first-line treatment to VAP patients caused by MRSA. Nevertheless, some studies have described *S. aureus* strains with decreased susceptibility to vancomycin (vancomycin intermediate-resistant *S. aureus*, VISA). The acquired-resistance of MRSA to vancomycin is related to acquire mutations that appear in MRSA during vancomycin therapy [62, 63]. More recently, studies describing MRSA strains with high-level vancomycin resistance (vancomycin-resistant *S. aureus*, VRSA) were described. The mechanism of resistance is associated to the presence of transposon Tn1546, acquired from vancomycin-resistant *Enterococcus faecalis*, which is known to alter cell wall structure and metabolism, but the resistance mechanisms in VISA and VRSA isolates are less well defined [62].

Antibiotic options for Gram-negative coverage are more varied and must contain two anti-pseudomonal antibiotics from different classes in the presence of risk factors for MDR pathogens for the initial treatment of suspected VAP. If the patient does not present risk factors for MDR pathogens, only one anti-pseudomonas drug should be prescribed [61].

The frequency of infections caused by *P. aeruginosa* has increased in combination with the morbidity and mortality among hospitalized patients, all of which are exacerbated by antimicrobial resistance. Studies have demonstrated that resistance to carbapenems, aminoglycosides, and fluoroquinolones has increased gradually over the past few years, as well as episodes caused by MDR strains. Many *P. aeruginosa* isolates display an intrinsic reduced susceptibility to several antibacterial agents, as well as a tendency to develop resistance during therapy, especially in carbapenem-resistant strains. The most common mechanism of imipenem resistance in *P. aeruginosa* is a combination of chromosomal AmpC production and porin alterations. It also produces extended-spectrum β-lactamases (ESBLs) and can harbor other antibiotic resistance enzymes such as *K. pneumoniae* carbapenemases (KPC) and imipenem metallo-β-lactamases. β-Lactamase production, especially ESBLs, remains the main factor to acquired β-lactam resistance [52, 64, 65].

*K. pneumoniae* may present two major types of antibiotic resistance: (1) expression of ESBLs, which make them resistant to cephalosporins and monobactams and (2) the expression of carbapenemases that make *K. pneumoniae* resistant to almost all available β-lactams, including carbapenems. The first reported of carbapenemase by *K. pneumoniae* was in the USA, in 1996, which was designated KPC. Currently four classes of carbapenemases (classes A–D) have already been described and KPCs are classified into class A. To date, 16 KPC class A variants have already been identified. In addition to KPCs, *K. pneumoniae* strains may carry other forms of carbapenemases, such as class B metallo-β-lactamases (such as New Delhi's metallo-β-lactamase NDM-1 enzymes) and OXA class. In addition to β-lactamases, mutations in outer membrane proteins (OMPs) may also make the bacterium more resistant to β-lactams, particularly if it was in combination with the expression of a carbapenemase [66].

*A. baumannii* is also considered an emerging cause of nosocomial outbreaks, especially by MDR strains in ICUs. The most significant mechanism of carbapenem resistance in *A. baumannii* is the production of carbapenemases, which can be either intrinsic or acquired. Carbapenems have been considered the agents of choice for infections caused by susceptible pathogens, but the rapid increase in carbapenem resistance rates has complicated this issue. Other mechanisms include: changes in OMPs, penicillin-binding proteins, and efflux pumps; resistance to aminoglycosides, mediated by aminoglycoside phosphotransferases, acetyltransferases, and adenyltransferases; resistance to quinolones, polymyxins, tetracyclines, among others [28].

A recent cohort study of bacteremia associated with pneumonia found that inappropriate initial antibiotic treatment seems to be the most important independent determinant of mortality and is the only identified mortality predictor amenable to intervention [67]. These Gram-negative bacteria are responsible for increasing numbers of infections encountered in hospitals, particularly among immunocompromised patients, and community-acquired infections are also increasing in prevalence. Furthermore, the impact of *P. aeruginosa* and *A. baumannii* resistance on health systems is a major concern in hospitals worldwide.

## 6. Laboratory diagnosis

The diagnosis of VAP is usually based on clinical, radiographic, and microbiological criteria. Microbiological diagnosis is important in the management of VAP, since early diagnosis can influence clinical outcomes. The usual methods for microbiological diagnosis are based on quantitative or semiquantitative culture, but the results can take 48 h or more to be available. The Gram stain method has been used as screening of infection and to guide initial antibiotic therapy. However, utility of microscopy examination of respiratory secretions is still controversial.

Molecular methods can also be used to obtain results more quickly and initiate rational antibiotic therapy of patients with VAP. Many method formats are available for the detection of target genes for microbial identification and also for the detection of antimicrobial resistance genes.

### 6.1. Culture

Semiquantitative culture of endotracheal aspirates (ETA) is the recommended microbiological procedure to diagnose VAP, since it is more sensitive and can be done more rapidly. Other biological specimens have been used, including the ones obtained by invasive sampling, such as: bronchoalveolar lavage (BAL), blind bronchial sampling (mini-BAL), and protected specimen brush (PSB). Blood cultures should also be performed for all patients with suspected VAP. In all cases, samples should be obtained before the patients initiate antibiotic therapy [61].

The main problem with the semiquantitative culture of ETA is that its high sensitivity promotes the unnecessary prescription of antibiotics to some patients. In the case of quantitative cultures of lower respiratory tract secretions, the following threshold cut-offs are usually applied to diagnosis true infection: ETA $10^5$–$10^6$, BAL $10^4$, and PSB $10^3$ CFU/mL. This strategy may lead to false-negative results and worse clinical outcomes in some patients [61].

### 6.2. Gram stain

The Gram stain of respiratory specimens can provide rapid information regarding morphological aspects of the bacterial pathogen and whether it is Gram-positive or Gram-negative. Additionally, microscopic examination may reveal whether the smear is suggestive of infection. It is generally accepted as active infection when the biological sample has more than 25 neutrophils and less than 10 epithelial cells per 10× low-power field.

A decision strategy based on the results of Gram stain was proposed to assist the clinician in the empirical prescription of antibiotics [68]:

- **If the Gram stain of the ETA is negative:** Antibiotic prescription can wait until the microbiological culture result is available, since it is very unlikely that the patient have VAP.
- **If the Gram stain of PSB is positive**: The antibiotic therapy can be initiated and based on the result of Gram stain, since it is very likely that the patient has VAP. Later, it can be adjusted according to the culture result.
- **If the Gram stain of PSB is negative and the Gram stain of the ETA is positive:** The antibiotic therapy may only be initiated depending on the severity of the patient's clinical condition or when the VAP is confirmed by the culture.

Nevertheless, the utility of Gram staining in the diagnosis of VAP and as a guide for the antibiotic empirical therapy of VAP is a very controversial subject. It is usually accepted that this old diagnostic tool has a high negative predictive value, i.e., VAP is unlikely with a negative Gram stain [69].

### 6.3. Molecular methods

Several molecular-based methods have been proposed for the detection of respiratory pathogens that offer a reliable diagnosis, with high sensitivity and specificity. Most of them are nucleic acid-based amplification methods that identify, simultaneously, multiple and specific target gene sequences (multiplex assays) of a wide range of bacterial species and resistance genes [70, 71].

Considering that the etiology of the VAP is very different from the community-acquired pneumonia, some main potential gene targets are *mecA* gene in *S. aureus*; $bla_{VIM}$ and $bla_{IMP}$ genes in *P. aeruginosa*; $bla_{OXA}$ genes in *Acinetobacter* spp.; and $bla_{KPC}$ gene in members of the Enterobacteriaceae family, in addition to the detection of *Stenotrophomonas maltophilia* [72].

Currently, a variety of platforms or systems are available to identify respiratory pathogens using distinct technologies. Some molecular diagnostic systems detect a small number of microorganisms, such as GeneXpertMRSA/SA that detects MRSA and MSSA. On the other hand, IRIDICA and MALDI-TOFI can detect a wide range of pathogens and resistance markers. **Table 2** shows the major commercial systems available to detect respiratory pathogens, including bacteria, viruses, and fungi.

Depending on the methods, the advantages of molecular methods include rapid results; detection of very low amounts of gene sequences; target sequences to identify the agent and/

| Systems | No. of pathogens/markers | Technology |
|---|---|---|
| Abbot IRIDICA System | 780 bacteria, 200 fungi, 13 viruses, and 4 resistance markers | PCR/ESI-MS |
| Accelerate PhenoTest™ BC kit | 27 bacteria and 2 yeasts and AST | FISH |
| Amplidiag® CarbaR+VRE | 5 carbapenemase and 2 vancomycin-resistance markers | Multiplex RT-PCR |
| CE-IVD HAI BioDetection kit | 12 most common nosocomial pathogens and 15 resistance markers | NSG |
| Curetis Unyvero™ | 16 bacteria, 1 fungus, 18 resistance markers | PCR |
| FilmArray® Respiratory Panel | 17 viruses and 3 bacteria | Multiplex RT-PCR |
| FTD Bacterial pneumoniae HAP | Detection and quantification of *K. pneumoniae* and *P. aeruginosa* | Multiplex RT-PCR |
| GeneXpertMRSA/SA | Only MRSA and MSSA | RT-PCR |
| MALDI-TOFI | Wide spectrum of bacteria and fungi | MS |
| NxTAG® Respiratory Pathogen Panel | 18 viruses and 3 bacteria | Multiplex RT-PCR |
| R-Biopharm RIDA® GENE-kits | *mecA/mecC*, SCCmec cassette, and *S. aureus* | Multiplex RT-PCR |
| Verigene® Respiratory Pathogens Flex Test | Up to 13 viruses and 3 bacteria (customized) | Multiplex RT-PCR |

AST: antimicrobial susceptibility testing; FISH: fluorescence *in-situ* hybridization; MALDI-TOF: matrix-assisted laser desorption/ionization time-of-flight; MRSA: methicillin resistant *S. aureus*; MSSA: methicillin sensitive *S. aureus*; MS: mass spectrometry; NGS: next-generation sequencing; PCR: polymerase chain reaction; PCR/ESI-MS: PCR-electrospray ionization mass spectrometry; RT-PCR: real time-PCR.

**Table 2.** Commercial molecular systems for detection of respiratory pathogens and resistance markers.

or the resistance gene markers; possibility to search for multiple agents and resistance markers; direct detection in clinical specimens; and higher sensitivity. On the other hand, among important drawbacks are: most of them are qualitative, risk of contamination, high costs, and lack of validation.

### 6.4. Exhaled breath metabolomics

Recent advances in diagnostic technologies have pointed to metabolomics as an emerging and faster method to aid in the diagnosis of various diseases, such as cancer, asthma, among others. The procedure can be performed with samples such as plasma and also with noninvasive samples, such as exhaled air and saliva. Results can return within a matter of hours, compared with days of conventional culture. In the case of exhaled air, the method consists in determining the profile of volatile organic compounds (VOCs) emitted by the patient through respiration [73]. These metabolic degradation products present in the expired air are derived from the patient and the pathogen. The VOC profile is detected through sensitive procedures such as nuclear magnetic resonance spectroscopy [74] and gas chromatography-mass spectrometry [75]. Studies in patients with VAP have allowed the determination of distinct VOC patterns in clinical cases associated to different pathogens, showing good correlation with the microbiological culture and offer great potential as biomarkers [76, 77].

Major drawbacks of this method include: (i) the sampling methodology, which should enable to sample from beyond the endotracheal tube and hence to exclude air from the upper respiratory tract; (ii) discovery of more pathogen-specific metabolites; and (iii) the need of trained personnel to operate the analytical methodology by gas chromatography-mass spectrometry apparatus.

## 7. Final considerations

One of the main problems of VAP is the lack of a gold standard for rapid and reliable diagnosis. Mortality associated with VAP remains high, mainly because of the increasing prevalence of MDR pathogens and their resistance profiles vary depending on the patient group and the hospital setting. However, significant progress has been obtained in the development of systems or platforms for molecular detection of respiratory pathogens, which are feasible to be applied to the routine diagnosis of VAP. Additionally, metabolic profiling of exhaled breath will aim to speed up the process after refinement of the sampling methodology and discovery of highly discriminatory biomarkers. With the validation and implementation of these methods for diagnosis, probably a more adequate control of VAP will be obtained. Especially, because the early and appropriate use of antibiotics may result in reduced mortality among patients under mechanical ventilation. Although, it is important to observe the guidelines for patient management, antibiotic therapy must be based on local prevalence and microbiology data.

## Author details

Valério Monteiro-Neto[1,2*], Lídio G. Lima-Neto[1], Afonso G. Abreu[1] and Cinara Regina A. V. Monteiro[1]

*Address all correspondence to: valerio.monteiro@ceuma.br

1 Ceuma University, São Luís, Brazil

2 Federal University of Maranhão, São Luís, Brazil

## References

[1] Cilloniz C, Martin-Loeches I, Garcia-Vidal C, San Jose A, Torres A. Microbial etiology of pneumonia: Epidemiology, diagnosis and resistance patterns. International Journal of Molecular Sciences. 2016;**17**(12):2120. DOI: 10.3390/ijms17122120

[2] Ewig S, Welte T, Chastre J, Torres A. Rethinking the concepts of community-acquired and health-care-associated pneumonia. Lancet Infectious Diseases. 2010;**10**(4):279-287. DOI: 10.1016/S1473-3099(10)70032-3

[3] American Thoracic Society, Infectious Diseases Society of America. Guidelines for the management of adults with hospital-acquired, ventilator-associated, and healthcare-associated pneumonia. American Journal of Respiratory and Critical Care Medicine. 2005;**171**(4):388-416. DOI: 10.1164/rccm.200405-644ST

[4] Blot S, Koulenti D, Dimopoulos G, Martin C, Komnos A, Krueger WA, et al. Prevalence, risk factors, and mortality for ventilator-associated pneumonia in middle-aged, old, and very old critically ill patients*. Critical Care Medicine. 2014;**42**(3):601-609. DOI: 10.1097/01.ccm.0000435665.07446.50

[5] Charles MP, Kali A, Easow JM, Joseph NM, Ravishankar M, Srinivasan S, et al. Ventilator-associated pneumonia. The Australasian Medical Journal. 2014;**7**(8):334-344. DOI: 10.4066/AMJ.2014.2105

[6] Hunter JD. Ventilator associated pneumonia. BMJ. 2012;**344**:e3325. DOI: 10.1136/bmj.e3325

[7] Nair GB, Niederman MS. Ventilator-associated pneumonia: Present understanding and ongoing debates. Intensive Care Medicine. 2015;**41**(1):34-48. DOI: 10.1007/s00134-014-3564-5

[8] Safdar N, Crnich CJ, Maki DG. The pathogenesis of ventilator-associated pneumonia: Its relevance to developing effective strategies for prevention. Respiratory Care. 2005;**50**(6):725-739; discussion 39-41

[9] Inchai J, Pothirat C, Liwsrisakun C, Deesomchok A, Kositsakulchai W, Chalermpanchai N. Ventilator-associated pneumonia: Epidemiology and prognostic indicators of 30-day mortality. Japanese Journal of Infectious Diseases. 2015;**68**(3):181-186. DOI: 10.7883/yoken.JJID.2014.282

[10] Gupta S, Boville BM, Blanton R, Lukasiewicz G, Wincek J, Bai C, et al. A multicentered prospective analysis of diagnosis, risk factors, and outcomes associated with pediatric ventilator-associated pneumonia. Pediatric Critical Care Medicine. 2015;**16**(3):e65-e73. DOI: 10.1097/PCC.0000000000000338

[11] Hudcova J, Craven DE. Ventilator-associated pneumonia. In: Siempos II, editor. Hospital-Acquired Pneumonia. London: Future Medicine Ltd; 2013. pp. 49-65

[12] Charles MP, Easow JM, Joseph NM, Ravishankar M, Kumar S, Umadevi S. Incidence and risk factors of ventilator associated pneumonia in a tertiary care hospital. The Australasian Medical Journal. 2013;**6**(4):178-182. DOI: 10.4066/AMJ.2013.1627

[13] Tan B, Zhang F, Zhang X, Huang YL, Gao YS, Liu X, et al. Risk factors for ventilator-associated pneumonia in the neonatal intensive care unit: A meta-analysis of observational studies. European Journal of Pediatrics. 2014;**173**(4):427-434. DOI: 10.1007/s00431-014-2278-6

[14] Chastre J, Fagon JY. Ventilator-associated pneumonia. American Journal of Respiratory and Critical Care Medicine. 2002;**165**(7):867-903. DOI: 10.1164/ajrccm.165.7.2105078

[15] Gil-Perotin S, Ramirez P, Marti V, Sahuquillo JM, Gonzalez E, Calleja I, et al. Implications of endotracheal tube biofilm in ventilator-associated pneumonia response: A state of concept. Critical Care. 2012;**16**(3):R93. DOI: 10.1186/cc11357

[16] Gu H, Ren D. Materials and surface engineering to control bacterial adhesion and biofilm formation: A review of recent advances. Frontiers of Chemical Science and Engineering. 2014;**8**(1):20-33. DOI: 10.1007/s11705-014-1412-3

[17] Polívková M, Hubáček T, Staszek M, Švorčík V, Siegel J. Antimicrobial treatment of polymeric medical devices by silver nanomaterials and related technology. International Journal of Molecular Sciences. 2017;**18**(2):419. DOI: 10.3390/ijms18020419

[18] Ramasamy M, Lee J. Recent nanotechnology approaches for prevention and treatment of biofilm-associated infections on medical devices. BioMed Research International. 2016;**2016**:17. DOI: 10.1155/2016/1851242

[19] Siempos, II, Ntaidou TK, Filippidis FT, Choi AM. Effect of early versus late or no tracheostomy on mortality and pneumonia of critically ill patients receiving mechanical ventilation: A systematic review and meta-analysis. The Lancet Respiratory Medicine. 2015;**3**(2):150-158. DOI: 10.1016/S2213-2600(15)00007-7

[20] Wang L, Li X, Yang Z, Tang X, Yuan Q, Deng L, et al. Semi-recumbent position versus supine position for the prevention of ventilator-associated pneumonia in adults requiring mechanical ventilation. Cochrane Database of Systematic Reviews. 2016;(1):CD009946. DOI: 10.1002/14651858.CD009946.pub2

[21] Panigada M, Berra L, Greco G, Stylianou M, Kolobow T. Bacterial colonization of the respiratory tract following tracheal intubation-effect of gravity: An experimental study. Critical Care Medicine. 2003;**31**(3):729-737. DOI: 10.1097/01.CCM.0000049943.01252.E5

[22] Gastmeier P, Sohr D, Geffers C, Ruden H, Vonberg RP, Welte T. Early- and late-onset pneumonia: Is this still a useful classification? Antimicrobial Agents and Chemotherapy. 2009;**53**(7):2714-2718. DOI: 10.1128/AAC.01070-08

[23] Restrepo MI, Peterson J, Fernandez JF, Qin Z, Fisher AC, Nicholson SC. Comparison of the bacterial etiology of early-onset and late-onset ventilator-associated pneumonia in subjects enrolled in 2 large clinical studies. Respiratory Care. 2013;**58**(7):1220-1225. DOI: 10.4187/respcare.02173

[24] Ferrer M, Difrancesco LF, Liapikou A, Rinaudo M, Carbonara M, Li Bassi G, et al. Polymicrobial intensive care unit-acquired pneumonia: Prevalence, microbiology and outcome. Critical Care. 2015;**19**:450. DOI: 10.1186/s13054-015-1165-5

[25] Park DR. The microbiology of ventilator-associated pneumonia. Respiratory Care. 2005;**50**(6):742-763; discussion 63-5

[26] Jones RN. Microbial etiologies of hospital-acquired bacterial pneumonia and ventilator-associated bacterial pneumonia. Clinical Infectious Diseases. 2010;**51**(Suppl 1):S81-S87. DOI: 10.1086/653053

[27] Resende MM, Monteiro SG, Callegari B, Figueiredo PM, Monteiro CR, Monteiro-Neto V. Epidemiology and outcomes of ventilator-associated pneumonia in northern Brazil: An analytical descriptive prospective cohort study. BMC Infectious Diseases. 2013;**13**:119. DOI: 10.1186/1471-2334-13-119

[28] Giamarellou H, Antoniadou A, Kanellakopoulou K. *Acinetobacter baumannii*: A universal threat to public health? International Journal of Antimicrobial Agents. 2008;**32**(2):106-119. DOI: 10.1016/j.ijantimicag.2008.02.013

[29] Joly-Guillou ML. Clinical impact and pathogenicity of *Acinetobacter*. Clinical Microbiology and Infection. 2005;**11**(11):868-873. DOI: 10.1111/j.1469-0691.2005.01227.x

[30] Peleg AY, Seifert H, Paterson DL. *Acinetobacter baumannii*: Emergence of a successful pathogen. Clinical Microbiology Reviews. 2008;**21**(3):538-582. DOI: 10.1128/CMR.00058-07

[31] Cerqueira GM, Peleg AY. Insights into *Acinetobacter baumannii* pathogenicity. IUBMB Life. 2011;**63**(12):1055-1060. DOI: 10.1002/iub.533

[32] Doi Y, Murray GL, Peleg AY. *Acinetobacter baumannii*: Evolution of antimicrobial resistance-treatment options. Seminars in Respiratory and Critical Care Medicine. 2015;**36**(1):85-98. DOI: 10.1055/s-0034-1398388

[33] Podschun R, Ullmann U. *Klebsiella* spp. as nosocomial pathogens: Epidemiology, taxonomy, typing methods, and pathogenicity factors. Clinical Microbiology Reviews. 1998;**11**(4):589-603

[34] Schroll C, Barken KB, Krogfelt KA, Struve C. Role of type 1 and type 3 fimbriae in *Klebsiella pneumoniae* biofilm formation. BMC Microbiology. 2010;**10**:179. DOI: 10.1186/1471-2180-10-179

[35] Jagnow J, Clegg S. *Klebsiella pneumoniae* MrkD-mediated biofilm formation on extracellular matrix- and collagen-coated surfaces. Microbiology. 2003;**149**(Pt 9):2397-2405. DOI: 10.1099/mic.0.26434-0

[36] Munoz-Price LS, Poirel L, Bonomo RA, Schwaber MJ, Daikos GL, Cormican M, et al. Clinical epidemiology of the global expansion of *Klebsiella pneumoniae* carbapenemases. Lancet Infectious Diseases. 2013;**13**(9):785-796. DOI: 10.1016/S1473-3099(13)70190-7

[37] Pan YJ, Lin TL, Chen YH, Hsu CR, Hsieh PF, Wu MC, et al. Capsular types of *Klebsiella pneumoniae* revisited by *wzc* sequencing. PLoS One. 2013;**8**(12):e80670. DOI: 10.1371/journal.pone.0080670

[38] Shon AS, Bajwa RP, Russo TA. Hypervirulent (hypermucoviscous) *Klebsiella pneumoniae*: A new and dangerous breed. Virulence. 2013;**4**(2):107-118. DOI: 10.4161/viru.22718

[39] Li B, Zhao Y, Liu C, Chen Z, Zhou D. Molecular pathogenesis of *Klebsiella pneumoniae*. Future Microbiology. 2014;**9**(9):1071-1081. DOI: 10.2217/fmb.14.48

[40] Pan YJ, Lin TL, Hsu CR, Wang JT. Use of a Dictyostelium model for isolation of genetic loci associated with phagocytosis and virulence in *Klebsiella pneumoniae*. Infection and Immunity. 2011;**79**(3):997-1006. DOI: 10.1128/IAI.00906-10

[41] Evrard B, Balestrino D, Dosgilbert A, Bouya-Gachancard JL, Charbonnel N, Forestier C, et al. Roles of capsule and lipopolysaccharide O antigen in interactions of human monocyte-derived dendritic cells and *Klebsiella pneumoniae*. Infection and Immunity. 2010;**78**(1):210-219. DOI: 10.1128/IAI.00864-09

[42] Lawlor MS, Handley SA, Miller VL. Comparison of the host responses to wild-type and *cpsB* mutant *Klebsiella pneumoniae* infections. Infection and Immunity. 2006;**74**(9):5402-5407. DOI: 10.1128/IAI.00244-06

[43] Regueiro V, Campos MA, Pons J, Alberti S, Bengoechea JA. The uptake of a *Klebsiella pneumoniae* capsule polysaccharide mutant triggers an inflammatory response by human airway epithelial cells. Microbiology. 2006;**152**(Pt 2):555-566. DOI: 10.1099/mic.0.28285-0

[44] Regueiro V, Moranta D, Frank CG, Larrarte E, Margareto J, March C, et al. *Klebsiella pneumoniae* subverts the activation of inflammatory responses in a NOD1-dependent manner. Cellular Microbiology. 2011;**13**(1):135-153. DOI: 10.1111/j.1462-5822.2010.01526.x

[45] Campos MA, Vargas MA, Regueiro V, Llompart CM, Alberti S, Bengoechea JA. Capsule polysaccharide mediates bacterial resistance to antimicrobial peptides. Infection and Immunity. 2004;**72**(12):7107-7114. DOI: 10.1128/IAI.72.12.7107-7114.2004

[46] Bachman MA, Lenio S, Schmidt L, Oyler JE, Weiser JN. Interaction of lipocalin 2, transferrin, and siderophores determines the replicative niche of *Klebsiella pneumoniae* during pneumonia. MBio. 2012;**3**(6): e00224-11. DOI: 10.1128/mBio.00224-11

[47] Bachman MA, Oyler JE, Burns SH, Caza M, Lepine F, Dozois CM, et al. *Klebsiella* pneumoniae yersiniabactin promotes respiratory tract infection through evasion of lipocalin 2. Infection and Immunity. 2011;**79**(8):3309-3316. DOI: 10.1128/IAI.05114-11

[48] Russo TA, Shon AS, Beanan JM, Olson R, MacDonald U, Pomakov AO, et al. Hypervirulent *K. pneumoniae* secretes more and more active iron-acquisition molecules than "classical" *K. pneumoniae* thereby enhancing its virulence. PLoS One. 2011;**6**(10):e26734. DOI: 10.1371/journal.pone.0026734

[49] Berra L, Sampson J, Wiener-Kronish J. *Pseudomonas aeruginosa*: Acute lung injury or ventilator-associated pneumonia? Minerva Anestesiologica. 2010;**76**(10):824-832

[50] Gellatly SL, Hancock RE. *Pseudomonas aeruginosa*: New insights into pathogenesis and host defenses. Pathogens and Disease. 2013;**67**(3):159-173. DOI: 10.1111/2049-632X.12033

[51] Kerr KG, Snelling AM. *Pseudomonas aeruginosa*: A formidable and ever-present adversary. Journal of Hospital Infection. 2009;**73**(4):338-344. DOI: 10.1016/j.jhin.2009.04.020

[52] Sievert DM, Ricks P, Edwards JR, Schneider A, Patel J, Srinivasan A, et al. Antimicrobial-resistant pathogens associated with healthcare-associated infections: Summary of data reported to the National Healthcare Safety Network at the Centers for Disease Control and Prevention, 2009-2010. Infection Control and Hospital Epidemiology. 2013;**34**(1):1-14. DOI: 10.1086/668770

[53] Sadikot RT, Blackwell TS, Christman JW, Prince AS. Pathogen-host interactions in *Pseudomonas aeruginosa* pneumonia. American Journal of Respiratory and Critical Care Medicine. 2005;**171**(11):1209-1223. DOI: 10.1164/rccm.200408-1044SO

[54] Kipnis E, Sawa T, Wiener-Kronish J. Targeting mechanisms of *Pseudomonas aeruginosa* pathogenesis. Médecine et Maladies Infectieuses. 2006;**36**(2):78-91. DOI: 10.1016/j.medmal.2005.10.007

[55] Kantyka T, Pyrc K, Gruca M, Smagur J, Plaza K, Guzik K, et al. *Staphylococcus aureus* proteases degrade lung surfactant protein A potentially impairing innate immunity of the lung. Journal of Innate Immunity. 2013;**5**(3):251-260. DOI: 10.1159/000345417

[56] Foster TJ, Geoghegan JA, Ganesh VK, Hook M. Adhesion, invasion and evasion: The many functions of the surface proteins of *Staphylococcus aureus*. Nature Reviews, Microbiology. 2014;**12**(1):49-62. DOI: 10.1038/nrmicro3161

[57] Soong G, Martin FJ, Chun J, Cohen TS, Ahn DS, Prince A. *Staphylococcus aureus* protein A mediates invasion across airway epithelial cells through activation of RhoA GTPase signaling and proteolytic activity. Journal of Biological Chemistry. 2011;**286**(41):35891-35898. DOI: 10.1074/jbc.M111.295386

[58] Archer GL. *Staphylococcus aureus*: A well-armed pathogen. Clinical Infectious Diseases. 1998;**26**(5):1179-1181

[59] Thammavongsa V, Kim HK, Missiakas D, Schneewind O. Staphylococcal manipulation of host immune responses. Nature Reviews. Microbiology. 2015;**13**(9):529-543. DOI: 10.1038/nrmicro3521

[60] Zhang C, Guo L, Chu X, Shen L, Guo Y, Dong H, et al. Presence of the Panton-Valentine Leukocidin Genes in Methicillin-Resistant *Staphylococcus aureus* is associated with severity and clinical outcome of hospital-acquired pneumonia in a Single Center Study in China. PLoS One. 2016;**11**(6):e0156704. DOI: 10.1371/journal.pone.0156704

[61] Kalil AC, Metersky ML, Klompas M, Muscedere J, Sweeney DA, Palmer LB, et al. Management of adults with hospital-acquired and ventilator-associated pneumonia: 2016 Clinical Practice Guidelines by the Infectious Diseases Society of America and the American Thoracic Society. Clinical Infectious Diseases. 2016;**63**(5):e61-e111. DOI: 10.1093/cid/ciw353

[62] Gardete S, Tomasz A. Mechanisms of vancomycin resistance in *Staphylococcus aureus*. Journal of Clinical Investigation. 2014;**124**(7):2836-2840. DOI: 10.1172/JCI68834

[63] Hafer C, Lin Y, Kornblum J, Lowy FD, Uhlemann AC. Contribution of selected gene mutations to resistance in clinical isolates of vancomycin-intermediate *Staphylococcus aureus*. Antimicrobial Agents and Chemotherapy. 2012;**56**(11):5845-5851. DOI: 10.1128/AAC.01139-12

[64] Kaye KS, Pogue JM. Infections caused by resistant Gram-negative bacteria: Epidemiology and management. Pharmacotherapy. 2015;**35**(10):949-962. DOI: 10.1002/phar.1636

[65] Potron A, Poirel L, Nordmann P. Emerging broad-spectrum resistance in Pseudomonas aeruginosa and *Acinetobacter baumannii*: Mechanisms and epidemiology. International Journal of Antimicrobial Agents. 2015;**45**(6):568-585. DOI: 10.1016/j.ijantimicag.2015.03.001

[66] Paczosa MK, Mecsas J. *Klebsiella pneumoniae*: Going on the offense with a strong defense. Microbiology and Molecular Biology Reviews. 2016;**80**(3):629-661. DOI: 10.1128/MMBR.00078-15

[67] Guillamet CV, Vazquez R, Noe J, Micek ST, Kollef MH. A cohort study of bacteremic pneumonia: The importance of antibiotic resistance and appropriate initial therapy? Medicine (Baltimore). 2016;**95**(35):e4708. DOI: 10.1097/MD.0000000000004708

[68] Blot F, Raynard B, Chachaty E, Tancrede C, Antoun S, Nitenberg G. Value of Gram stain examination of lower respiratory tract secretions for early diagnosis of nosocomial pneumonia. American Journal of Respiratory and Critical Care Medicine. 2000;**162**(5):1731-1737. DOI: 10.1164/ajrccm.162.5.9908088

[69] O'Horo JC, Thompson D, Safdar N. Is the gram stain useful in the microbiologic diagnosis of VAP? A meta-analysis. Clinical Infectious Diseases. 2012;**55**(4):551-561. DOI: 10.1093/cid/cis512

[70] Lung M, Codina G. Molecular diagnosis in HAP/VAP. Current Opinion in Critical Care. 2012;**18**(5):487-494. DOI: 10.1097/MCC.0b013e3283577d37

[71] Mothershed EA, Whitney AM. Nucleic acid-based methods for the detection of bacterial pathogens: Present and future considerations for the clinical laboratory. Clinica Chimica Acta. 2006;**363**(1-2):206-220. DOI: 10.1016/j.cccn.2005.05.050

[72] Tenover FC. Developing molecular amplification methods for rapid diagnosis of respiratory tract infections caused by bacterial pathogens. Clinical Infectious Diseases. 2011;**52**(Suppl 4):S338-S345. DOI: 10.1093/cid/cir049

[73] Beale DJ, Jones OA, Karpe AV, Dayalan S, Oh DY, Kouremenos KA, et al. A review of analytical techniques and their application in disease diagnosis in breathomics and salivaomics research. International Journal of Molecular Sciences. 2016;**18**(1):24

[74] Motta A, Paris D, Melck D, De Laurentiis G, Maniscalco M, Sofia M, et al. Nuclear magnetic resonance-based metabolomics of exhaled breath condensate: Methodological aspects. European Respiratory Journal. 2012;**39**(2):498-500

[75] Ibrahim B, Basanta M, Cadden P, Singh D, Douce D, Woodcock A, et al. noninvasive phenotyping using exhaled volatile organic compounds in asthma. Thorax. 2011;**66**: 804-809. DOI: 10.1136/thx.2010.156695

[76] Filipiak W, Beer R, Sponring A, Filipiak A, Ager C, Schiefecker A, et al. Breath analysis for in vivo detection of pathogens related to ventilator-associated pneumonia in intensive care patients: A prospective pilot study. Journal of Breath Research. 2015;**9**(1):016004

[77] Fowler SJ, Basanta-Sanchez M, Xu Y, Goodacre R, Dark PM. Surveillance for lower airway pathogens in mechanically ventilated patients by metabolomic analysis of exhaled breath: A case-control study. Thorax. 2015;**70**(4):320-325

# Advancing in the Direction of Right Solutions: Treating Multidrug-Resistant Pneumonia

Manu Chaudhary, Gazalla Ayub and Anurag Payasi

Additional information is available at the end of the chapter

http://dx.doi.org/10.5772/intechopen.69979

**Abstract**

Worldwide, antibiotic resistance is a major contemporary public health threat due to rapid emergence of resistant bacteria and endangering the efficacy of antibiotics. There are significant number of reports on clinical failure of β-lactam and β-lactamase inhibitor combination and even carbapenems due to various carbapenem resistance mechanisms. The increasing rate of the antibiotic resistance and its impact on treatment failure encouraged us to study newly reported concept of antibiotic adjuvant entities (AAEs) by which the increasing failure rate of antibiotics can be controlled. These AAEs have been developed for both Gram-positive and Gram-negative multidrug-resistant (MDR) infections. Elores (ceftriaxone + sulbactam with adjuvant ethylenediaminetetraacetic acid (EDTA)) and Potentox (cefepime + amikacin with adjuvant potassium chloride) are the AAEs for Gram-negative MDR pathogens each catering to a different type of resistance and Vancoplus (ceftriaxone + vancomycin with adjuvant L-arginine), another AAE, can help us to last longer in the war against antibiotic-resistant Gram-positive bugs particularly which cause complicated lower respiratory tract infection (LRTI) leading to pneumonia. These new antibiotic additions (Elores, Potentox, and Vancoplus) to the current armamentarium to treat MDR infections, including pneumonia, can help us combat against antimicrobial resistance more efficiently.

**Keywords:** antibiotic resistance, pneumonia, Elores, Potentox, Vancoplus

## 1. Introduction

Pneumonia commonly described as infection of lungs is classified according to where or how it is acquired: community-acquired, healthcare-associated, hospital-acquired, or ventilator-associated pneumonia [1, 2]. According to the area of lung affected, pneumonia can be lobar pneumonia, bronchial pneumonia, and acute interstitial pneumonia [2]. Pneumonia can be

INTECH
open science | open minds

© 2017 The Author(s). Licensee InTech. This chapter is distributed under the terms of the Creative Commons Attribution License (http://creativecommons.org/licenses/by/3.0), which permits unrestricted use, distribution, and reproduction in any medium, provided the original work is properly cited.

bacterial, viral, and less commonly fungal [3]. In the pediatric age group, pneumonia may additionally be classified as non-severe, severe, or very severe depending on the signs and symptoms [4].

## 2. Definitions

Hospital-acquired pneumonia (HAP) or nosocomial pneumonia refers to any pneumonia contracted by a patient in a hospital at least 48–72 h after being admitted. Community-acquired pneumonia (CAP) is defined as pneumonia acquired outside a hospital or a long-term care facility. It occurs within 48 h of hospital admission or in a patient presenting with pneumonia who does not have any of the characteristics of healthcare-associated pneumonia. The nosocomial pneumonia, which is associated with mechanical ventilation for a duration of more than 48 h, is termed as ventilator-associated pneumonia (VAP), whereas the healthcare-associated pneumonia is defined as the pneumonia occurring in non-hospitalized patients having contact with the healthcare system.

## 3. Epidemiology

From 1930s, prior to the discovery of antibiotic, till date pneumonia remains the major cause of death among all age groups accounting for four million deaths annually. The rate of death is highest among children aged less than 5 years worldwide [5]. According to a study conducted by Farooqui et al. [6], 3.6 million (3.3–3.9 million) episodes of severe pneumonia and 0.35 million (0.31–0.40 million) all-cause pneumonia deaths occurred in children younger than 5 years in India. Furthermore, 0.56 million (0.49–0.64 million) severe episodes of pneumococcal pneumonia and 105,000 (92,000–119,000) pneumococcal deaths occurred in India. According to American Thoracic Society/Infectious Diseases Society of America (ATS/IDSA), 2005, HAP had a crude mortality rate of 30–70% with an estimated attributable mortality rate to pneumonia between 27 and 50%. According to some estimates, VAP contributes up to 50–85% of all cases of nosocomial pneumonia [7, 8]. Furthermore, it mainly occurs in intensive care unit (ICU) patients where they most often require ventilator support, amounting to 9–27% of all mechanically ventilated patients [8]. It is estimated that four million cases of CAP occur annually in the United States, of which 20–25% are severe enough to warrant hospitalization [9]. Pneumonia is responsible for about 1.6 million deaths among children aged <5 years in Africa and South-East Asia regions [10, 11]. HAP and VAP are important causes of mortality and morbidity, which continue to baffle the treating physicians in today's era of MDR.

## 4. Economic burden

Pneumonia is one of the most common causes of economic burden across the globe involving great exploitation of health resources. World Health Organization (WHO) has indicated

http://dx.doi.org/10.5772/intechopen.69979

that more death of children occurs due to pneumonia than any other diseases. According to a study conducted in India [11], the average cost per patient not put on ventilator is INR 27,123, whereas the cost associated with ventilated patient is almost twice INR 44,812. Ventilator support is the most expensive intervention adding to the cost of care followed by the cost of antibiotics and investigations and still making the patient more prone to complicated infections like biofilm. Thus, the disease adds significantly to the cost of hospital care and to the length of hospital stay. The situation does not seem to improve as antibiotic pipeline is virtually dry and the resistance appears to be further mounting in most parts of the world as per the latest Center for Disease Dynamics, Economics and Policy (CDDEP) reports.

## 5. Etiology

The etiology of pneumonia in high-income countries is different than in low-income countries [12, 13]. It has been reported that viruses contribute to 30–67% cases of CAP in developed countries and are more frequently identified in children aged less than 1 year than in those aged above 2 years [12]. Bacteria are more frequently identified with increasing age, resulting in mixed infections being less common with age [12].

Respiratory syncytial virus (RSV) is the prime cause of viral pneumonia in children admitted to hospital in developing countries, followed by influenza A and B, parainfluenza, human metapneumovirus, and adenovirus [13]. The bacterial pathogens causing pneumonia include *Pseudomonas aeruginosa, Haemophilus influenza* type b, *Acinetobacter baumannii, Klebsiella pneumoniae, Escherichia coli, Staphylococcus aureus*, methicillin-resistant *S. aureus* (MRSA), and *Streptococcus pneumoniae* [8, 14, 15].

## 6. Diagnosis

The outline for the diagnosis of pneumonia is highlighted in WHO/UNICEF Integrated Management of Childhood Illness (IMCI) guidelines. Fever and cough are the most common ones. Fever is present in 65–90% and cough in 75–96% of patients with pneumonia. Other typical respiratory complaints include sputum production, dyspnea, and chest pain [16]. In a hospital, there are numerous investigations available including radiography and microbiological methods to investigate pneumonia.

## 7. Treatments

The treatment of pneumonia depends on the age, the severity of illness, the likely causative agents, and their resistance patterns. Guidelines recommended the use of third- and fourth-generation cephalosporins, BL + BLI (β-lactam + β-lactamase inhibitor) combinations, and even carbapenems for the management of Gram-negative infections and vancomycin/linezolid for the management of Gram-positive infections.

## 8. Antibiotic resistance

Worldwide, antibiotic resistance is a major contemporary public health threat due to rapid emergence of resistant bacteria and endangering the efficacy of antibiotics [17]. In 2014, the WHO warned that the antibiotic resistance crisis is becoming extremely serious [18] and is attributed to the overuse and misuse of these medications, as well as a lack of new drug development by the pharmaceutical industry [19]. Different molecular mechanisms are responsible for the development of antimicrobial resistance such as alteration of bacterial cell permeability, acquisition of extended spectrum β-lactamase production (ESBLs), and metallo-β-lactamases (MBLs), bacterial biofilm formation, activation of efflux pump, bacterial conjugation, and curli fiber formation [17, 20–25].

In India, the prevalence of ESBL producing organisms among Gram-negative pathogens was up to 73.5% [26]. Similarly, the prevalence of MBLs is also increasing at an immense rate [27, 28]. Scores of reports highlighting antibiotic resistance because of efflux pump in bacteria is increasing significantly [29]. Outer membrane permeability and β-lactamase are key factor for the resistance of bacteria to antibiotics [30]. The increasing rate of the biofilm problem and its impact on antibiotic resistance triggered us to think new means which could disrupt the biofilm formation by inhibiting bacterial adhesion and curli formation.

There are significant number of reports on the clinical failure of β-lactam and β-lactamase inhibitor combination and even carbapenems due to various carbapenem resistance mechanisms. A number of studies have demonstrated the decreased susceptibility of Enterobacteriaceae to cephalosporins and other drugs [31, 32]. The ESBLs enzyme confers resistance not only to broad-spectrum cephalosporins, including oxymino-β-lactam antibiotics, but also to other commonly used antibiotics, including aminoglycosides and quinolone [33, 34]. Overexpression of efflux pump is often associated with extrusion of most of the β-lactam antibiotics, leading to decreased susceptibility of antibiotics [35].

A decreased susceptibility rates of *P. aeruginosa* and *A. baumannii* to β-lactams including carbapenems has been reported in various countries [36–38]. Failure of vancomycin and linezolid could be attributed to the emergence of VRSA (vancomycin-resistant *S. aureus*), hGISA (hetrogeneous glycopeptide intermediate *S. aureus*) [39, 40]. This has raised a huge unmet need in the search for novel resistance-breaking therapies. Besides the above factors, inappropriate selection of empiric broad-spectrum antibiotics stretches the length of treatment and causes emergence of antibiotic resistance.

In view of the above background, the increasing rate of the antibiotic resistance and its impact on treatment failure encouraged us to study newly reported concept of antibiotic adjuvant entity by which the increasing failure rate of antibiotics can be controlled. Adjuvants are commonly used chemical entities which do not possess antibacterial activity of their own but help antibiotic in breaking one or more mechanisms of resistance and accelerate antibiotic effectiveness making AAEs as empiric choice [41]. Information regarding the prevalence of antimicrobial resistance in pathogens can be used for selecting an optional treatment. Earlier studies have supported the combination therapy of two or more drugs in combination with adjuvant (which are usually non-antibiotic in nature) as a suitable approach to reduce the frequency of antibiotic resistance [24].

A few of such synergistic novel antimicrobial adjuvant entities, their mechanisms, and clinical outcomes, which can revolutionize the future, will be discussed in this book chapter. These AAEs have been developed for both Gram-positive and Gram-negative multidrug-resistant infections. Elores (ceftriaxone + sulbactam with adjuvant EDTA) and Potentox (cefepime + amikacin with adjuvant potassium chloride (KCl)) are the AAEs for Gram-negative MDR pathogens each catering to a different type of resistance, and Vancoplus (ceftriaxone + vancomycin with adjuvant L-arginine), another AAE, can help us to last longer in the war against antibiotic-resistant Gram-positive bugs particularly which cause complicated LRTI leading to pneumonia (HAP/CAP/VAP/HCAP).

### 8.1. CSE1034 (Elores)

CSE1034 is a novel combination of third-generation cephalosporin "ceftriaxone," an irreversible β-lactamase inhibitor "sulbactam," and non-antibiotic adjuvant Antibiotic Resistance Breaker (ARB) "disodium edetate." Due to synergistic action of the inhibition of cell wall by ceftriaxone accompanied by the specific inhibition of β-lactamases by β-lactam component produced by common Gram-negative and Gram-positive pathogens, this drug has been reported to be affective against multiple types of MDR organisms. CSE1034 has proven activity against a wide range of ESBL and MBL producing Gram-negative pathogens and is used as a treatment option for a multitude of bacterial infections.

#### *8.1.1. Mechanism of action*

Ceftriaxone acts by binding to penicillin-binding proteins (PBPs) which are transpeptidases that catalyze the cross-linking of the peptidoglycan polymers synthesizing cell wall and subsequently inhibiting bacterial cell wall synthesis. The cell wall of bacteria consists of pentapeptide units attached to a polysaccharide backbone with alternating units of N-acetylglucosamine (NAG) and N-acetylmuramic acid (NAM). PBPs act on a terminal D-alanyl-D-alanine moiety on a pentapeptide unit and catalyze the formation of a peptide bond between the penultimate D-alanine and a glycine unit on an adjacent peptidoglycan strand. The ceftriaxone structure is the mimic of D-alanyl-D-alanine moiety and the PBPs wrongly attack the β-lactam ring in ceftriaxone, which leads to the inactivation of PBPs. As the peptidoglycan synthesis is essential to maintain bacterial cell wall integrity, so the inhibition of PBPs leads to damage and destruction of the cell wall and ultimately in cell lysis.

Sulbactam is a potent, highly specific inhibitor of a wide variety of β-lactamases including penicillinases and cephalosporinases produced commonly by different strains of bacteria and chromosomally mediated enzymes induced in some strains of *Klebsiella, Enterobacter*, and *Serratia* species to degrade antibiotics. By forming a protein complex with β-lactamases produced by bacterial strains resistant to ceftriaxone, the full potential of ceftriaxone is restored by the addition of sulbactam. Sulbactam not only potentiates the antibacterial activity of ceftriaxone against ESBL-producing pathogens but also exhibits a moderate antibacterial activity.

Disodium edetate is a non-antibiotic adjuvant acts as ARB which chelates the divalent metal ions particularly zinc that functions as a cofactor for carbapenemases. As zinc is necessary for the MBL activity, thus EDTA activity makes MBL-producing organisms susceptible toward Elores [24, 25, 42, 43]. Disodium edetate also chelates divalent metal ions located in the outer membrane causing destabilization of outer membrane and thus resulting in enhanced penetration of drugs inside the bacterial cells. Moreover, CSE1034 downregulates acrA, acrB, tolC, mexA, and mexB genes in MexA-MexB-OprM efflux pump, which in turn enhances the susceptibility of Gram-negative bacteria (GNB) toward CSE1034 which overexpress this efflux transporter.

#### *8.1.2. Activity spectrum*

Elores has a broad spectrum of activity against both Gram-positive and Gram-negative bacteria pathogens. It is reported to be active against both ESBL and MBL producing organisms, including *E. coli, K. pneumoniae, Acinetobacter* spp., and *Pseudomonas* spp. Susceptibility data from various parts of India were collected from various clinical samples (including urine, pus, sputum, bronchoalveolar lavage, and endotracheal fluid); this AAE is very promising. The prevalence of resistance to Elores in ESBL and MBL organisms is reported to be less in various parts of India. The drug has been approved by the Drug Controller General of India (DCGI) for the treatment of various bacterial infections caused by the susceptible isolates of *K. pneumoniae, K. oxytoca, E. coli, P. aeruginosa, Acinetobacter* spp., *S. pneumoniae,* and *S. aureus*. A number of randomized phase 3 comparative trials, prospective, retrospective, and case studies have demonstrated the efficacy of Elores in the treatment of infections pertaining to respiratory tract, skin and skin structure, genitourinary tract, musculoskeletal, and gastrointestinal tract when compared with carbapenems and BL-BLIs showed very promising results [24, 25, 42]. These various published susceptibility reports suggest the use of Elores empirically in HAP and VAP caused due to MDR ESBL and MBL-producing Gram-negative pathogens [44]. A number of studies including randomized phase 3 trials, prospective, retrospective, and case studies validate the safety and efficacy of CSE1034. A phase 3 trial reports published in 2013 showed significantly high improved efficacy of CSE1034 compared to ceftriaxone in LRTI patients [45, 46]. Based on the safety and efficacy data, Elores is recommended as a carbapenem-sparer antibiotic. CSE1034 has shown to be effective and safe in moderate to severe HAP and VAP patients. CSE1034 has shown promising results in sepsis as monotherapy as well as along with colistin [47, 48]. CSE1034 was found to be safe with no serious adverse event was reported in phase 3 trial and post-marketing surveillance studies. Overall, CSE1034 is found to be well tolerated in adult population.

### **8.2. Potentox**

With regard to Potentox for pneumonia, first of all, let's see what this unique AAE offers. Potentox is a synergistic antibiotic combination of cefepime and amikacin and potassium chloride. Cefepime is the fourth-generation broad-spectrum cephalosporin. It is frequently used as first-line empirical therapy for healthcare-associated infections, including those caused by suspected Gram-negative bacteria. Cefepime has relatively low propensity for degradation by ESBLs compared to other cephalosporins. Cefepime also remains active against infections due to AmpC-producing organisms. Amikacin is one of the most commonly used aminoglycosides and it has the highest recommendation from IDSA 2016 for usage in nosocomial pneumonia cases as an empirical antibiotic in the combination protocol against nosocomial pneumonia. Potentox (cefepime + amikacin) is not just the most active combination in vitro [23, 49] but also has demonstrated efficacy in vivo as the most active combination [50, 51].

#### 8.2.1. Mechanism of action

Amikacin, which belongs to aminoglycoside antibiotic group, blocks the production of protein by binding irreversibly to the four nucleotides of 16S rRNA of 30S ribosomal subunit of the pathogenic organism. This region where amikacin binds is known to interact with the wobble base in the anti-codon of tRNA. Thus, amikacin interferes with the tRNA acceptor site and prevents the formation of initiation complex with messenger RNA. This leads to misreading of mRNA so incorrect amino acids are inserted into the polypeptide leading to nonfunctional or toxic peptides and the breakup of polysomes into nonfunctional monosomes.

Cefepime, a fourth-generation cephalosporin, is bactericidal and has the same mode of action as other β-lactam antibiotics. It disrupts the synthesis of the peptidoglycan layer of bacterial cell wall which is important for cell wall structural integrity.

Potassium chloride is a metal halide salt composed of potassium and chloride that is used as an adjuvant in Potentox. Interestingly, Potentox due to adjuvant potassium chloride exhibits activity against Quinolone-resistant Gram-negative pathogens, the prevalence of which is rising alarmingly in developing countries.

#### 8.2.2. Activity spectrum

Both cefepime and amikacin individually have become a victim of high level of resistance [52]. This is where precisely, Potentox is used in combating these multidrug-resistant pathogens as Potentox has demonstrated in vitro and in vivo activity against these resistant isolates to which cefepime and amikacin are resistant individually. Global surveillance studies demonstrate that the actual acquired fluoroquinolone resistance rates are highly variable and are as high as almost 100%, particularly in Asia, whereas resistance rates in Europe and North America range from <10% in rural areas to >30% which is still pretty high. This highlights the importance of Potentox use to target multiple drug resistance effectively which developed both in community and in hospital settings.

Multi-centric randomized comparative open-labeled phase 3 trial of synergistic antibiotic combination of cefepime and amikacin versus cefepime alone was conducted in nosocomial pneumonia and showed superiority of Potentox in efficacy over cefepime alone.

Potentox and Elores can serve as a true carbapenem sparer as medically important Gram-negative bacteria are developing resistance very fast against this valuable class of antibiotic. In the era of antimicrobial resistance, the judicious use of different antimicrobials in a balanced fashion can help us in preserving these antibiotics for longer duration.

### 8.3. Vancoplus

While we look for HAP/VAP due to Gram-positive bacteria, methicillin-resistant *S. aureus* is a big concern and empirical antibiotic therapy should cover MRSA whenever factors increase the likelihood of MRSA. Now, MRSA is not confined to western countries only. A network of microbiology laboratories (Indian Network for Surveillance of Antimicrobial Resistance—INSAR) at premier medical colleges and hospitals in India was formed with support from the World Health Organization. In an article published in 2013, INSAR reported that MRSA prevalence in India is to the tune of 40% which shows that MRSA is a significant problem for India too.

Vancoplus is a novel AAE of ceftriaxone and vancomycin along with L-arginine as adjuvant caters to all types of mixed infection especially MRSA, VRSA, VISA, and hGISA [43].

### *8.3.1. Mechanism of action*

The vancomycin plays its bactericidal role primarily through inhibiting cell wall biosynthesis. Specifically, vancomycin forms hydrogen bond interactions with the terminal D-alanyl-D-alanine moieties of the N-acetylmuramic acid- and N-acetylglucosamine-peptide subunits and thus prevents their incorporation into the peptidoglycan matrix, a major component of Gram-positive cell walls. Additionally, vancomycin is known to alter bacterial-cell-membrane permeability and RNA synthesis. No cross-resistance is known to occur between vancomycin and other antibiotics. The mechanism of action of ceftriaxone is already discussed in Elores drug section.

### *8.3.2. Activity spectrum*

Earlier, the natural glycopeptide vancomycin was considered the drug of choice to treat MRSA infections. However, the concerns regarding the efficacy of vancomycin against MRSA including poor bactericidal activity and high recurrence rates are increasing [53]. Stevens and Moise Broder have reported in two studies, published in CID 2004 and 2006, respectively, that MRSA treatment failure rate is associated with higher vancomycin minimum inhibitory concentration (MIC). Higher vancomycin MIC is associated with higher mortality in HAP/VAP due to MRSA. We have started witnessing vancomycin resistance, either in the intermediate range or in the full-resistance range, even in India. Among high-risk MRSA bacteremia patients, Sakoulas et al. [54] documented treatment failure rates of 44% when vancomycin MICs were <0.5 μg/ml and of 90% when vancomycin MICs were 1–2 μg/ml ($p$ = 0.01) [54]. Although many other drugs including tigecycline, linezolid, and daptomycin have also been approved and represent alternate antibiotic therapy to vancomycin, no study has reported the superiority in terms of efficacy and safety of these drugs over vancomycin [55]. These clinical challenges necessitate finding alternative effective empirical solutions for the management of MRSA infections and/or mixed infections. It will be prudent to start empirically with an antibiotic which shows MIC in the susceptibility range and works effectively at lower MIC also and that is what Vancoplus offers due to double insult caused by both ceftriaxone and vancomycin. Besides this, Vancoplus effectively helps in preventing and breaking biofilm which is a very frequent problem in intubated nosocomial pneumonia patients [23].

European Antimicrobial Resistance Surveillance Network (EARS-Net) data show that the occurrence of methicillin-resistant *S. aureus* was stabilizing in several European countries; still the percentage of MRSA among all *S. aureus* isolates remained above 25% in seven of the 29 EU/EEA reporting countries. The risk factor in ICU patients increases with an increased length of stay and patients with catheter or other devices. In such cases, Vancoplus is a highly reliable product because it takes care of mixed Gram-negative and Gram-positive infections effectively. Although both these drugs have known incompatibility when given individually and needs infusion line flushing or advised to be given contralaterally, the presence of adjuvant not only potentiates the activity of duo but also makes them compatible [56]. It has been observed that when two non-compatible drugs are administered due to medical urgency with due precautions, still there exists certain degree of degradation of one of the drug molecules in vivo resulting in lesser efficacy than expected. Vancoplus overcomes this challenge effectively.

Additionally, one of the biggest challenges in the management of *S. aureus* infection including all resistant versions is the management of virulence factors. Panton Valentine Leukocidin (PVL) and δ-toxin, alpha toxins are responsible for cell lysis including human erythrocytes, neutrophils, as well as various mammalian cells. β-Lactams may even induce the production of cytolysins and other virulence-related exoproteins when inadequately used for treating MRSA, which potentially worsens clinical outcomes. In the treatment of meningitis particularly it becomes added taxing issue to prevent neuronal cell damage which is caused by virulence factors generated by pathogens even if treated. Here, Vancoplus offers additional protection by neutralizing toxins secreted by pathogen and reducing sequelae drastically and makes the product highly beneficial for immune-compromised patients [23].

In a nut shell, a number of agencies (Infectious Diseases Society of America/American Thoracic Society, US FDA and SWAB, Asia Pacific Society for Critical Care Medicines, European Society of Intensive Care Medicines, Indian Society of Critical Care Medicines, etc.) have issued guidelines for the treatment of CAP/HAP/HCAP, CUTI/sepsis and the management of other critical ICU infections. The concept of antibiotic adjuvant entity is new and will take time to be a part of these guidelines. The author has tried to share the latest and emerging trends in MDR infection management with proven efficacy and safety in millions of patients across various developing economies. The world has now started talking about adjuvant therapy and soon these therapies will be part of standard critical infection management program. These new antibiotic additions (Elores, Potentox, and Vancoplus) to the current armamentarium to treat MDR infections including pneumonia can help us combat against antimicrobial resistance more efficiently due to presence of ARB as adjuvant.

### 8.4. Adjuvant therapy to treat secondary bacterial superinfections caused by influenza and other respiratory viruses

Viral influenza is very common in community and is often mistreated with antibiotics. Antibacterial drugs are not meant for viral infections and misuse leads to creation of resistant bacterial species. Viral-bacterial co-infections in humans are well documented. Viral infections often lead to bacterial superinfections. Bacterial superinfections accompanied by influenza and other respiratory virus infections contribute to the significant morbidity and mortality particularly among elderly and young children.

Bacterial infection could be concomitant with influenza viral infection as a result of an enhanced pneumonic illness or may happen soon following influenza virus has been widely cleared from the lungs, when the host seems to be more susceptible to bacterial infection [57, 58].

Morbidity and mortality have been recognized to be greater in cases of influenza-associated bacterial infection in all age groups [59]. The increase in influenza infection during winter is often associated with a rise in cases of community-acquired pneumonia. The most common causes of CAP are *S. pneumoniae, S. aureus*, and *H. influenzae. S. pneumoniae* is the most frequently isolated pathogen associated with influenza [60], although deaths, especially in children, are also associated with *S. aureus* infection, as highlighted by the recent emergence of community-acquired methicillin-resistant *S. aureus* [61]. Besides influenza, other respiratory viruses, such as coronavirus, adenovirus, and respiratory syncytial virus, are also associated with pneumonia [62].

The mechanisms of superinfection are very complex process. Several reports indicate that changes due to virus in the respiratory tract prime the upper airway and lung make way for subsequent bacterial infection. Super bacterial infections are accompanied by virus-induced cytopathology, leading to immunological impairment, which could be caused in part by the overproduction of inflammatory cytokines [63]. Transformation of the immune response by curtailing the capacity of the host to clear bacteria may contribute to the severity of the resulting infection [64]. Earlier studies on animal model have demonstrated that influenza predisposes to bacterial pneumonia [63, 65, 66]. It has been reported with 7–21 days of lag time for the onset of bacterial infection following seasonal influenza. However, shorter times from onset to death have been noticed in pandemic periods [67–69].

### 8.5. Antibiotic adjuvants potentiate anti-inflammatory properties of antibiotics

There is limited information on the effectiveness of adjuvant therapy for the treatment of bacterial complications of influenza. In a very recent study [70], explored the adjuvant effect of polyactin (PA), an inactivated trivalent influenza virus (ITIV) with or without PA or MF59 was instilled intranasally once a week in BALB/c mice. Results showed that PA is a novel mucosal adjuvant for intranasal vaccination with the inactivated trivalent influenza vaccine that has safe and effective mucosal adjuvanticity in mice and successfully induces both serum and mucosal antibody responses and a cell-mediated response.

The inflammatory response of viral infections results in the excessive production of reactive oxygen species (ROS) in the cells and tissues, and antioxidant system cannot neutralize them. Imbalance in this protective mechanism can lead to the damage of cellular molecules such as DNA, proteins, and lipids [71]. Moreover, the role of ROS in inflammation has been investigated vigorously by earlier authors [72, 73]. ROS are thought to be key signaling molecules in the progression of inflammatory disorders. It induces inflammation by the induction of COX-2, inflammatory cytokines (TNF$\alpha$, interleukin 1 (IL-1), and IL-6), chemokines (IL-8 and CXCR4), and pro-inflammatory transcription factors (NF-$\kappa$B) [74]. Inflammatory cytokines trigger inflammation, causing the immune response to weaken which may help to increase the risk of bacterial infection. This rise in inflammatory markers with infection is a cascade reaction and is not easily broken only by antibiotics. Adjuvants have a major role to play here. Buret [75] reported that some antibiotics, such as the 16-membered macrolide tilmicosin, may generate anti-inflammatory benefits by modulating the production of pro-inflammatory mediators, and by inducing neutrophil apoptosis. Many studies have highlighted that adjuvants co-administered with antibiotics reduce the oxidative stress, which in turn reduce inflammation [76, 77]. Dwivedi et al. [78] reported that AAE used for 21 days, the levels of antioxidant enzymes (superoxidase dismutase, catalase, glutathione reductase, glutathione peroxidase), along with xanthine oxidase, lipid peroxidation, myeloperoxidase (MPO) levels, hepatic, and renal parameters were significantly improved in plasma and tissues of the AAE-treated group indicating antioxidant or free radical scavenging properties [50].

Osteomyelitis is an infection and inflammation in bone which is primarily caused by *S. aureus* and *S. epidermidis* and the levels of cytokines (TNF$\alpha$ and IL-6) is increased in osteomyelitis [79]. Dwivedi et al. [80] demonstrated that the combination of antibiotic along with adjuvant significantly improved the inflammatory cytokines (TNF$\alpha$ and IL-6), malondialdehyde (MDA), and myeloperoxidase in animal osteomyelitis infection model. From the earlier explanation, it may be concluded that compounds or drugs along with adjuvant generating both antibacterial and anti-inflammatory effects are likely to be most effective at treating bacteria-induced inflammatory syndromes.

## Author details

Manu Chaudhary, Gazalla Ayub and Anurag Payasi*

*Address all correspondence to: ccmb@vmrcindia.com

Venus Medicine Research Centre, Hill Top Industrial Estate, Jharmajri EPIP, Bhatoli Kalan, India

## References

[1] American Thoracic Society, Infectious Diseases Society of America. Guidelines for the management of adults with hospital-acquired, ventilator-associated, and healthcare-associated pneumonia. American Journal of Respiratory and Critical Care Medicine. 2005;**171**:388-416

[2] Sharma S, Maycher B, Eschun G. Radiological imaging in pneumonia: Recent innovations. Current Opinion in Pulmonary Medicine. 2007;**13**(3):159-169

[3] Dunn L. Pneumonia: Classification, diagnosis and nursing management. Nursing Standard (Royal College of Nursing (Great Britain). 1987, 2005;**19**(42):50-54

[4] World Health Organization. Pocket Book of Hospital Care for Children: Guidelines for the Management of Common Illnesses with Limited Resources. Geneva: World Health Organization; 2005. p. 72

[5] Black RE, Cousens S, Johnson HL, Lawn JE, Rudan I, Bassani DG, et al. Global, regional, and national causes of child mortality in 2008: A systematic analysis. Lancet. 2010; **375**(9730):1969-1987

[6] Farooqui H, Jit M, Heymann D, Zodpey S. Burden of severe pneumonia, pneumococcal pneumonia and pneumonia deaths in Indian states: Modelling based estimates. PLoS One. 2015;**10**(6):e0129191

[7] Hunter JD. Ventilator associated pneumonia. British Medical Journal. 2012;**344**:e3325

[8] Oliveira MS, Prado GV, Costa SF, Grinbaum RS, Levin AS. Ampicillin/sulbactam compared with polymyxins for the treatment of infections caused by carbapenem-resistant Acinetobacter spp. Journal of Antimicrobial Chemotherapy. 2008;**61**(6):1369-1375

[9] Centers for Disease Control and Prevention Web Site. Pneumonia. Available from: http://www.cdc.gov/nchs/FASTATS/pneumonia.htm [Accessed: February 6, 2010]

[10] Kabra SK, Lodha R, Pandey RM. Antibiotics for community-acquired pneumonia in children. The Cochrane Database of Systematic Reviews. 2013;**4**(6):CD004874

[11] Kateel R, Adhikari P, Rajm S. Cost and antibiotic utilization of pneumonia patients in intensive care unit. Journal of Applied Pharmaceutical Science. 2016;**6**(02):087-090

[12] Harris M, Clark J, Coote N, Fletcher P, Harnden A, McKean M, Thomson A. British Thoracic Society guidelines for the management of community acquired pneumonia in children: Update 2011. Thorax. 2011;**66**(2):ii1-23

[13] Rudan I, Boschi-Pinto C, Bioglay Z, Mulholland K, Campbell H. Epidemiology and etiology of childhood pneumonia. Bulletin of the World Health Organization. 2008;**86**(5):408-416

[14] Moreira MR, Filho PPG. Multidrug-resistant pathogens causing ventilator-associated pneumonia: Risk factors, empirical antimicrobial therapy and outcome of patients in an intensive care unit (ICU) of a Brazilian university hospital. International Journal of Medicine and Medical Sciences. 2012;**4**(9):204-210

[15] Kalanuria AA, Zai W, Mirski M. Ventilator-associated pneumonia in the ICU. Critical Care. 2014;**18**:208

[16] Bochud PY, Moser F, Erard P, Verdon F, Studer JP, Villard G, Cosendai A, Cotting M, Heim F, Tissot J, Strub Y, Pazeller M, Saghafi L, Wenger A, Germann D, Matter L, Bille J, Pfister L, Francioli P. Community-acquired pneumonia. A prospective outpatient study. Medicine (Baltimore). 2001;**80**:75-87

[17] Chaudhary M, Payasi A. Prevalence of heterogeneous glycopeptide intermediate resistance in methicillin-resistant *Staphylococcus aureus*. American Journal of Infectious Diseases. 2013;**9**(3):63-470

[18] Ventola CL. The antibiotic resistance crisis: Part 1: Causes and threats. Pharmacy and Therapeutics. 2015;**40**(4):277-283

[19] Gould IM, Bal AM. New antibiotic agents in the pipeline and how they can help overcome microbial resistance. Virulence. 2013;**4**(2):185-191

[20] Askoura M, Mottawea W, Abujamel T, Taher I. Efflux pump inhibitors (EPIs) as new antimicrobial agents against *Pseudomonas aeruginosa*. Libyan Journal of Medicine. 2011;**13**:6

[21] Chaudhary M, Kumar S, Payasi A. A novel approach to combat acquired multiple resistance in *Escherichia coli* by using EDTA as efflux pump inhibitor. Journal of Microbial and Biochemical Technology. 2012;**4**(6):126-130

[22] Chaudhary M, Payasi A. Sulbactomax prevents antimicrobial resistance development by inhibition of conjugal transfer of F plasmids. International Journal of Drug Development & Research. 2012;**4**(1):337-345

[23] Chaudhary M, Payasi A. Resistance patterns and prevalence of the aminoglycoside modifying enzymes in clinical isolates of gram negative pathogens. Global Journal of Pharmacology. 2014;**8**(1):73-79

[24] Kumar M, Chaudhary S, Makkar MK, Garg N, Chugh S. Comparative antimicrobial efficacy evaluation of a new product Elores against meropenem on Gram-negative isolates. Asian Journal of Pharmaceutical Clinical Research. 2015;**8**:1-4

[25] Arora S, Munshi N. Comparative assessment of antibiotic susceptibility pattern of Gram negative pathogens isolated from intensive care unit patients in Pune. British Microbiology Research Journal. 2015;**10**(2):1-9

[26] Dalela G. Prevalence of extended spectrum β-lactamase (ESBL) producers among Gram negative bacilli from various clinical isolates in a tertiary care hospital at Jhalawar, Rajasthan, India. Journal of Clinical and Diagnostic Research. 2012;**6**:182-187

[27] Bora A, Ahmad G. Detection of NDM-1 in clinical isolates of *Klebsiella pneumoniae* from Northeast India. Journal of Clinical and Diagnostic Research. 2012;**6**:794-800

[28] Uma KR, Srinivasa RR, Suchismita S, Shashikala P, Kanungo R, Jayachandran S, Prashanth K. Phenotypic and genotypic assays for detecting the prevalence of metallo-b-lactamases in the clinical isolates of *Acinetobacter baumannii* from a south Indian tertiary care hospital. Journal of Medical Microbiology. 2009;**58**:430-435

[29] Levy SB. Active efflux mechanisms for antimicrobial resistance. Antimicrobial Agents and Chemotherapy. 1992;**36**:695-703

[30] Hancock REW, Wong PGW. Compounds which increase the permeability of the *Pseudomonas aeruginosa* outer membrane. Antimicrobial Agents and Chemotherapy. 1984;**26**:48-52

[31] Wani KA, Thakur MA, Fayaz AS, Fomdia A, Gulnaz B, Maroof P. Extended spectrum β-lactamase mediated resistance in *Escherichia coli* in a tertiary care hospital. International Journal of Health Sciences. 2009;**3**:155-163

[32] Kibret M, Abera B. Antimicrobial susceptibility patterns of *E. coli* from clinical sources in northeast Ethiopia. African Health Sciences. 2011;**11**:S40–S45

[33] Pitout JD. Infections with extended-spectrum beta-lactamase producing Enterobacteriaceae: Changing epidemiology and drug treatment choices. Drugs. 2010;**70**:313-333

[34] Endimiani A, Paterson DL. Optimizing therapy for infections caused by Enterobacteriaceae producing extended-spectrum β-lactamases. Seminars in Respiratory and Critical Care Medicine. 2007;**28**:646-655

[35] Yu EW, Aires JR, Nikaido H. AcrB multidrug efflux pump of *Escherichia coli*: Composite substrate-binding cavity of exceptional flexibility generates its extremely wide substrate specificity. Journal of Bacteriology. 2003;**85**:5657-5664

[36] Owlia P, Azimi L, Gholami A, Asghari B, Lari AR. ESBL and MBL mediated resistance in *Acinetobacter baumannii*: A global threat to burn patients. Infez Med. 2012;**20**:182-187

[37] Mansoor T, Musani MA, Khalid G, Kamal M. *Pseudomonas aeruginosa* in chronic suppurative otitis media: Sensitivity spectrum against various antibiotics in Karachi. Journal of Ayub Medical College. 2009;**21**:120-123

[38] Tripathi P, Banerjee G, Saxena S, Gupta M K, Ramteke PW. Antibiotic resistance pattern of *Pseudomonas aeruginosa* isolated from patients of lower respiratory tract infection. African Journal of Microbiology Research. 2011;**5**:2955-2959

[39] Kirby A, Graham R, Williams NJ, Wootton M, Broughton CM, Alanazi M, et al. *Staphylococcus aureus* with reduced glycopeptide susceptibility in Liverpool, UK. Antimicrobial Chemotherapy. 2010;**65**:721-724

[40] Chaudhary M, Payasi A. Changing trends of commonly used intensive care unit antibiotics due to differential membrane permeability in resistant *Escherichia coli* collected in EASE programme. Journal of Microbial and Biochemical Technology. 2013;**5**:084-087

[41] Beranal P, Molina-Santiago C, Daddaoua A, Llamas MA. Antibiotic adjuvants identification and clinical use. Microbial Biotechnology. 2013;**6**(5):445-449

[42] Sahu M, Sanjith S, Bhalekar P, Keny D. Waging war against extended spectrum beta lactamase and metallobetalactamase producing pathogens—novel adjuvant antimicrobial agent CSE1034—an extended hope. Journal of Clinical and Diagnostic Research. 2014;**8**(6):DC20–DC23

[43] Chaudhary M, Patnaik SK, Payasi A. Inhibition of Panton Valentine Leukocidin toxin indeed neutrophil cell lysis by Vancoplus in methicillin-resistant *Staphylococcus aureus* infections. American Journal of Infectious Diseases. 2014;**10**(4):154-163

[44] Bhatia P, Mir MA. A new fixed dose combination of ceftriaxone + sulbactam + disodium edetate for definitive treatment of infections due to piperacillin/tazobactam resistant bacteria: A retrospective efficacy and pharmacoeconomic study. British Journal of Medicine and Medical Research. 2016;**15**(4):1-14

[45] Chaudhary M, Payasi A. A randomized, open label, prospective, multicenter phase III clinical trial of Elores in lower respiratory tract and urinary tract infections. Journal of Pharmacy Research. 2013;**6**:409-413

[46] Chaudhary M, Payasi A. Clinical, microbial efficacy and tolerability of Elores, a novel antibiotic adjuvant entity in ESBL producing pathogens: Prospective randomized controlled clinical trial. Journal of Pharmacy Research. 2013;**7**:275-280

[47] Verma S. A retrospective study to evaluate the efficacy of a new antibiotic adjuvant entity (β-lactam/β-lactamase inhibitor/adjuvant disodium edetate combination) for management of sepsis. Research Journal of Infectious Diseases. 2015;**3**:1-7

[48] Agarwal VK, Bansal A, Pujani M, Jawa M, Mahajan P, Jain A. A retrospective comparative study to evaluate the use of a new betalactam + betalactamase inhibitor (ceftriaxone + sulbactam + disodium edetate) in comparison to meropenem in the management of Gram-negative bacterial sepsis. Tropical Journal of Medical Research. 2016;**19**(1):5-10

[49] Chaudhary M, Payasi A. A solution to combat aminoglycoside and quinolone resistant gram negative organisms. International Journal of Current Research. 2015;**7**(6):17006-17011

[50] Dwivedi VK, Soni A, Chaudhary M, Singh CP, Shrivastava SM. Fixed-dose combination of cefepime plus amikacin (Potentox) inhibits pneumonia infection. Experimental Lung Research. 2009;**35**(7):621-629

[51] Dwivedi VK, Soni A, Payasi A, Ahmed A, Singh SP, Chaudhary M. Potentox reduces biochemical and inflammatory response in osteomyelites infection. International Journal of Osteoporosis and Metabolic Disorders. 2011;**4**(1):26-36

[52] Shahid M, Malik A. Resistance due to aminoglycoside modifying enzymes in *Pseudomonas aeruginosa* isolates from burns patients. Indian Journal of Medical Research. 2005;**122**:324-332

[53] Liu C, Bayer A, Cosgrove SE, Daum RS, Fridkin SK, Gorwitz RJ, Kaplan SL, Karchmer AW, Levine DP, Murray BE. Clinical practice guidelines by the Infectious Diseases Society of America for the treatment of methicillin-resistant *Staphylococcus aureus* infections in adults and children. Clinical Infectious Diseases. 2011;**52**:e18-e55

[54] Sakoulas G, Moise-Broder PA, Schentag J, Forrest A, Moellering RC Jr, Eliopoulos GM. Relationship of MIC and bactericidal activity to efficacy of vancomycin for treatment of methicillin-resistant *Staphylococcus aureus* bacteremia. Journal of Clinical Microbiology. 2004;**42**:2398-2402

[55] Wunderink RG, Mendelson MH, Somero MS, Fabian TC, May AK, Bhattacharyya H, Leeper KV Jr, Solomkin JS. Early microbiological response to linezolid vs vancomycin in ventilator-associated pneumonia due to methicillin-resistant *Staphylococcus aureus*. Chest. 2008;**134**(6):1200-1207

[56] Chaudhary A, Kumar S, Bansal R, Payasi A. Synergy of a novel antibiotic adjuvant entity against multi drug resistant methicillin-resistant *Staphylococcus aureus* and heterogeneous glycopeptide-intermediate Staphylococcus aureus. Journal of Pharmacy Research. 2013;**7**:781–e786

[57] Small C-L, Shaler CR, McCormick S, Jeyanathan M, Damjanovic D, Brown EG, Arck P, Jordana M, Kaushik C, Ashkar AA, Xing Z. Influenza infection leads to increased susceptibility to subsequent bacterial superinfection by impairing NK cell responses in the lung. Journal of Immunology. 2010;**184**:2048-2056

[58] Hament JM, Kimpen JL, Fleer A, Wolfs TF. Respiratory viral infection predisposing for bacterial disease: A concise review. FEMS Immunology and Medical Microbiology. 1999;**26**:189-195

[59] Seki M, Kosai K, Yanagihara K, Higashiyama Y, Kurithara S, Izumikawa K, Miyazaki Y, Hirakata Y, Tashiro T, Hohno S. Disease severity in patients with simultaneous influenza and bacterial pneumonia. Internal Medicine. 2007;**46**:953-958

[60] Brundage JF. Interactions between influenza and bacterial respiratory pathogens: Implications for pandemic preparedness. The Lancet Infectious Diseases. 2006;**6**:303-312

[61] Finelli L, Fiore A, Dhara R, Brammer L, Shay DK, Kamimoto L, Fry A, Hageman J, Gorwitz R, Bresee J, Uyeki T. Influenza-associated pediatric mortality in the United States: Increase of *Staphylococcus aureus* coinfection. Pediatrics. 2008;**122**:805-811

[62] Pavia AT. What is the role of respiratory viruses in community acquired pneumonia; what is the best therapy for influenza and other viral causes of CAP? Infectious Disease Clinics of North America. 2013;**27**:157-175

[63] Beadling C, Slifka MK. How do viral infections predispose patients to bacterial infections? Current Opinion in Infectious Diseases. 2004;**17**:185-191

[64] McCullers JA. Insights into the interaction between influenza virus and pneumococcus. Clinical Microbiology Reviews. 2006;**19**:571-582

[65] Loving CL, Brockmeier SL, Vincent AL, Palmer MV, Sacco RE, Nicholson TL. Influenza virus coinfection with bordetella bronchiseptica enhances bacterial colonization and host responses exacerbating pulmonary lesions. Microbial Pathogens. 2010;**49**:237-245

[66] Diavatopoulos DA, Short KR, Price JT, Wilksch JJ, Brown LE, Briles DE, Strugnell R, Wijburg OL. Influenza A virus facilitates *Streptococcus pneumoniae* transmission and disease. FASEB Journal. 2010;**24**:1789-1798

[67] Grabowska K, Hogberg L, Penttinen P, Svensson A, Ekdahl K. Occurrence of invasive pneumococcal disease and number of excess cases due to influenza. BMC Infectious Diseases. 2006;**6**:58

[68] Sachedina N, Donaldson LJ. Paediatric mortality related to pandemic influenza A H1N1 infection in England: An observational population based study. The Lancet. 2010;**376**:1846-1852

[69] Lee EH, Wu C, Lee EU et al. Fatalities associated with the 2009 H1N1 influenza a virus in New York City. Clinical Infectious Diseases. 2010;**50**:1498-1504

[70] Ren S-T, Zhang X-M, Sun P-F, Sun L-J, Guo X, Tian T, Zhang J, Guo Q-Y, Li X, Guo L-J, Che J, Wang B, Zhang H. Intranasal immunization using mannatide as a novel adjuvant for an inactivated influenza vaccine and its adjuvant effect compared with MF59. PLoS One. 2017;**12**(1):e0169501

[71] Ďuračková Z. Some current insights into oxidative stress. Physiological Research. 2010;**59**:459-469

[72] Mittal M, Siddiqui MR, Tran K, Reddy SP, Malik AB. Reactive oxygen species in inflammation and tissue injury. Antioxidants & Redox Signaling. 2014;**20**(7):1126-1167

[73] Berlett BS, Stadtman ER. Protein oxidation in aging, disease, and oxidative stress. Journal of Biological Chemistry. 1997;**272**:20313-20316

[74] Gupta SC, Hevia D, Patchva S, Park B, Koh W, Aggarwal BB. Upsides and downsides of reactive oxygen species for cancer: The roles of reactive oxygen species in tumorigenesis, prevention, and therapy. Antioxidants & Redox Signaling. 2012;**16**:1295-322

[75] Buret AG. Immuno-modulation and anti-inflammatory benefits of antibiotics: The example of tilmicosin. Canadian Journal of Veterinary Research. 2010;**74**(1):1-10

[76] Dwivedi VK, P. Kumar, Chaudhary M. Comparative study of CSE 1034 and ceftriaxone in pneumonia induced rat. Clinical and Experimental Pharmacology. 2012;**2**:1

[77] Kaulmann A, Bohn T. Bioactivity of polyphenols: Preventive and adjuvant strategies toward reducing inflammatory bowel diseases—promises, perspectives, and pitfalls. Oxidative Medicine and Cellular Longevity. 2016;**2016**:29

[78] Dwivedi VK, Bhatnagar A, Chaudhary M. Protective role of ceftriaxone plus sulbactam with VRP1034 on oxidative stress, hematological and enzymatic parameters in cadmium toxicity induced rat model. Interdisciplinary Toxicology. 2012;**5**(4):192-200

[79] Kopf M, Baumann H, Freer G, Freudenberg M, Lamers M, Kishimoto T, Zinkernazel R, Bleuthmann H, Kohler G. Impaired immune and acute phase responses in IL-6 deficiency mice. Nature. 1994;**368**:339-342

[80] Dwivedi VK, Soni A, Payasi A, Ahmad A, Shambhu PS, Chaudhary M. Potentox Reduces Biochemical and Inflammatory Response in Osteomyelitis Infection. International Journal of Osteoporosis and Metabolic Disorders. 2011;**4**: 26-36

Section 3

# Idiopathic and Viral Etiologies of Pneumonia

Chapter 7

# Interstitial Pneumonia Associated with Connective Tissue Disease: A Comprehensive Overview and an Insight into the Pathogenesis

Akira Takeda and Yoshiki Ishii

Additional information is available at the end of the chapter

http://dx.doi.org/10.5772/intechopen.70864

**Abstract**

Interstitial pneumonia (IP) refers to involvement of the lung parenchyma by varying degrees of inflammation and fibrosis, in contrast to airspace disease typically seen in bacterial pneumonia. IP lies in the center of a heterogenous group of diffuse interstitial lung diseases (ILDs), either idiopathic or linked to underlying disorders. One of the major categories of disorders frequently associated with IP is a connective tissue disease (CTD), in which autoimmune-mediated tissue injury leads to multiple organ impairment. Today, IP represents the most critical pulmonary complication in CTD, resulting in significant morbidity and mortality. Despite growing understanding of the pathology of IPs, as well as the accumulating knowledge from both basic and clinical studies of CTDs, the pathogenesis of CTD-associated IP remains unclear. This chapter will provide an overview of the general understanding of ILD and illustrate the current state of knowledge on IP associated with CTD, in order to fully comprehend the entirety of its complex pictures. Moreover, we will propose a new insight into the immune pathogenesis of CTD-IP by presenting evidence which robustly indicates that T cells trigger initial development of IP in polymyositis/dermatomyositis, suggesting potential approaches for controlling such particular T cells in therapeutic interventions for IP.

**Keywords:** interstitial pneumonia, interstitial lung disease, connective tissue disease, polymyositis/dermatomyositis, T lymphocyte, T cell receptor, antigen-driven mechanisms

## 1. Introduction

The term "Interstitial pneumonia" (IP) is used to describe noninfectious, inflammatory lung disorders characterized by the histologic abnormalities with diffuse interstitial fibrosis involving alveolar walls. In contrast to airspace disease typically seen in bacterial pneumonia, IP

INTECH
open science | open minds

© 2018 The Author(s). Licensee InTech. This chapter is distributed under the terms of the Creative Commons Attribution License (http://creativecommons.org/licenses/by/3.0), which permits unrestricted use, distribution, and reproduction in any medium, provided the original work is properly cited.

refers to involvement of the lung parenchyma by varying combination of fibrosis and inflammation [1, 2]. IP is included in the "interstitial lung disease" (ILD), i.e., a heterogenous group of diffuse parenchymal lung disorders, either idiopathic or associated with injurious or inflammatory causes, in which the major site of damage is the lung interstitium [3]. Customarily, the designations IP and ILD are sometimes used interchangeably. To be accurate, however, ILD comprises a broader range of lung diseases which involves the pulmonary interstitium, including drug-induced pneumonitis and eosinophilic pneumonia, etc. Primarily, IP refers to the particular disease entities which belong to idiopathic interstitial pneumonia (IIP) defined by the 2002 and 2012 American Thoracic Society/European Respiratory Society (ATS/ERS) classification [1–4]. IIP was categorized into several forms of IPs, afterward each histopathologic pattern of which has been applied to the ILD associated with underlying diseases as well; the details of these will be described later.

From the pathophysiological perspective, the pulmonary interstitium consists of area with minimal connective tissue matrix between the capillaries and the alveolar space that allows close apposition of gas and blood flow leading to efficient gas exchange. If any injury from a specific exposure of chemicals or proteins, an autoimmune-mediated inflammation, or unknown etiology occurs and persists, the lung may respond to the damage by repairing process with increased interstitial tissue resulting in histological remodeling. Thus, ILDs may cause serious pulmonary dysfunction, which is often associated with substantial morbidity and poor prognosis.

ILD comprises a variety of disorders with diverse backgrounds. A part of ILD has no identifiable underlying cause and is regarded as idiopathic, whereas it is often associated with a specific environmental exposure or with underlying diseases such as connective tissue disease (CTD) [1]. The CTDs are a group of systemic, inflammatory, autoimmune disorder, in which autoimmune-mediated tissue injury leads to multiple organ impairment including respiratory system. Today, IP or ILD is one of the most serious pulmonary complications associated with CTDs, resulting in significant morbidity and mortality [5]. Despite growing, understanding of the details of pathology in IPs, as well as accumulating evidences which support an association between IP with CTD and the presence of autoantibodies, the pathogenesis of CTD-associated IP remains unclear.

During the last years, we have been exploring the possible involvement of adaptive immunity in the pathogenesis of IP associated with CTDs, and we found intriguing evidence which strongly suggests a pivotal role of T cells in triggering the development of pulmonary alveolitis through antigen-driven immune responses in early stage IP [6, 7]. In this chapter, first, we will overview the current concepts of ILD as well as CTD-associated IP, in order to comprehend the whole picture including pathological features. Then, novel findings demonstrated in our recent studies of IP associated with polymyositis/dermatomyositis will be discussed.

## 2. Understanding of interstitial lung disease

### 2.1. The concept of interstitial lung disease

ILD, also known as diffuse parenchymal lung disease (DPLD), is a generic term encompassing a broad spectrum of heterogenous lung disorders, either idiopathic or associated with injurious or inflammatory causes, in which the major site of damage is the lung interstitium [1–3]. Because of the nature of DPLD which involves the interstitium, the ILDs share common radiologic, pathologic, and clinical manifestations. Clinically, exertional dyspnea and nonproductive cough are most common manifestations. Bilateral inspiratory fine crackles, most prominent at the lung bases, are usually audible on auscultation. Clubbed fingers characterized by hypertrophy and enlargement of the distal phalanges of the hands are often seen and reported in 30–50% of patients with IPF (idiopathic pulmonary fibrosis; to be mentioned later) [8]. Clinical features suggestive of rheumatic disorders, such as arthralgia, Raynaud's phenomenon, and skin manifestations, might be observed in the setting of an underlying CTD. The plain chest radiograph shows reduced lung volumes with bilateral reticular or reticulonodular opacities. High-resolution computed tomography (HRCT), which offers better definition of the characteristic details of lung parenchyma, can reveal usually bilateral, peripheral, and basilar predominant abnormalities with reticulonodular infiltrates, often with honeycombing and cystic changes by IP type to be described later. Although chest radiography is less useful than HRCT in the detailed evaluation, it is helpful for evaluating disease distribution and its serial change during patient follow up [8]. Physiologically, the patients demonstrate diminished diffusion capacity (decreased DLco) with usually restrictive impairment in pulmonary function tests.

### 2.2. Classification of interstitial lung disease

**Figure 1** provides an overview of the classification of ILD, based on the 2002 and 2012 the American Thoracic Society/European Respiratory Society (ATS/ERS) classification statements [1–3]. Briefly, ILDs consist of disorders of known causes (underlying diseases, environmental, or drug related) as well as disorders of unknown causes. The latter include idiopathic interstitial pneumonias (IIPs), granulomatous lung disorders (e.g., sarcoidosis), and other forms of orphan ILD, i.e., lymphangioleiomyomatosis (LAM), pulmonary Langerhans cell histiocytosis/histiocytosis X (PLCH), and eosinophilic pneumonia. Thus, the ILDs comprise a variety of disorders with diverse backgrounds. Whereas a part of ILD has no identifiable underlying cause, often, it is associated with a specific environmental exposure or with underlying CTD [5]. ILDs are classified according to specific clinical, radiological, and histopathological features. The ILDs, however, frequently have similar clinical features. As ILDs are often uneasy to distinguish each other, the updated guidelines in the 2013 ATS/ERS classification statement underlined the importance of multidisciplinary diagnosis (MDD) facilitated by professional experts [2, 3]. Adequate presentation and discussion of clinical and radiological data are essential for an accurate MDD. Among diagnostic modalities, high-resolution computed tomography (HRCT) makes it possible to characterize ILD with great precision. Surgical lung biopsy also remains the gold standard for evaluation of ILD.

### 2.3. Classification of idiopathic interstitial pneumonia

As noted above, if ILD is found to have no association with specific causes, such as chemical exposure, underlying systemic diseases, or genetic causes, the disease is classified as "idiopathic interstitial pneumonia" (IIP). IIPs are a heterogenous group of nonneoplastic disorders involving damage to the lung parenchyma with varying patterns of inflammation and fibrosis. The interstitium includes the space between epithelial and endothelial basement membranes and is the primary site of injury in IIPs. Frequently affecting not only the interstitium, but IIPs

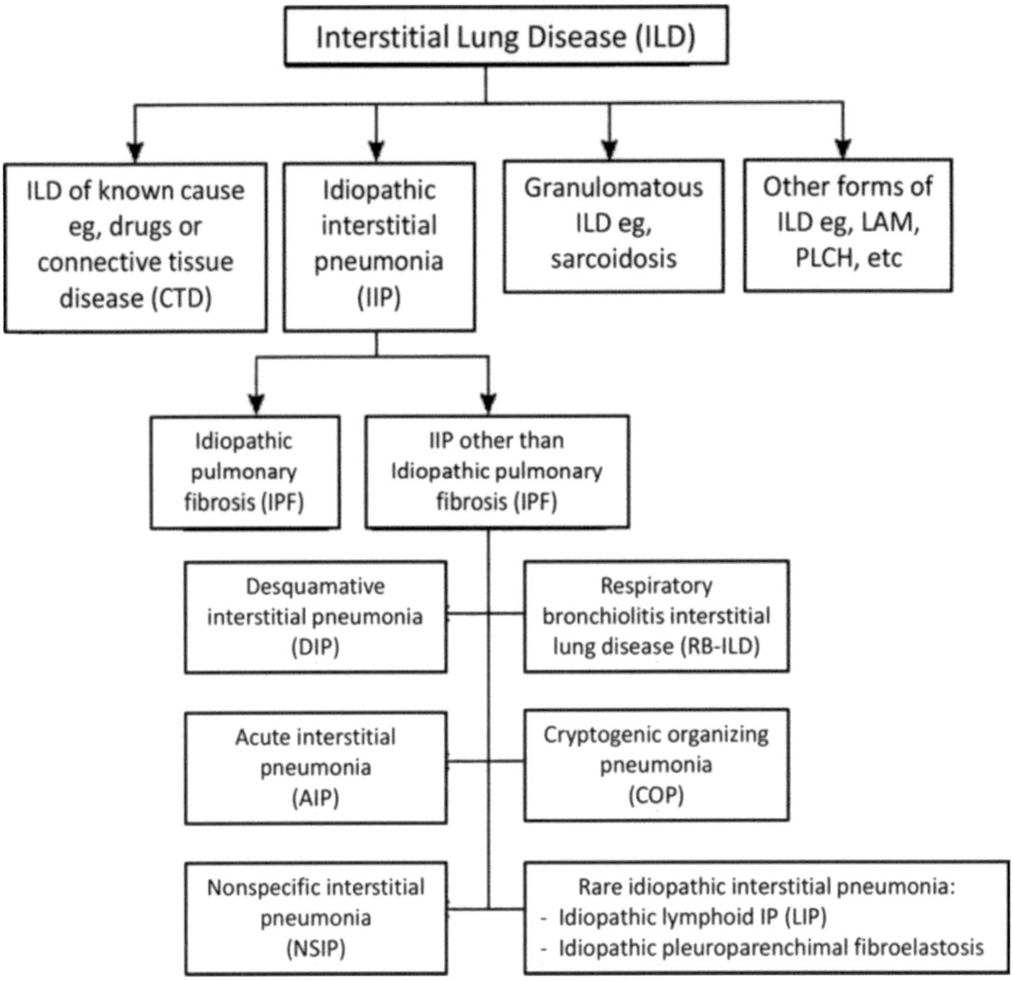


**Figure 1.** Classification of interstitial lung disease. Interstitial lung diseases (ILDs), also termed as diffuse parenchymal lung diseases (DPLDs), consist of disorders of known causes (connective tissue diseases, environmental, or drug related) as well as disorders of unknown cause. The latter include idiopathic interstitial pneumonias (IIPs), granulomatous lung disorders (e.g., sarcoidosis), and other forms of interstitial lung disease (ILD) including lymphangioleiomyomatosis (LAM), pulmonary Langerhans cell histiocytosis/histiocytosis X (PLCH), and eosinophilic pneumonia. The idiopathic interstitial pneumonias (IIPs) are further categorized as idiopathic pulmonary fibrosis (IPF), nonspecific interstitial pneumonia (NSIP), cryptogenic organizing pneumnia (COP), acute interstitial pneumonia (AIP), respiratory bronchiolitis interstitial lung disease (RB-ILD), or desquamative interstitial pneumonia (DIP). Lymphoid interstitial pneumonia (LIP) is occasionally associated with other disease processes, such as connective tissue diseases or immunosuppression while idiopathic LIP is rare.

may also involve the airspace, peripheral airways, and vessels, along with their respective epithelial and endothelial linings [1, 2].

As shown in **Figure 1**, the IIPs are further categorized into "idiopathic pulmonary fibrosis" (IPF), "nonspecific interstitial pneumonia" (NSIP: further subdivided into cellular and fibrotic NSIP), "cryptogenic organizing pneumonia" (COP), "acute interstitial pneumonia" (AIP), "respiratory bronchiolitis interstitial lung disease" (RB-ILD), or "desquamative interstitial pneumonia" (DIP) [1, 2]. "Lymphoid interstitial pneumonia" (LIP) is occasionally associated with other processes, such as connective tissue diseases or immunosuppression, while idiopathic LIP is rare. Among the IIPs, idiopathic pulmonary fibrosis (IPF) is the most common prototypic IIP. "Usual interstitial pneumonia" (UIP) is the pathologic pattern of lung injury seen in IPF. Categorization of major IIP and corresponding histological patterns defining each entity are shown in **Table 1** [2].

#### *2.3.1. The importance of HRCT findings in the classification and diagnosis of interstitial lung disease*

The ATS/ERS/JRS/ALAT 2011 guidelines for IPF have assigned a primary diagnostic role to HRCT, and the HRCT criteria outlined was the same as those in the revised guideline published in 2015 [8–10]. The diagnosis of IPF should be based on the exclusion of other known causes of ILDs (environmental exposures, drugs, and CTDs) and presence of UIP on HRCT; UIP is characterized on HRCT by the presence of reticular abnormalities with subpleural and basal distribution, honeycombing with or without traction bronchiectasis, and absence of features inconsistent with UIP such as extensive ground-glass opacities, diffuse mosaic attenuation, profuse micronodules, and consolidations. Certain HRCT features predict histopathologic patterns of the different forms of ILD. **Table 2** outlines the classification of histological and corresponding radiological patterns defining each entity of IIP, which is also applicable to CTD-associated ILD, to be explained later [5, 11].

| Category | Clinical–radiologic–pathologic diagnoses | Associated radiologic and/or pathologic morphologic patterns |
|---|---|---|
| Chronic fibrosing IP | Idiopathic pulmonary fibrosis (IPF) | Usual interstitial pneumonia (UIP) |
| | Idiopathic nonspecific interstitial pneumonia (NSIP) | Nonspecific interstitial pneumonia (NSIP) |
| Smoking-related IP* | Respiratory bronchiolitis-interstitial lung disease (RB-ILD) | Respiratory bronchiolitis-ILD (RB-ILD) |
| | Desquamative interstitial pneumonia (DIP) | Desquamative interstitial pneumonia (DIP) |
| Acute/subacute IP | Cryptogenic organizing pneumonia (COP) | Organizing pneumonia (OP) |
| | Acute interstitial pneumonia (AIP) | Diffuse alveolar damage (DAD) |

Definition of abbreviation: IP = interstitial pneumonia.

*Desquamative interstitial pneumonia can occasionally occur in nonsmokers.

Adapted from Travis et al. [2].

**Table 1.** Categorization of major IIP.

## 3. Clinical landscape of interstitial lung disease in connective tissue disease

The connective tissue disease (CTD) is a systemic, inflammatory, autoimmune disorder characterized by immune-mediated multiple organ dysfunction. The category of CTD includes a variety of diseases: rheumatoid arthritis (RA), systemic lupus erythematosus (SLE), systemic sclerosis (Scleroderma, SSc), polymyositis/dermatomyositis (PM/DM), and a group of vasculitides. The CTD-related disorders such as Sjögren's syndrome (SS), mixed connective tissue disease (MCTD), etc., are also captured under the extended umbrella of CTD, as they share similar features. Involvement of the respiratory system occurs in those diseases and may be often major contributor to significant morbidity and mortality [5]. The clinical presentation is variable, ranging from cough, dyspnea, pleuritic pain to abnormal diffuse lung shadows on chest X-ray, in addition to clinical features suggestive of rheumatic disorders, i.e., arthralgia, Raynaud's phenomenon, and skin rashes. Some patients may have presentations dominated by pulmonary manifestations over those of autoimmune disease. Thus, it is crucial for physicians to carefully evaluate the evidence of underlying CTDs in all patients who present with ILD.

### 3.1. Prevalence of ILD

ILD, especially IP, is one of the most common and clinically important complications of the various CTDs and the CTD-related disorders of which the most often implicated disorders

| Pattern | Histology | CT features |
|---|---|---|
| UIP | Subpleural and peripheral fibrosis. Temporal and spatial heterogeneity. Scattered *fibroblastic foci* and honeycombing are key features | Basal, subpleural reticulation and honeycombing; traction bronchiectasis; little, if any, ground-glass attenuation |
| NSIP | Uniform interstitial involvement by variable degrees of degrees of fibrosis and inflammation. Honeycombing is rare | Bilateral patchy ground-glass opacities admixed with reticulation and traction bronchiectasis/bronchiolectasis. Little or no honeycombing. Usually, predominantly basal |
| OP | Connective tissue plugs within small airways and air spaces (Masson bodies). In its "pure" form, little or no inflammation or fibrosis in the surrounding interstitium | Airspace consolidation, with a predominantly basal/peripheral or peribronchovascular distribution. Bands with air bronchograms and a perilobular pattern can also be seen |
| DIP | Extensive macrophage accumulation within the distal air spaces. Mild interstitisal involvement | Patchy ground-glass opacities. Microcystic change can be seen within the ground-glass, Basal, peripheral distribution frequent |
| LIP | Bronchiolocentric lymphoid tissue hyperplasia | Ground-glass attenuation is the predominant finding, with thin-walled cysts frequently present. Lung nodules and septal thickening may also be seen |
| RB-ILD | Bronchiolocentric macrophage accumulation. Mild bronchiolar fibrosis | Centrilobular nodules, ground glass opacities. Diffuse or upper lung distribution |
| DAD | In the acute phase: hyaline membrane, edema. In the organizing phase: airspace and interstitial organization | Acute phase: diffuse ground-glass opacities and consolidation in dependent areas. Organizing phase: reticular pattern, traction bronchiectasis and architectural distortion |

Abbreviation: DIP, desquamative interstitial pneumonia; NSIP, non-specific interstitial pneumonia; UIP, usual interstitial pneumonia; OP, organizing pneumonia; DAD, diffuse alveolar damage; RB-ILD, respiratory bronchiolitis interstitial lung disease; LIP, lymphocytic interstitial pneumonia.

Adapted from de Lauretis et al. [11].

**Table 2.** Classification of histological and radiological patterns for IP.

are SSc, RA, PM/DM, Sjögren's syndrome (SS), mixed connective tissue disease (MCTD), and SLE, according to prevalence [12, 13]. The frequency of ILD in CTDs is presented in **Table 3** [12]. Essentially, as every component of the lungs is a potential target for CTDs, there is a wide variety of pulmonary manifestations associated with the diseases [13].

### 3.2. Multidisciplinary diagnostic approach

Though the prevalence of ILD in CTDs varies based on patient selection and methods used for detection, the percentage appears to be higher than previously regarded. ILD may precede the extrapulmonary manifestations of CTD as a *forme fruste* of systemic disease, in some patients by years, while the rheumatic symptoms predate ILD in others [14–16]. Sometimes, it makes the distinction between idiopathic pulmonary fibrosis (IPF) and CTD-related ILD difficult [11, 16]. Despite similarities in clinical and pathologic presentation, the prognosis and treatment of CTD-associated ILD can differ greatly from that of other forms of ILD such as IPF [13, 16, 17]. Therefore, early detection of pulmonary involvement and early accurate diagnosis of CTDs are both important for initiating appropriate intervention. The multidisciplinary diagnostic team (MDD team), including a pulmonologist, a pathologist, and a rheumatologist, can contribute to it; a report indicates that 50% of patients referred with an initial concern for IPF had their diagnosis changed to a CTD-ILD after combined evaluation by the specialists [12].

The evaluation of ILD in patients with CTD is complex due to the heterogeneity of CTDs, the varied types and severity of ILD, and also the fact that ILD may be identified at any point in time in these patients. Fischer, et al. emphasize the importance of cross-disciplinary collaboration and thorough evaluations, which are needed either when CTD patients develop ILD or when encountering ILD patients with possible occult CTD [18]. The detection of occult CTD in patients with "idiopathic" ILD requires careful attention to historical clues, subtle physical examination findings, and autoantibody profiles, as well as radiologic and histopathological features. Such evaluation can be optimized by a multidisciplinary approach in collaboration with specialists including radiologists, pathologists, and rheumatologists. The standard clinical approach for evaluating patients with ILD for CTDs is well summarized by Vij R and Strek ME in their review [5].

| Connective tissue disease | Frequency of ILD | Patterns |
|---|---|---|
| Systemic sclerosis | 45% (clinically significant) | NSIP 80–90%, UIP 10–20%, OP, DAD |
| Rheumatoid arthritis | 5–58% | UIP 50–60%, NSIP 30–60%, OP, LIP, DAD, DIP |
| Polymyositis/dermatomyositis | 30–70% | NSIP, OP, UIP, DAD |
| Sjögren's syndrome | Up to 25% | NSIP, OP, UIP, LIP |
| Systemic lupus erythematosus | 2–8% | NSIP, OP, UIP, DAD |
| Mixed connective tissue disease | 20–60% | NSIP, OP, UIP, DAD |

Modified from Castelino et al. [12].

**Table 3.** Features of ILD associated with CTD.

### 3.3. Laboratory tests and biomarkers

Since the spectrum of ILD associated with CTD is broad, careful evaluation for autoantibodies or other serologic tests in conjunction with clinical features of autoimmune disease is crucial [19, 20]. Because of the variable incidence and outcome of ILD in CTD, biomarkers including autoantibodies are critical for diagnosis, prognosis, patient subtyping, and predicting response to treatment. Major autoantibodies and serologic tests commonly available for the evaluation of CTD-ILDs include antinuclear antibody (ANA), anti-double-stranded DNA, anti-ribonucleoprotein (anti-RNP) antibody, anti-Smith (anti-Sm) antibody, anti-scleroderma-70 (Scl-70) antibody, anti-Ro (SS A), anti-La (SS B), anti-Jo-1 antibody, rheumatoid factor (RF), and anti-cyclic citrullinated peptide antibody (ACPA) [5].

Some of the established biomarkers include lung epithelium-specific proteins [20]. Evidence indicates that repetitive injuries to alveolar epithelial cells (AEC) and airway Club cells trigger an exaggerated wound healing response. During the process, while AEC type I cells undergo apoptosis, regenerated hyperplastic AEC type II cells produce a vast array of cytokines, growth factors, and release surfactant proteins and mucins [21]. Surfactant proteins (SP-A and SP-D) and KL-6 in the serum are useful biomarkers, which have been well established for various ILDs. SP-D and SP-A, secreted by AEC II and airway Club cells, are surfactant lipoproteins and phospholipids which stabilize alveolar surface tension, playing an important role in the lung host defense system [22]. SP-D serum levels are more sensitive than SP-A in detecting ILD as defined by CT but less specific [23]. KL-6 is a high-molecular-weight mucin-like glycoprotein, now classified as MUC1, which is highly expressed by AEC II and bronchiolar epithelial cells and increases following cellular injury and/or regeneration [24]. KL-6 has profibrotic and antiapoptotic effects on lung fibroblasts [25]. Serum KL-6 has been shown to be elevated not only in IIP but also in CTD-ILD, as well as hypersensitivity pneumonitis, drug-induced pneumonitis, etc. [24, 26].

There are a number of principal autoantibodies which have been validated for the clinical use. Antinuclear antibody (ANA) determined by an immunofluorescence assay is most versatile, presenting with several major patterns; mainly homogeneous (associated with ANAs against double strand (ds) DNA in SLE and histones), speckled/peripheral (less specific), and nuclear (most often associated with limited scleroderma). ANA titer higher than 1–160 is regarded as significant in most laboratories [27]. When using enzyme immunoassay (EIA) and enzyme-linked immunosorbent assay (ELISA) for ANAs, we can detect single autoantigens such as dsDNA, Smith antigen, scleroderma (Scl-70) (also termed topoisomerase-1), SSA/Ro, SSB/La, etc. [27]. Some of the recent, newly developed autoantibodies with distinct clinical and immunological characteristics will be explained later.

### 3.4. Undifferentiated connective tissue disease (UCTD) and interstitial pneumonia with autoimmune features (IPAF)

Besides classical, well-established CTDs, increasing attention has been paid to pulmonary involvement in undifferentiated CTD (UCTD) [15, 17, 28–30]. UCTD has been generally defined as a condition that presents with signs and symptoms suggestive of CTDs along with positive ANA but does not fulfill any rheumatology classification criteria for specific CTDs [30, 31]. Mosca et al. reported that 60% of patients with UCTD remain undifferentiated. When evolution to defined CTD occurs, it usually does within the first 5 years of disease. UCTD may develop into any of the CTDs, most often into SLE [29]. There are a large number of patients, in whom the IP appears to be the lone part for the clinically predominant manifestation of an occult CTD with subtle clinical features that suggest an autoimmune process but not meet established criteria for CTD, raising a controversy over the strategies for identification and classification of these patients. Well-organized prospective studies have been needed to better understand this entity of the lung disease and distinguish it from the ILD with well-defined CTD or IIP. Proposed terminology to classify such patients includes "undifferentiated CTD" [31], "lung-dominant CTD" [15], and "autoimmune-featured ILD" [32]. Recently, the "ATS/ERS Task Force on Undifferentiated Forms of CTD-associated ILD" created consensus regarding the nomenclature and classification criteria for patients with IIP and features of autoimmunity and proposed the term "interstitial pneumonia with autoimmune features" (IPAF). The classification criteria require evidence of IP and are organized around three central domains: a clinical domain consisting of specific extra-thoracic features, a serologic domain consisting of specific autoantibodies, and a morphologic domain consisting of specific chest imaging, histopathologic, or pulmonary physiologic features [33]. Currently, it is not yet clear whether IPAF is a distinct phenotype of ILD or simply a part of IIP. Adopting IPAF classification may provide platform for the future study of a more uniform cohort, and prospective survey will be needed in determining efficacy of therapy and outcomes for the patients [34].

## 4. Pulmonary histopathology in connective tissue disease

The underlying pathology in CTD-associated ILD can be dominated by inflammation or fibrosis or by a combination of both with distinct radiologic and histopathologic patterns [12]. Classification of histological and radiological patterns developed for IIPs is applied to CTD-ILD [1, 5, 11]. The radiological and corresponding histological patterns defining each entity of CTD-associated IP are summarized in **Table 2** [11]. Although there is substantial histological overlap among the pulmonary manifestations of different CTDs and with other etiologies, certain histologic patterns may favor one CTD over another, and occasionally distinctive histologic clues may be present [35, 36]. It is possible in many cases to confirm CTD-ILD and guide patient management using histologic features. Pulmonary histopathology is thus helpful, and surgical lung biopsy remains the gold standard for evaluation of CTD-associated ILD [35]. ILD can present acutely or chronically, with acute presentations being more common in SLE and PM/DM. Histological patterns of CTD-associated IP include, most frequently, nonspecific interstitial pneumonia (NSIP), usual interstitial pneumonia (UIP), organizing pneumonia (OP), diffuse alveolar damage (DAD), and lymphocytic interstitial pneumonia (LIP). By contrast, desquamative interstitial pneumonia (DIP) and respiratory bronchiolitis-associated interstitial pneumonia (RB-ILD) are uncommon forms of IP in CTD. Both, typically affecting cigarette smokers, share overlapping clinicopathological features and have a relatively better prognosis than UIP.

### 4.1. Nonspecific interstitial pneumonia (NSIP)

In the history of classification, the recognition that the cases of ILD exist from which lung biopsy samples do not fit into any well-defined histologic patterns of idiopathic IP led to proposals of the terms "unclassified interstitial pneumonia" by Kitaichi in 1990 [37] and "nonspecific interstitial pneumonia/fibrosis (NSIP)" by Katzenstein and Fiorelli in 1994 [38]. This novel concept has helped to identify a group of ILDs with a more favorable prognosis and which needs to be distinguished from IPF/UIP, while also having different characteristics from DIP, AIP, and COP [1]. Katzenstein, in her large study of 64 such cases, utilized the descriptive term "nonspecific interstitial pneumonia/fibrosis (NSIP)," which was characterized by varying proportions of interstitial inflammation and fibrosis that appeared to be occurring over a single time span (i.e., a temporally uniform process). NSIP may have varying etiologies, including underlying CTD as well as organic dust or other exposures [38]. Subsequent intensive studies in collaboration with pathologists and radiologists have endorsed its differentiation from other types of IP, gaining the term NSIP, a broad acceptance [39, 40]. NSIP pattern of lung injury, itself further subdivided into cellular and fibrotic NSIP, is the most common pattern of IP in all CTDs except for RA, in which UIP pattern pathology may be more common [41, 42]. NSIP lung injury is characterized by diffuse, although often variable, alveolar septal thickening due to collagen deposition. The amount of associated interstitial inflammation varies, but in most cases, it consists of mild patchy lymphoplasmacytic infiltrate. Although NSIP is not a pattern specific to CTD-IP, there are several histologic clues which support CTD, and when found, make the diagnosis of CTD-IP more likely [35].

- Involvement of multiple lung components: concurrent involvement of alveolar septal interstitium, airways, vessels, and pleura is an important clue to the diagnosis of CTD-IP and can be helpful in differentiation of it from IPF.
- Interstitial fibrosis with overlapping NSIP and UIP: a histologic overlap of UIP and NSIP patterns is frequently shown in CTD, although similar findings may be seen in some variants of chronic hypersensitivity pneumonia, etc.
- Lymphoid aggregates: formation of prominent lymphoid aggregates, often with germinal centers, is a characteristic feature of CTD-IP, classically seen in RA and Sjögren's syndrome.

### 4.2. Usual interstitial pneumonia (UIP)

UIP is the prototype of histopathology which characterizes IPF, a chronic form of idiopathic interstitial lung disease [1, 2]. UIP pattern is often encountered in CTD-IP, with more prevalence in advanced cases. This pattern is classically identified by its patchy nature (spatial heterogeneity) and chronic active appearance (temporal heterogeneity). Fibrosis is accentuated in the subpleural regions with microscopic honeycombing observed as irregular airspaces surrounded by dense fibrosis. Fibroblast foci (regions of new fibrosis) are found at the interface between central and peripheral regions [35]. While primary UIP pattern is found in 13–56% of RA-ILD cases, some studies have reported that the most frequent histologic pattern of ILD among RA patients is NSIP, followed closely by UIP, accounting for 30–67% and 13–57% of RA-ILD, respectively [36]. Studies of PM/DM-ILD identified an UIP pattern in 5–33% of cases.

In SSc-ILD, UIP pattern was found in 15% in one study and 26% in another. UIP pattern has also been reported in 17% of Sjögren's syndrome cases in a study. Whereas idiopathic pulmonary fibrosis (IPF) is a progressively deteriorating ILD, in which the characteristic histological pattern of IPF is UIP; interestingly, a UIP pattern is associated with a significantly better survival in CTD compared to the IPF [43]. Histologically, CTD-associated UIP biopsies had fewer fibroblastic foci, smaller honeycombing spaces, higher numbers of germinal centers, and higher inflammation scores than IPF/UIP biopsies [44].

### 4.3. Diffuse alveolar damage (DAD)

Since 1935, when Louis Hamman and Arnold Rich described four patients with acute respiratory failure of unknown etiology, the existence of cases which manifest acute respiratory failure with bilateral lung infiltrates has been recognized [45]. All four patients died and were revealed at autopsy to have a distinctive pathology that in modern times is recognized as the organizing stage of diffuse alveolar damage (DAD). This acute idiopathic respiratory condition was subsequently given the eponym Hamman-Rich syndrome. Although the histology of DAD was described even earlier, the term of "diffuse alveolar damage" (DAD) was presented by Katzenstein, et al. in their comprehensive review with their own data [46]. They concluded that endothelial and alveolar cell injury leads to fluid and cellular exudation, with hyaline membranes and edema being well-known features.

The term "acute interstitial pneumonia" (AIP) was introduced in 1986 by Katzenstein et al. for cases identical to the Hamman-Rich syndrome to lay emphasis on the fact that the condition is an acute form of idiopathic interstitial lung disease, clinically and histologically distinct from chronic forms, the prototype of which is IPF [47]. The prognosis of AIP is dismal and the mortality high. Today, AIP is defined by the following key elements: acute onset of respiratory symptoms typically resulting in acute respiratory failure; bilateral lung infiltrates on radiographs; the absence of identifiable etiology; and histological documentation of DAD [1, 47, 48]. Whereas the term AIP is applied when DAD is of unknown etiology, similar injury due to a known cause is generally referred to as DAD (stating the cause or the underlying disease).

DAD is thus a histologic pattern of injury usually associated with a life-threatening acute or subacute presentation which often correlates with the clinical entity of acute respiratory distress syndrome (ARDS) [49]. In earliest phase, the histology of DAD comprises alveolar septal edema and fibrin deposition in airspace. Over hours to days, these changes are accompanied by fibroplasia in alveolar septa, accumulation of alveolar macrophages (including foam cells), and formation of hyaline membranes [50]. Organizing thrombi are often found in small to medium-sized arteries. Within days to weeks after injury, airspace plugs of organizing pneumonia and type II pneumocytes hyperplasia on alveolar surfaces become prominent, representing a histologic pattern described as "organizing DAD."

Besides AIP, infection is the most important etiology to exclude in patients in whom a diagnosis of AIP is clinically considered. Infectious etiology includes fungi, pneumocystis organisms, and viruses such as cytomegalovirus (CMV), etc. Despite prominent neutrophilia observed in bronchoalveolar lavage (BAL) fluid samples, there is usually a paucity of inflammatory cells on histologic sections in case of AIP. If prominent acute inflammation is seen, particularly in the airspaces, it raises suspicion of infection. Other clues to specific etiologies include viral cytopathic changes observed in some viral pneumonias (e.g., cytomegalovirus, respiratory syncytial virus, adenovirus); food or other foreign material (with or without giant cell reaction) suggesting aspiration; and prominent eosinophilia suggesting a primary eosinophilic disorder such as eosinophilic granulomatosis with polyangiitis (EGPA/Churg–Strauss syndrome) or acute eosinophilic pneumonia [35].

CTDs are another major group of diseases that may manifest pathologically as DAD. To identify CTD as an etiology of DAD in patients, exclusion of other possible cause must be established. Of note, DAD usually occurs in patients with established CTD-ILD but also can occasionally be the presenting manifestation of the disease [51]. In CTD patients who initially present with DAD, rheumatologic manifestations and serological tests should help to establish the correct diagnosis. In patients with CTD on immunosuppressive therapy, infectious etiology and drug toxicity should be considered as a potential cause of DAD. In SLE, cases of diffuse alveolar hemorrhage commonly show histological features of DAD [52]. In PM/DM, an older case series found DAD pattern in 4 of 15 cases (27%); a more recent series identified DAD in 2 of 70 cases (3%), possibly reflecting improvements in diagnosis and treatment of this disease [53, 54]. A study suggests that DAD is more common in DM-ILD than in PM-ILD [55]. In RA, one study reported primary DAD pattern found in 2 of 33 cases (6%) [56]. In a more recent study of CTD-associated DAD, RA accounted for five of nine cases; in four cases, DAD occurred in patients with established, pre-existing RA-ILD, whereas one manifested as a de novo presentation [51].

### 4.4. Organizing pneumonia (OP)

While OP is characterized by fibrosis and chronic inflammation like IP, it differs in that the reaction affects predominantly the airspaces rather than the interstitium; this disorder is not an interstitial process [57]. However, many include OP in the classification of IP [40]. OP is histologically characterized by consolidation of airspaces by rounded branching polypoid plugs of granulation tissue [35]. This airspace organization is usually found in the alveoli as well as terminal airways. Pure involvement of airways is rare, and thus, it should raise suspicion of a primary small airway disease. Alveolar macrophages with foamy cytoplasm are often found; however, this nonspecific finding may also be observed in cases of aspiration or drug toxicity. Usually, there are not abundant neutrophils in the histology of OP. If prominent inflammation, particularly involving the airspaces, is found, it should raise suspicion of infection as a cause. Also, when eosinophils are prominent in the airspace, suspicion of a primary eosinophilic disorder, e.g., EGPA/Churg-Strauss syndrome, eosinophilic pneumonia, etc., or a drug adverse reaction must be raised. Overall, a predominant OP pattern, if encountered, accounts for a broad range of differential diagnosis to be considered, which include CTD, infectious pneumonia (particularly viral or atypical bacterial), aspiration, and drug toxicity. Thus, after all diagnostic exclusion is made, cryptogenic organizing pneumonia (COP) is determined as the diagnosis.

In many cases of CTD, the associated ILD may demonstrate focal lesions of OP pattern superimposed on a background of the other patterns of IP, frequently seen in NSIP. Therefore, true OP is less common in CTD-ILD. Among the RA-ILD, one study reported a primary OP pattern in 2 of 18 cases of RA-ILD (11%), and another stated 6 of 40 cases (15%) [42, 56]. Of note, OP can occasionally be the inaugural manifestation of RA [58]. In PM/DM-ILD, OP is common; OP as the primary pattern was present in 6 of 15 cases (40%) in one series, 5 of 13 (38%) in another [53, 59]. In a study of cases with Sjögren's syndrome reported, OP was found in 4 of 18 biopsies (22%) in the series [51]. By contrast, OP is a very rare manifestation in SSc; detected only in 1 of 80 cases in a large series [60].

### 4.5. Lymphocytic interstitial pneumonia (LIP)

The term "lymphocytic interstitial pneumonia" (LIP) refers to a pattern of IP in cases with diffuse and marked thickening of alveolar septal interstitium predominantly by dense lymphocytic infiltrate [61]. The infiltrate is polyclonal and may be admixed with variable numbers of plasma cells and macrophages. Germinal centers are frequently present. Histologically, LIP overlaps with follicular bronchiolitis and nodular lymphoid hyperplasia. When present, LIP pattern may raise concern for a possible lymphoproliferative process, which should be ruled out using appropriate immunohistochemical studies and flow cytometric analyses [35]. It should be noted that LIP has been associated with some viral infections, particularly human immunodeficiency virus. Classically, LIP was well-recognized in Sjögren's-associated ILD, where it was initially reported in at least 25% of cases based on a series of 12 biopsies [62]. A more recent study identified LIP primary pattern in 3 of 18 cases of Sjögren's-ILD (17%) [51].

## 5. Characteristic of interstitial lung disease in major connective tissue disease

### 5.1. Interstitial lung disease in systemic sclerosis

SSc is recognized as the CTD with the highest prevalence of ILD, ranging from 40 to 80%, depending on the modalities used for ascertainment [63]. The frequency of ILD varies according to patient selection, subsets of skin disease extent and ethnicity. In a large autopsy study, ILD was the most common pulmonary lesion in SSc, being found in >70% of the cases, and arteriolar thickening, described as medial hypertrophy or concentric intimal proliferation, was the most specific lesion in the lungs suggestive of pulmonary hypertension, being noted in 29% of the patients [64]. SSc, classically "scleroderma," is defined by the presence of major criteria; i.e., skin thickening proximal to metacarpo-phalangeal joints and minor criteria; i.e., sclerodactyly, esophageal involvement, and lung fibrosis [65]. It is subdivided into a limited cutaneous form, including CREST (Calcinosis, Raynaud's syndrome, Esophageal dysmotility, Sclerodactyly, Telangiectasia) syndrome and a diffuse cutaneous form (diffuse SSc has skin sclerosis proximal to elbows and knees), with varying degrees of skin, esophageal, lung, cardiac, and vascular involvement. Both forms can be progressive in nature.

As mentioned above, pulmonary manifestations in SSc include ILD and vascular disorder manifesting as pulmonary arterial hypertension (PAH). Today, both pulmonary complications are the leading cause of morbidity and mortality in patients with SSc. In line with SSc as the vasculature disorder, ranging from Raynaud' s phenomenon to PAH and renal crisis, nailfold capillary microscopy is now a well-established measure to evaluate capillary damage or abnormality [66]. The capillary changes observed in digits can be a predictor of severe vascular complications, being helpful in recognizing early disease [67].

In the context of autoantibodies, anti-nuclear antibodies (ANA) are found in the majority of SSc patients although not in every case. In 2013, the novel classification criteria of American College of Rheumatology (ACR)/European League against Rheumatism (EULAR) collaborative initiative for SSc incorporated three major autoantibodies [68]. These antibodies with high specificity for SSc are against topoisomerase (ATA or anti Scl-70), anticentromere antibodies (ACA), and anti-RNA polymerase III (ARA). They are closely related to distinct disease patterns; anti-topoisomerase antibodies are strongly associated with ILD, whereas anticentromere antibodies are highly predictive of the absence of significant lung fibrosis but associated with development of pulmonary hypertension [69]. Anticentromere antibodies, which are frequently found among Caucasians (20–35%), are strongly indicative of a limited form disease referred as CREST syndrome [69]. The other major autoantibody, anti-RNA polymerase III, is linked to diffuse skin disease and renal crisis, with less significant lung fibrosis. This antibody has another aspect that may herald paraneoplastic SSc [70]. While almost all patients with anti-topoisomerase antibodies have some extent of ILD, more than half of the SSc patients with ILD are negative for this antibody.

The most common pattern of ILD in SSc is fibrotic NSIP which manifests as dense, paucicellular interstitial fibrosis that maintains the underlying architecture [60, 71, 72]. As the lung disease progresses, the areas of fibrosis may become confluent and appear as honeycomb. SSc patients may also present with typical UIP pattern with temporal and special heterogeneity, in contrast to the diffuse and uniform fibrosis of NSIP. In most SSc patients, ILD remains stable without treatment despite having some degree of lung fibrosis. However, some proportions of the SSc patients develop significant and progressive ILD. In SSc-associated ILD, placebo-controlled randomized trials, named the Scleroderma Lung Study (SLS) and the fibrosing alveolitis scleroderma trial (FAST), have been performed, suggesting certain effectiveness of immunosuppressive therapy in preventing further decline in patients with progressive ILD to be mentioned later [73, 74].

### 5.2. Interstitial lung disease in rheumatoid arthritis

RA is the most common CTD, occurring in 1–2% of the population, more frequently in women. Although RA is primarily characterized by synovial inflammation which leads an erosive inflammatory polyarthropathy, predominantly affecting the distal joints, extra-articular manifestations are seen in approximately half of patients with RA. Extra-articular manifestations include subcutaneous nodules, skin ulceration, scleritis/episcleritis, pericarditis, splenomegaly, and a variety of pleuro-pulmonary abnormalities.

Lung disease accounts for 10–20% of mortality in RA, second only to cardiac disease [75–77]. Airway, pleural, vascular, and parenchymal involvement can occur in RA patients, as well as pulmonary disorders indirectly associated with RA such as opportunistic infections and drug-induced lung disease. All pleuro-pulmonary manifestations in RA are more common in males;

ILD affects men twice as commonly as women. The prevalence of ILD ranges widely from 5 to 58% in various reports [78–80]. It is difficult to confirm the exact prevalence because it depends on modalities of ascertainment and patient selection such as autopsy, hospital, and community-based studies. In a study of 36 patients with new onset RA, abnormalities consistent with ILD were found in 58% of patients; physiology 22%, chest X ray 6%, HRCT 33%, BAL 52%, and 99mTc-DTPA radionuclide scan 15% [81]. Smoking is a significant risk factor for ILD; an odds ratio of 3.8 for ILD was observed in RA patients with a smoking history >25 pack years [82].

In the context of histological patterns, the predominant ILD histology in RA patients is NSIP (cellular or, more commonly, fibrotic NSIP), followed closely by UIP, accounting for 30–67% and 13–57% of RA-associated ILD, respectively [42, 44, 59, 83–85]. Some studies have noted greater incidence of UIP histology in RA-ILD found in up to 56% of patients in a series [42]. These NSIP and UIP patterns are followed by organizing pneumonia (OP). There is evidence suggesting that a UIP pattern may be associated with a worse survival than fibrotic NSIP in cases of RA, in contrast with the other CTDs. A pattern of DAD/acute interstitial pneumonia (AIP) is infrequent but may occur as fulminant ILD manifestation of RA, which can develop in a previously normal lung or as the presenting pattern of a previously undiagnosed ILD. The characteristic CT pattern of DAD includes widespread ground glass with/without areas of dependent consolidation, although a similar pattern could represent opportunistic or viral infection and acute heart failure.

### 5.3. Interstitial lung disease in polymyositis/dermatomyositis

Idiopathic inflammatory myopathy (IIM), a group of systemic autoimmune disorders that affect skeletal muscles and other organs, comprises three major categories: polymyositis (PM), dermatomyositis (DM), and inclusion body myositis (IBM). PM and DM are sometimes recognized together as they share similar clinical signs and symptoms with exception of cutaneous manifestations such as "heliotrope rash" on the upper eyelids, "mechanic's hands" on the fingers, and "Gottron papules" on the dorsal surface of the hands seen in DM. Pathologically, however, these are distinct entities; PM is T cell-mediated diseases, where CD8-positive cytotoxic T cells invade muscle fibers expressing MHC class I antigens, whereas DM is characterized by a complement-mediated microangiopathy [86–88].

The diagnosis of PM/DM is made on the basis of clinical features and examinations, which include symmetrical proximal muscle weakness, elevated serum muscle enzymes, characteristic electromyographic alterations, muscle biopsy histopathology consistent with myositis, and for DM, typical cutaneous manifestations mentioned above and less-specific skin rashes. Moreover, muscle magnetic resonance imaging (MRI) and ultrasound (US) have been also introduced in the diagnostic work up of patients with inflammatory myopathies. Classification criteria for PM/DM date back to initial publications by Medsger et al. [89]. Since, in 1975, Bohan and Peter classified myositis, their criteria have been widely used [90, 91]. However, it demonstrated poor specificity and cannot distinguish PM from IBM or some forms of dystrophies for instance. Thus, several diagnostic criteria for inflammatory myopathies have been proposed with little acceptance, including recent muscle-biopsy-based diagnostic criteria [92]. Further prospective studies are required to develop improved and universal classification criteria.

Several neuromuscular diseases which may mimic PM/DM and should be considered in the differential diagnosis include drug or toxic myopathies (alcohol, colchicine, statins, etc.), endocrine myopathies (hyper-hypothyroidism), metabolic myopathies, mitochondrial myopathies, muscular dystrophies, infectious myositis, neuropathies, paraneoplastic syndromes, other connective tissue disorders, amyloidosis, and sarcoidosis [93]. Muscular dystrophies, where an increase of creatine kinase (CK), electrodiagnostic, and bioptic abnormalities similar to PM/DM may be present, can be distinguished from DM/PM by the positive family history, the relatively early insidious onset, and slow progression. Iatrogenic myopathy is secondary to corticosteroids use, where CK is normal and the histological examination shows atrophic changes of muscle fibers. Other diseases to consider in the differential diagnosis are endocrine or dysionemia-induced myopathies. Rheumatic polymyalgia (polymyalgia rheumatica) is characterized by normal CK and histological absence of inflammatory abnormalities. Infectious myositis especially viral and parasitic myositis are characterized by a diffuse muscular involvement and a subacute or chronic course. Bacterial myositis is localized and acute. Among other rare inflammatory myopathies, nodular focal myositis is considered as a variant of PM/DM and may present at onset (As localized, a differential diagnosis with muscular cancers and/or thrombophlebitis must be considered). Eosinophilic myositis, characterized by muscle eosinophil infiltrate, may be part of a hypereosinophilic syndrome (pneumonia, endocardial and myocardial fibrosis, and peripheral neuropathy, etc.) or be associated with eosinophilic fasciitis. Granulomatous myositis can be isolated or in the context of granulomatous syndromes, such as sarcoidosis or Crohn's disease; the main histological finding is the presence of granulomatous lesions which may contain epithelioid cells, histiocyte, and Langerhans giant cells. In the differential diagnoses of IBM, polyneuropathy and amyotrophic lateral sclerosis have also to be considered [93, 94].

Concerning extra-muscular involvement, respiratory disease is a major cause of morbidity and mortality in PM/DM [53, 95–100]. PM/DM-associated pulmonary disorders may manifest as ILD and as a consequence of respiratory muscle weakness leading to hypoventilation or aspiration pneumonia. ILD is the most common extra-muscular complication in PM/DM and have been recognized in 30–70% of the patients [100–102]. The reported prevalence varies depending on the modalities or tests for detection and patient selections. Since Tazelaar et al. reported a histopathological study of lung biopsy specimens in patients with PM/DM in terms of treatment responses and survivals, histopathology fairly serves relevant clinical decisions [53]. As for the prevalence of the different histopathologic patterns, NSIP is by far the most frequent finding, followed by DAD, UIP, and OP [54, 103–107]. Our study with HRCT scans of 14 cases of histologically proven NSIP associated with PM/DM showed that the predominant features were of reticular and/or ground-glass opacities with or without consolidation. Reticular and ground-glass opacities predominated in the lower zone of each lung, and consolidation predominated at the lung periphery [108].

In the context of subtypes of PM/DM, the following concepts of amyopathic dermatomyositis and anti-synthetase syndrome warrant particular attentions.

### 5.4. Amyopathic dermatomyositis

Clinically amyopathic dermatomyositis (CADM), which is characterized by the cutaneous findings of DM with no muscle involvement or only minimal weakness, affects approximately 20% of patients with DM [109, 110]. Patients with CADM have a greater risk of developing ILD, especially prone to rapidly progressive lung disease corresponding to DAD [111, 112]. Anti-melanoma differentiation-associated gene 5 (MDA5) antibodies (also referred to as anti-CADM-140 antibodies) were identified in the serum from patients with CADM by firstly immunoprecipitation assays [113]. The presence of anti-MDA5 antibodies is strongly associated with DM, especially with CADM, and rapidly progressive ILD, which are thus associated with particularly poor clinical outcomes.

### 5.5. Anti-synthetase syndrome (ASS)

A subset of patients may manifest a clinical syndrome known as "anti-synthetase syndrome (ASS)," which is characterized by the presence of one of the anti-aminoacyl-t-RNA synthetase (ARS) antibodies such as anti-Jo-1, anti-PL-7, anti-PL-12, anti-EJ, anti-OJ, and anti-KS, together with stigmata of PM/DM including myositis, ILD, polyarthritis, fever, Raynaud's phenomenon, and mechanic's hand [114, 115]. Anti-Jo-1, the first anti-ARS antibody, is the best understood of the anti-synthetase antibodies, with a strong correlation with ILD in patients with PM/DM; the incidence of ILD approaches 90% [116, 117].

### 5.6. Myositis-specific autoantibodies and myositis-associated autoantibodies

Circulating autoantibodies directed against nuclear or cellular components are frequently detected in patients with PM or DM. These antibodies are categorized into two groups; one is specific to PM/DM, whereas the other is found in overlap syndrome with myositis. Targoff et al. designated these two categories of autoantibodies as "myositis-specific antibodies; MSAs" and "myositis-associated antibodies; MAAs," respectively [114]. Classical autoantibodies such as anti-aminoacyl transfer RNA synthetases (ARS) antibodies, anti-signal recognition particle (SRP) antibodies [118, 119], and Mi-2 antibodies are classified as MSAs, where especially anti-Mi-2 antibodies are DM specific [120]. Later, the new DM specific antibodies have been disclosed. These include the antibodies directed against melanoma differentiation–associated gene5 (MDA5) (anti-CADM-140 antibody, mentioned above) [113, 121, 122], transcriptional intermediary factor-1-gamma (anti-p155 antibody) [123, 124], NXP-2 (anti-NMP-2 antibody) [125, 126], and small ubiquitin-like modifier activating enzyme (anti-SAE antibody) [127]. Usually, MSAs are distinct, and their presence is mutually exclusive.

Because of their strong associations with a pattern of clinical features, such as myopathy, skin lesions, and ILD, these novel autoantibodies are useful biomarkers for classifying disease subgroups, predicting future organ involvement, and forecasting the prognosis of patients with PM/DM [114, 128–131]. The autoantibodies are detectable in PM/DM; both MSA and MAA are listed and summarized in **Table 4** [102]. The pathogenetic mechanisms of expression of such autoantibodies are still awaited to be illuminated.

| Autoantibodies | Antibody target | Frequency in polymyositis/ADM/ JDM % | Frequency of ILD in adult /juvenile myositis % | Clinical spectrum | |
|---|---|---|---|---|---|
| | | | | In adulthood | In childhood |
| **Myositis- specific autoantibodies (MSA)** | | | | | |
| *Anti-t-RNA synthetase* | | 29/20/5 | | | |
| Anti-Jo1 (PL1) | Histidyl-ARS | 21/11/<3 | 66/63 | Arthralgia, fever, RP, mechanic's hand, puffy finger | Arthralgia, fever, RP, mechanic's hand, sclerodactyly |
| Anti- PL7 | Threonyl-ARS | 5/2/<1 | 84/63 | | |
| Anti- PL12 | Alanyl-ARS | 2/3/<1 | | | |
| Anti-KS | Asparaginyl-ARS | <1 | | | |
| Anti-OJ | Isoleucyl-ARS | <1 | | | |
| Anti-EJ | Glycyl-ARS | <1 | | | |
| Anti-SC | Lysyl-ARS | <1 | | | |
| Anti-JS | Glutaminyl-ARS | <1 | | | |
| Anti-YRS(Ha) | Tyrosyl-ARS | <1 | <1 | | |
| Anti-Zo | Phenylalanyl-ARS | <1 | | | |
| **Dermatomyositis Specific autoantibodies** | | | | | |
| Anti-Mi2 | Nucleosome remodeling deacetylase complex | 1/9/4–10 | 4/0 | Classical DM without extramuscular involvement | Mild or moderate JDM |
| Anti-NXP2(MJ,p140) | Nuclear matrix protein 2 | 10/0–3/12–25 | 0/25 | DM without extramuscular involvement, calcinosis | Mild or moderate JDM |
| Anti-MDA5(CADM-140) | Melanoma differentiation-associated gene encoding RNA helicase | <1/14–46/7 | Europe:60; Asia:90/ Europe:19; Asia:53 | Amyopathic DM, severe cutaneous ulcers, rapidly progressive ILD | Severe cutaneous ulcers, RP-ILP, mediastinal emphysema |
| Anti-TIF1γ(p1555/140) | Transcriptional intermediary factor 1γ | <1/10–30/14–29 | <10/3 | Cancer associated DM in 78% of cases | Mild or moderate JDM |

http://dx.doi.org/10.5772/intechopen.70864

| Autoantibodies | Antibody target | Frequency in polymyositis/ADM/ JDM % | Frequency of ILD in adult /juvenile myositis % | Clinical spectrum | |
|---|---|---|---|---|---|
| | | | | In adulthood | In childhood |
| **Other MSA** | | | | | |
| Anti-SRP | Signal recognition particle | 5/1/<3 | 15/0 | Necrotising myopathy | Severe JPM |
| Anti-HMGR(200-100) | 3-hydroxy-3-methylglu taryl-coenzyme A reductase | 10/<1/unknown | Unknown | Necrotising myopathy | Unknown |
| Anti-SAE | Small ubiquitin-like modifier activating enzymes | <1/5–10/1–9 | | DM | Unknown |
| **Myositis associated autoantibodies** | | | | | |
| Anti-RO/SSA | RNP complexes with small cytoplasmic RNAs(hy-RNA) | 12/13/0 | | | |
| Anti-U1RNP | 70 KDa,A and C polypeptides of U1 snRNP | 5/6/6 | 7 | DM, fever, RP, sclerodactyly | |
| Anti-PM/Scl(75 and 100 Kda) | PM/Scl complex encompassing C1D,PM-SCl-100 and PM-SCl-75 proteins of the human exosome | 6/9/4 | 38 | Fever, RP, sclerodactyly | |
| Anti-Ku | 80 and 70 KDa DNA binding dimeric protein | 2/1/0 | 27 | Fever, RP, sclerodactyly | |

ADM: adult dermatomyositis; JDM: juvenile dermatomyositis; ILD: interstitial lung disease; SRP: signal recognition particle; ARS: aminoacyl-t-RNA synthetase; RP: Raynaud's phenomenon; DM: dermatomyositis specific rash; RP-ILP: rapidly progressive ILD; JPM: juvenile poly myositis

Adapted from Lega et al. [120].

**Table 4.** Autoantibodies in polymyositis/dermatomyositis.

# 6. Pathogenesis of interstitial pneumonia associated with connective tissue disease

## 6.1. Classic mechanisms in the pathogenesis of interstitial pneumonia in connective tissue disease

Numbers of studies on the pathogenesis of IP have been performed in SSc as well as in mouse models of IP, providing evidence for plausible mechanisms that may lead to pulmonary fibrosis in CTD. This is natural because, among the whole CTDs, SSc has the highest prevalence of IP, and currently, the lung disease consists the major cause of death in patients with SSc, being shifted away from mortality due to renal crisis which was more common in the past. The high morbidity and mortality due to IP in SSc have been eliciting not only multidisciplinary clinical studies but also basic researches. Many lines of evidence acquired from the studies on SSc, and relevant researches on fibrosis have been implying the following potential scenario of classic mechanisms in the pathogenesis of CTD-IP [12, 132, 133].

### *6.1.1. Mediators eliciting and perpetuating interstitial pneumonia in systemic sclerosis*

The key mechanisms in CTD-IP involve an interplay between various cell types and humoral factors; the pathogenesis is initiated by microvascular injury, leading to endothelial cell damage and alveolar epithelial injury [12, 132, 133]. This is followed by activation of the coagulation cascade, release of various cytokines, e.g., IL-1, IL-4, IL-6, IL-13, chemokines, and lysophosphatidic acid (LPA), and growth factors including transforming growth factor beta (TGF-β), connective tissue growth factor (CTGF), and insulin-like growth factor (IGF-1), which leads to activation of fibroblasts, resulting in the development of fibrosis [12, 132, 134]. Many epithelial-derived factors influence the behavior of fibroblasts, with soluble mediators known to exhibit profibrotic activities [134]. The pivotal mediator of fibrosis is the multifunctional cytokine, TGF-β, which, along with platelet-derived growth factor, endothelin-1 (ET-1), plays a major role in the pathogenesis of SSc. There is evidence that epithelial-to-mesenchymal transdifferentiation (EMT) occurs in lung fibrosis, and this process is mediated by TGF-β and potentially ET-1 [135, 136]. TGF-β responses are mediated by canonical Smad signaling [137]. Binding of TGF-β to its receptor elicits signaling through phosphorylation and nuclear translocation of cytoplasmic Smad protein, triggering transcription of genes such as type I collagen, fibronectin, α-smooth muscle actin, and CTGF, which promote fibrogenesis [138]. ET-1 is a potent vasoconstrictor produced by endothelial cells, epithelial cells, and mesenchymal cells. ET-1 binds to ET-1A and ET-1B receptors, recruits fibroblasts, stimulates extracellular matrix production, and also stimulates TGF-β production in lung fibroblasts [139]. Elevated levels of ET-1 have been found in the blood vessels, lung, kidneys, and skin of SSc patients [140]. LPA is produced by activated platelets and fibroblasts. The LPA receptor is expressed in fibroblasts, endothelial cells, and epithelial cells. Both are involved in the development of lung fibrosis in mouse model of IPF, suggesting LPA mediates fibroblast recruitment [141]. IGFs have been implicated in pulmonary fibrosis because increased levels of IGF-1 are detected in the serum as well as in the BAL of SSc patients [142]. CTGF, also

http://dx.doi.org/10.5772/intechopen.70864

known as CCN2, which plays a pivotal role in the stimulation of extracellular matrix production and myofibroblast differentiation, is involved in angiogenesis and forming the connective tissue [143]. The levels are elevated in the skin and lungs from SSc patients as well as in the sera [144].

The earliest events of the parenchymal lung involvement in CTD include inflammation and associated alveolar epithelial injury which occurs due to undetermined causes or can be caused by some environmental pathogens. The alveolar epithelial damage and inflammation let resident fibroblasts of pulmonary interstitium to locate to the alveolar wall, and the fibroblasts become activated through a variety of mediators such as TGF-β [145, 146]. The activation of resident fibroblasts was shown to be induced by the recruitment of active TGF-β from the lung tissue [147]. The resident lung fibroblasts play a pivotal role in lung fibrosis, and they are considered to be a more primitive or less differentiated lineage of fibroblasts that are prepared for repair at injury response [148]. The recruitment of activated fibroblasts and myofibroblasts that produce large amount of extracellular matrix proteins occurs in the process. These population of cells are not only derived from resident interstitial fibroblasts but also come from circulating progenitor cells which include mesenchymal stem cells recruited from the bone marrow and cells of a monocyte lineage that localize to the lung [149]. Myofibroblasts persist as critical profibrotic cells in affected lung tissue. It is conceivable that minor injury and subsequent disease process lead to the development of a lung microenvironment prone to fibrosis. That series of events results in an accumulation of constituents of the extracellular matrix (ECM), which remodels normal tissue architecture, which in turn culminates in pulmonary organ failure. Essentially, the lung is primed to develop fibrosis in response to injury, and it is likely that the intrinsic response is more severe in CTDs than normal individuals. Thus, in SSc, such genetic or intrinsic differences can be reflected to the serological phenotypes such as the expression of autoantibodies. Patients with SSc having anti-topoisomerase antibodies are liable to develop significant lung fibrosis, while those with anti-RNA polymerase III antibodies are less [150].

#### *6.1.2. Involvement of immune mechanisms in interstitial pneumonia in systemic sclerosis*

The immune system is also implicated in the pathology of SSc. Several lines of evidence suggest that a specific population of activated T cells exhibiting type 2 helper T (Th2) phenotype potentially mediates tissue fibrosis, secreting IL-4 and IL-13 both of which activate fibroblasts and collagen production by inducing TGF-β [151]. In SSc, T cells with memory phenotype were found in lung biopsy specimens from patients with lung involvement [152]. In some studies reported, increased numbers of lung memory CD8 T cells are associated with more severe pulmonary fibrosis [153–155]. Luzina et al. have shown an increase in CD8 T cells in the lungs of SSc patients by using T cells isolated from BAL fluid and demonstrated that a subset of patients at higher risk of progressive lung disease had activated, long-lived CD8 T cells which could promote fibrosis through production of profibrotic factors such as IL-4 and oncostatin M, as well as activation of TGF-β [156]. Regulatory T cells (Tregs) which maintain self tolerance can be impaired in their ability to suppress CD 4 effector T cells [157]. Currently, the precise knowledge of the role of effector cells in innate and adaptive immune system in

SSc-associated IP is rather insufficient. More fundamental investigations in this aspect are needed to address to many queries as to the whole scenario of the development of IP in CTDs.

Besides, as concerns idiopathic pulmonary fibrosis (IPF), the latest evidence of immune mechanisms in IPF was reviewed in the recent literature, which includes involvement of both innate immunity and adaptive immunity at several levels of the processes toward development of fibrinogenesis in the human lung of IPF or in its model mice, as summarized in **Table 5** [158]. Briefly, in adaptive immune system, the role of T cells seems complex and subset dependent; Th2 and Th17 cells were shown to promote pulmonary fibrosis, although Th1, Th22, and γδ-T cells have been found to attenuate fibrotic disease. Treg and Th9 subsets have been proposed to exert both anti- and profibrotic effects. In innate immunity, M2 macrophages and neutrophils have been suggested to enhance pulmonary fibrosis, whereas M1 macrophages were assigned a protective role, but contradictory findings have also been described [158].

After all, a variety of studies on the pathogenesis of IPF have been conducted, and many experimental models were generated to explore the mechanisms. However, it is yet highly questionable whether the evidence provided from the studies of IPF is applicable to the etiology of CTD-associated IP. Furthermore, it is still unclear whether the animal models such as the mouse bleomycin model can truly replicate the autoimmune progressive forms of the ILDs seen in human CTDs.

### 6.2. A new insight into the pathogenesis of interstitial pneumonia in connective tissue disease: "T cells trigger interstitial pneumonia in polymyositis/dermatomyositis"

We have speculated that exploring the early immune phases of IP in the lung would be the most direct approach to understand the pathogensis before more complex secondary immune responses occur in the evolution of IP [6, 7]. PM/DM is one of the major CTD, of which the most critical problem is pulmonary involvement. As mentioned before, ILD, mainly IP, often severe and progressive, has been recognized in 30–70% of PM/DM patients and is frequently associated with a dismal prognosis. While the presence of myositis-specific autoantibodies, such as Jo-1 and activated T cell muscle infiltrates, suggests autoimmune mechanisms in the etiology of PM, the pathogenesis of the associated IP remains undefined. We encountered two cases of early-stage PM-associated IP, of which we had an opportunity of investigating the fresh lung tissues obtained by video-assisted thoracoscopic (VATS) biopsy performed for the sake of histopathological diagnosis toward treatment options. Since this is the clear and robust demonstration of the pivotal role of T cells in CTD-IP, we herein present the details of our study with two cases of early-stage PM-associated IP both suggesting that T cells contribute to the early phase of the development of IP. Lung tissue was utilized with the approval of the institutional review board.

#### *6.2.1. Analysis in cases of interstitial pneumonia associated with polymyositis/dermatomyositis*

Patient A was a 51-year-old woman with no tobacco history and no family history of lung diseases, referred to our clinic for evaluation of arthralgia and myalgia. At 49 years, the patient

| Cells and mediators | Description |
|---|---|
| Immune cells | |
| T cells | Th1 cytokines (IFN-Υ and IL-12) attenuate PF, Th2 cytokines (IL-4, IL-5 and IL-13) enhance PF, Th17 cells enhance PF, Tregs and Th9 (IL-9) have both pro- and antifibrotic roles in PF; Th22 (IL-22) and Υδ-T cells have an antifibrotic role in PF. |
| Macrophages | M1 marcrophages induce myofibroblast apoptosis and digest ECM by activation of MMPs. M2 macrophages recruit and activate fibroblast through TGF-β1 and PDGF secretion. M2 macrophages further produce TIMPs and inhibit degradation of ECM. Both Macrophages phenotypes (M1/M2) can exert pro- and antifibrotic effects. |
| Neutrophils | Neutrophils produce elastase, MMPs, and TIMPs. Neutrophil elastase activates TGF-β and recruits inflammatory cells to the lung, thereby promoting PF. |
| Fibrocytes | Fibrocytes produce ECM, cross-linking enzymes, chemokines, growth factors, and MMPs, and promote PF. Fibrocytes secrete paracrine mediators, which activate resident fibroblasts to promote PF. Fibroblasts can differentiate into fibroblasts and myofibroblasts. |
| Cytokines | |
| IL-1β | Profibrotic effects of IL-1β, mediated through IL-1R/MyD88 signaling pathway. |
| IL-13 | IL-13 differentiates human lung fibroblast to myofibroblast through a JNK-dependent pathway. |
| IL-17 | IL-17 interacts/cooperates with TGF-β signaling to promote PF. |
| TGF-β1 | TGF-β promote EMT through SMAD-2/3 signaling pathways. TGF-β1 induces PF through ERK, MAPK, PI3K/Akt, and Rho-like GTPase pathways. TGF-β1 differentiates fibroblasts into and increase ECM accumulation. |
| PDGF | PDGF stimulates fibroblasts and increase ECM gene expression in fibroblasts. |
| Chemokines | |
| CCL2 | CCL2 increase fibrocyte recruitment and differentiation into fibroblasts, resulting in excessive collagen deposition. CCL2 activates M2 macrophage activation and promote PF. |
| CCL17 | CCL17 promotes PF through the recruitment of CCR4^+ Th2 cells and alveolar macrophages. |
| CCL18 | CCL18 increase collagen production in lung fibroblasts through ERK1/2, PKCα, and Sp1/Smad3 signaling pathways. |
| CXCL 12 | CXCL 12 recruits fibrocytes and activates the Rac1/ERK and JNK signaling pathways to induce AP-1 activation and CTGF expression in fibroblasts |

Definition of abbreviations: Ap-1, activator protein 1; CCL, CC chemokine; CTGF, connective tissue growth factor; CXCL, CXC chemokine ligand; ECM, extracellular matrix; EMT, epithelial-mesenchymal transition; ERK, extracellular signal-regulated kinase; IL-1R1, IL-1 receptor 1; JNK, c-Jun N-terminal kinases; MAPK, mitogen-activated protein kinase; MMP, matrix metalloproteinase; MyD88, myeloid differentiation primary response gene 88; PDGF, platelet-derived growth factor; PF, pulmonary fibrosis; PI3K, phosphatidylinositol 3-kinase; PKC, protein kinase C; Rac 1, Ras-related C3 botulinum toxin substrate 1; SMAD, SMA/MAD homology; Sp1, specificity protein 1; TGF, transforming growth factor; TIMP, tissue inhibitors of metalloproteinase; Tregs regulatory T cells.

Adapted from Kolahian et al. [158].

**Table 5.** Possible immune mechanisms for pulmonary fibrosis.

noticed Raynaud's phenomenon and polyarthralgia, for which she was given low-dose prednisolone with clinical improvement. Two months before the referral, she developed polyarthralgia and myalgia. On physical examination, the patient had no skin lesions but presented with fine crackles audible on inspiration in both lower lung fields. Erythrocyte sedimentation rate (ESR) was 135 mm/hr, and C-reactive protein (CRP) level was 1.2 mg/dL (reference range: 0.0–0.4). Rheumatoid factors (RFs), speckled anti-nuclear factors (ANFs), and anti-histidyl-t-RNA synthetase (Jo-1) antibodies were positive, while anti-ribonucleoprotein (RNP) and anti-scleroderma-70 (scl-70) antibody assays were negative. Levels of lactate dehydrogenase (LDH, 798 IU/L) (reference range: 109–435), creatine kinase (CK, 559 IU/L) (reference range: 44–140), and myoglobin (120 ng/mL) (reference range: 28–60) were elevated. Muscle strength was nearly normal, but electromyogram showed myogenic patterns in the muscle groups of the upper limb girdle bilaterally. Muscle biopsy revealed lymphocyte infiltration into myofibrils and muscle atrophy, consistent with PM. Arterial blood gas analysis demonstrated a pH of 7.413; partial pressure of carbon dioxide ($PCO_2$), 44.6 Torr; partial pressure of oxygen ($PO_2$), 84.3 Torr; and bicarbonate ($HCO_3$-) concentration, 28.4 mmol/L. Pulmonary function tests revealed a restrictive pattern; vital capacity (VC) was 74.8%, and diffusing capacity (DLco) was 13.44 mL/min/mmHg (67.3%). Analysis of bronchoalveolar lavage fluid (BAL) showed 75% macrophages, 15% neutrophils, and 10% lymphocytes. Human leukocyte antigen (HLA) serotypes were as follows: A2, A26, B15, Cw1, Cw9, DR14, DR8, DR52, DQ7, and DQ6. Chest radiography and chest computed tomography (CT) revealed mild, subpleural, linear, and reticular opacities in posterior and lateral areas of both lungs (**Figure 2a**). The patient underwent video-assisted thoracoscopic (VATS) lung biopsy for histopathologic diagnosis and therapeutic planning. Biopsy specimens from anterior basal segment (S8) and lateral basal segment (S9) of the right lower lobe revealed an early usual IP (UIP) pattern, demonstrating heterogeneous lesions with residual air spaces and early fibrotic changes, surrounded by mild alveolitis with mononuclear cell infiltrations. Based on these clinical and histopathologic findings, the patient was diagnosed with interstitial pneumonia associated with PM. She was subsequently treated with methylprednisolone pulse therapy (1 g/day for 3 days) followed by oral prednisolone (30 mg/day). Over 10 months, the dose of prednisolone was tapered to 12.5 mg/day with excellent control of progression of pulmonary lesions and myositis.

Patient B was a 43-year-old woman, a lifetime nonsmoker, referred to our clinic for arthralgia and myalgia. The patient had developed Raynaud's phenomenon 6 months prior to this presentation. On physical examination, she had swollen fingers, with no skin rash. Fine crackles were heard on inspiration in the lower lung fields. No muscle weakness was apparent, but thorough examination revealed myositis. Laboratory data were as follows: LDH level, 616 IU/L; CK level, 410 IU/L; and CRP level, 0.4 mg/dL. Histological examination of muscle biopsy specimen showed mononuclear cell infiltrates in muscle tissue, consistent with PM. Assays for RF, anti-dsDNA antibodies, anti-Jo-1 antibodies, anti-centromere antibodies, and anti-scl-70 antibodies were negative. ANF (speckled pattern) and anti-ribonucleoprotein (RNP) antibodies were positive. Arterial blood gas analysis was unremarkable. Pulmonary function testing showed a restrictive pattern; VC, 70.6%, and DLco, 14.71 mL/min/mmHg (77.2%). BAL analysis demonstrated 67% macrophages, 11% neutrophils, and 22% lymphocytes. HLA serotypes were as follows: A24, A26, B15, B61, Cw10, DR9, DR53, and DQ9. Chest radiography and CT revealed subpleural and basilar linear and reticular opacities with ground glass attenuation (**Figure 2b**). Histopathological examination of lung specimens from VATS biopsy of superior (S4) and anterior basal (S8) segments of the left lower lobe disclosed a nonspecific IP (NSIP) pattern. Specimens showed mild and homogeneous changes with

http://dx.doi.org/10.5772/intechopen.70864

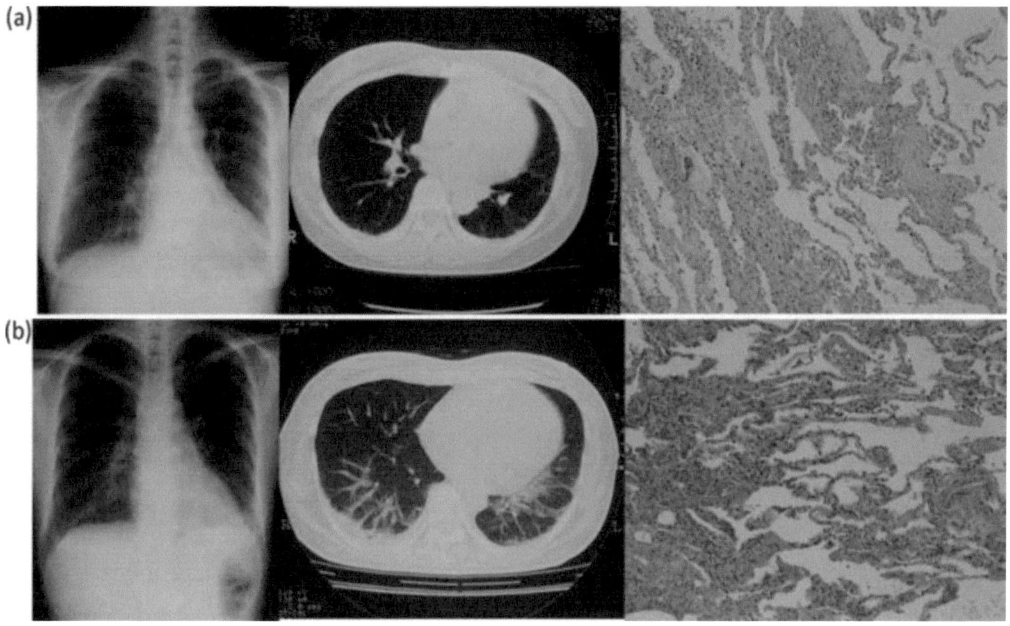


**Figure 2.** (a) Chest radiography, CT, and photomicrograph of patient A. Chest X-ray and HRCT of patient A show subpleural mild linear and reticular opacities in posterolateral lung. Lung biopsy from patient A depicts heterogeneous lesions including residual air spaces and early fibrotic changes with fibroblastic foci, mild alveolitis with thickened alveolar walls, and mononuclear cell infiltrations (hematoxylin and eosin stain, original magnification ×200). (b). Chest radiography, CT, and photomicrograph of patient B. Chest X-ray and HRCT of patient B show thickened interlobular septa with bibasilar and subpleural ground glass opacities. Lung biopsy from patient B depicts mild, homogeneous changes with partial inflammatory thickening of the alveolar wall, with granulation tissues in alveolar spaces, fibrosis, and inflammatory cell infiltrates (hematoxylin and eosin stain, original magnification ×200).

partial inflammatory thickenings of the alveolar wall, with granulation tissues in alveolar spaces, fibrosis, and inflammatory-cell infiltrations. Clinical and histopathologic findings lead to a diagnosis of IP associated with PM. She was subsequently given pulse therapy with methylprednisolone (1 g/day for 3 days) followed by oral prednisolone (50 mg/day), which was effective in ceasing active myositis and IP. When the dose of prednisolone had been tapered to 30 mg/day after 4 months, respiratory function testing showed that %VC and DLco had improved to 79.0% and 17.56 mL/min/mmHg (90.7%), respectively.

Immunohistochemical analysis was performed on lung-infiltrating cells utilizing biopsy specimens. Substantial infiltrations of mononuclear cells were noted in both patient A (UIP pattern) and patient B (NSIP pattern). The mononuclear cells were predominantly CD3+ T cells, accompanied by a subtle infiltration of B cells (CD20+), and a minimal number of monocytes (CD19+). Of infiltrating T cells, CD4+ cells were predominant compared to CD8+ cells in both cases. We then analyzed T cell receptor $\alpha$-chain variable region (TCR V$\alpha$) and TCR $\beta$-chain variable region (TCR V$\beta$) repertoires of T cells infiltrating the lung tissues using an adaptor ligation polymerase chain reaction (PCR)-based microplate hybridization assay [159]. Quantitative assay has been used in many previous studies, and accuracy and reproducibility of this assay have been validated [160, 161]. Briefly, total RNA was extracted with TRIzol

Reagent (Invitrogen, USA) from lung tissues obtained by VATS biopsy. Complementary DNA (cDNA) was synthesized with reverse transcriptase (Superscript II) and BSL-18E primer adaptor. Universal adaptor primers were ligated to the cDNA, and PCR was performed with the universal primer and primers specific for TCR Cα or Cβ chains. PCR products were biotinylated by amplification with 5′-biotin primer and the universal primer. The biotinylated PCR products were hybridized on microplate wells immobilized with various oligo probes specific for TCR Vα or Vβ region sequences. Finally, the amount of biotinylated product bound to each probe was measured by quantitative enzyme-linked immunosorbent assay (ELISA) with alkaline phosphatase streptavidin. The results of quantitative analysis of TCR Vα or TCR Vβ usage in patient A and B are shown in **Figure 3a** and **b**, respectively. The open column and solid column indicate the frequencies of TCR Vα/Vβ repertoires in the lung tissue and the peripheral blood lymphocytes (PBLs), respectively. We found that the usage of repertoires of TCR Vα/Vβ in the lung differed from those in PBL, with certain TCR V gene families detected more frequently from lung tissue. In patient A, TCR repertoires of VA2.1, VA8.1, VB4.1, and VB24.1 were predominantly expressed in the lung compared to PBL, while TCR V repertoires VA23.1 and VB13.1 were more frequently expressed in lung tissue from patient B. As expected, no TCR signals were detected on normal lung tissue obtained from patients without IP using the same method (data not shown).

#### *6.2.2. Discussion*

IP associated with PM/DM is recognized as a critical complication due to its association with poor disease prognosis. In this study, we investigated T cells infiltrates by analyzing the TCR repertoire usage in lung tissue in two patients with PM-associated early IP. Both patients showed marked lymphocytes aggregates, predominantly CD3+ T cells, at IP lesion sites. In addition, the analysis of TCR Vα/Vβ repertoire usage indicated a modest accumulation of T cells expressing selected TCR V-gene segments, which differed distinctly from those of PBL. These findings strongly suggest pathogenic involvement of organ-specific oligoclonal T cell accumulation in development of PM-associated IP. Since TCR diversifies with disease progression due to the phenomenon of "determinant spreading" in which autoreactive T cell responses, initiated by a single antigenic epitope, evolve into multiepitopic responses, we considered it important to perform TCR analysis from lung tissue in the earliest stage of IP [162]. Regarding differences in predominant TCR V gene usage between the two cases, we suspect this is due to HLA differences. A previous study on lung TCR repertoire in patients with PM by Englund et al. reported selective TCR V gene usage, characterized by a panel of TCR-specific monoclonal antibodies on flow cytometry [163]. However, that study used BAL fluid rather than lung tissue in which infiltrating T cells may be more directly involved in the disease process. Although we also tried to analyze TCR repertoire from BAL fluid, the data were inconclusive due to lack of TCR signals along with background noise from RNA debris. To our knowledge, this is the first robust demonstration of the presence of selective TCR V gene usage and its differential expression in lung tissues of patients with PM using both lung biopsy tissue from early IP and PBL. Because our study involved only two cases, these findings should be confirmed in a larger study. However, we believe these findings strongly suggest that T cells which are recruited into the lung may be exposed to autoantigens, selectively expanding by antigen-driven responses. Further studies are needed to identify T cell epitopes

http://dx.doi.org/10.5772/intechopen.70864

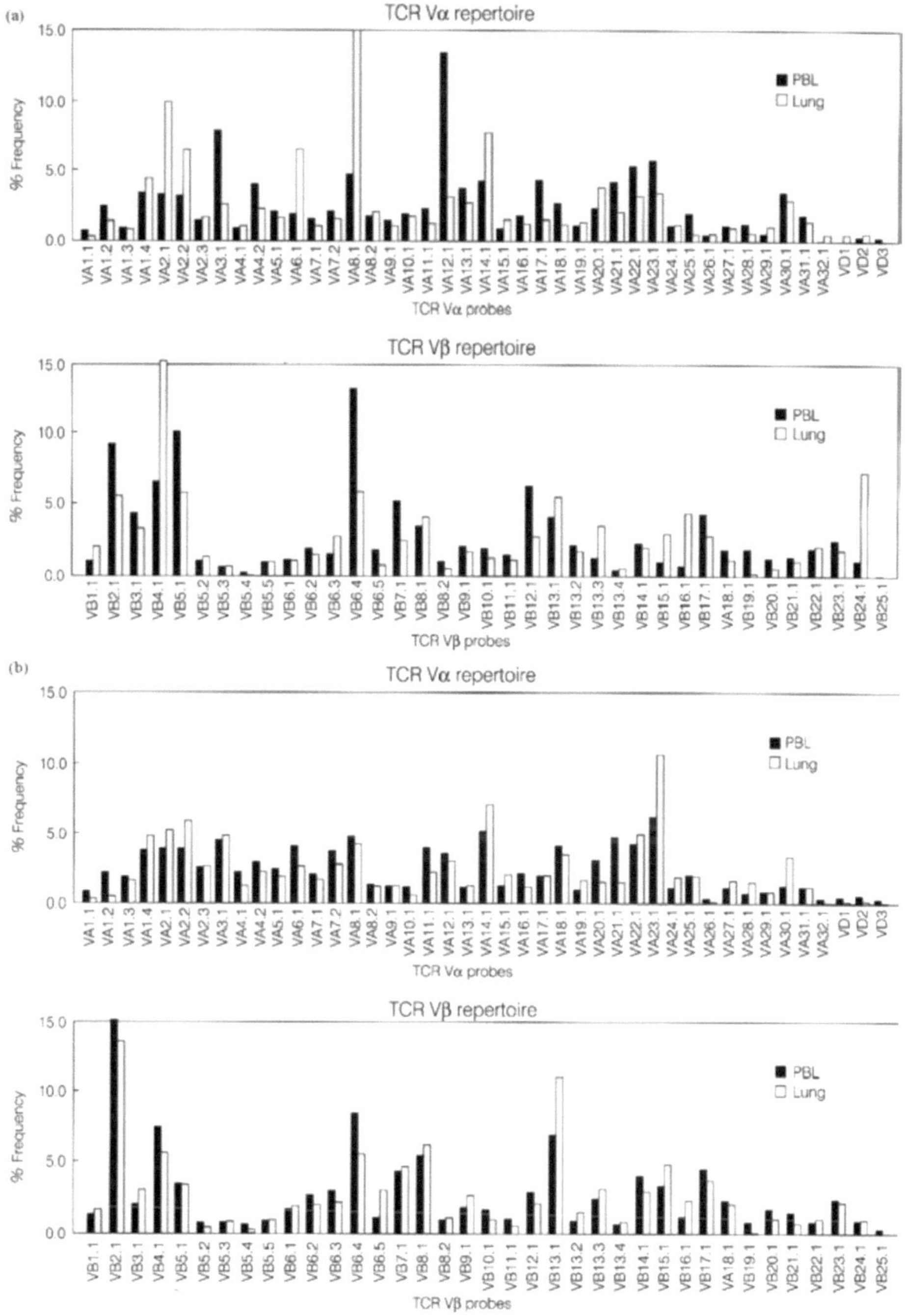


**Figure 3.** (a) Quantitative analysis of TCR repertoires: TCR Vα gene usage (top) and TCR Vβ gene usage (bottom) in patient A. Solid and open bars indicate frequencies of TCR Vα/Vβ repertoires in PBL and lung tissue, respectively. VA2.1 and VA8.1 and VB4.1 and VB24.1 repertoires predominate in lung tissue compared with PBL. (b). Quantitative analysis of TCR repertoires: TCR Vα gene usage (top) and TCR Vβ gene usage (bottom) in patient B. Solid and open bars indicate frequencies of TCR Vα/Vβ repertoires in PBL and lung tissue, respectively. VA23.1 and VB13.1 repertoires are more frequent in lung tissue compared with PBL.

of the pathogenic antigens, which may potentially lead to the development of antigen-specific, molecular-targeted therapies, such as the induction of anergy by peptide analogues similar in structure to culprit antigens [164, 165].

Thus, as a result, the T cell receptor (TCR) repertoire study combined with histological analysis demonstrated substantial CD3+ T cell lung infiltrates with specific oligoclonal TCR usage that differed from those in PBL, suggesting a pivotal role for T cells in the pathogenesis of PM-associated IP via antigen-driven immune mechanisms.

## 7. Management of interstitial pneumonia associated with connective tissue disease

Because of the wide variation in manifestations of ILD in the autoimmune disease of CTD, no simple management strategy is adequate for every possible clinical setting. While a part of patients with CTD-associated ILD have limited and stable disease, not always requiring treatment, the significant proportions have severe and progressive disease which necessitates prompt and appropriate treatment. Essentially, nevertheless, general therapeutic principles in CTDs can be applied to many situations including acute and chronic disease. These include use of corticosteroids, azathioprine (AZA), cyclophosphamide (CYC), methotrexate (MTX), mycophenolate mofetil (MMF), and calcineurin inhibitors [13]. Although there are no specific guidelines for the management of CTD-ILD, general strategies recommended for IPF of IIP are also often applied in some cases of CTD-ILD. Emerging treatments with effects in IPF, e.g., Pirfenidone (a pyridine showing both anti-inflammatory and anti-fibrotic effects) and Nintedanib (a small-molecule tyrosine kinase inhibitor targeting VEGF-, FGF-, PDGF-receptors) may offer additional treatment options, though the efficacy has not been evaluated in CTD-ILD [166]. Basically, in contrast to the dismal prognosis in IPF/UIP of IIP with a median survival since diagnosis of 2–3 years, clinical experience in managing patients has taught us that immunosuppressive drugs in CTD-associated ILDs are capable of benefiting a significant proportion of patients, particularly those with certain histological patterns of disease.

With regard to the clinical study, there have been only two randomized placebo-controlled trials investigating the effect of immunosuppressive treatment in SSc-associated ILD. Briefly, the Scleroderma Lung Study (SLS) and the Fibrosing Alveolitis Scleroderma Trial (FAST), evaluated CYC (given orally at 2 mg/kg for 1 year in SLS and intravenously at a dose of 600 mg/m$^2$ monthly for 6 months, followed by oral AZA for the following 6 months in FAST) for SSc-ILD [72, 73]. Both studies found a slower decline in forced vital capacity (FVC) in the CYC group compared with placebo. Intravenous CYC elicited a lower rate of bone marrow toxicity, severe infections, and gonadal failure compared to oral administration, likely due to higher cumulative dose acquired by daily oral administration [167]. Six months after quitting of immunosuppressant, the recovery in FVC fell into baseline, suggesting the requirement of prolonged immunosuppression therapy to maintain stability of lung function [168]. However, it should be noted that, despite studies supporting the benefit of CYC therapy in preventing deterioration in the lung function and premature death in patients with SSc–ILD, recent systematic review and meta-analysis of RCTs and observational prospective cohort studies failed to validate any clinically significant improvement in pulmonary function in SSc patients treated with CYC [169, 170].

In PM/DM-associated ILD, high-dose steroid is often the first-line drug, although no definite therapeutic recommendation for the disease has been established yet. The other drugs most frequently used are AZA, MMF, hydroxychloroquine, MTX, CYC, and calcineurin inhibitors, e.g., cyclosporine A (CSA) and tacrolimus (TAC). Rituximab, anti-CD20 monoclonal antibody therapy, has lately emerged as a promising remedy of biologics in patients who have failed conventional immunosuppression treatments [171, 172]. Among a variety of immunosuppressants, the efficacy of calcineurin inhibitors for the treatment of PM/DM-associated ILD should be highlighted. CSA, which inhibits T cell proliferation and T cell-mediated cytokine productions at the transcriptional level, has begun to be used for PM/DM-ILD since the 1980s [173–175]. In 1998, the first nation-wide survey for the treatment with CSA in IP associated with CTDs was conducted in Japan, and the efficacy of a combination therapy with CSA and corticosteroids in PM/DM associated IP was indicated [176]. A number of retrospective and open-label studies have supported the benefit of CSA for the treatment of ILD with PM/DM [177–181]. Takada et al. published a retrospective multicenter study of 38 cases with acute ILD with PM/DM, whereas it was shown that the combination therapy with CSA and corticosteroids started from the early phase of ILD is superior to corticosteroid monotherapy [178]. Today, calcineurin inhibitors are widely used especially in Japan as both an induction and maintenance therapy for PM/DM-ILD, generally resulting in favorable prognostic outcomes. The appropriate serum concentration of CSA to ensure a maximal effect as well as to avoid toxicity in patients with PM/DM-ILD should reach approximately 150 ng/mL and1000 ng/mL, at trough and at 2 hours after administration, respectively [179]. Another calcineurin inhibitor, TAC, which is a 100-fold potent T cell inhibitor compared to CSA, was also introduced into the treatment for PM/DM-ILD, and its efficacy and tolerability have been demonstrated in retrospective studies and case series since the report by Oddis et al. in 1999 [182–185]. Ochi, et al. described a superior effect of TAC used in two myositis patients with progressive ILD who failed CYC and corticosteroid treatment but successfully recovered with TAC, showing significant improvement in symptoms and radiologic changes [183]. The appropriate tacrolimus trough level for the treatment of ILD in PM/DM patients have not been established by clinical trials, but it is usually set as 5–20 ng/mL on the basis of data from renal and bone marrow transplantation [186].

Given the treatment-effect heterogeneity of the lung disease observed in PM/DM, it is important to prepare novel therapeutics for the challenging cases of ILD which are refractory to conventional formulas. Recently, Suda et al. reported the effectiveness of multitarget therapy for the ILD in two cases of anti-MDA5 antibody-positive DM which is known to be associated with progressive ILD and sometimes has a lethal outcome despite strong immunosuppressive therapy including CYC [187]. They used TAC and mizoribine (MZR, an inosine monophosphate dehydrogenase inhibitor) in combination with corticosteroids. MZR is a nucleoside of the imidazole class, with the same mechanism as MMF: selective inhibition of lymphocyte proliferation by blocking inosine monophosphate dehydrogenase [188]. The safety and steroid-sparing effects of MZR have been shown in various CTDs, and the efficacy of multitarget therapy using TAC and MZR was reported for systemic lupus erythematosus [189, 190].

## 8. Conclusions

Despite increased recognition of CTD-associated ILD and its prognostic significance, the pathologic mechanisms that lead to the considerable pulmonary changes are not yet fully defined, and thus, the only limited progress has been so far made in the therapeutic domains. Immunosuppression therapy remains the mainstay of treatment for CTD-ILD. To generate significant advances in therapeutic intervention strategy, fundamental understanding of the pathogenesis of CTD-ILD is essential. As noted, we had an opportunity to carefully study the cases of early-stage IP associated with PM by utilizing lung biopsy tissue and PBLs. The T cell receptor (TCR) repertoire study combined with histological analysis demonstrated substantial CD3+ T cell lung infiltrates with specific oligoclonal TCR usage that differed from those in PBL, suggesting a pivotal role for T cells in the pathogenesis of PM-associated IP via antigen-driven immune responses. The results imply potential elucidation of specific antigen(s) that oligoclonal, lung-infiltrating T cells recognize, which may provide novel insights into the development of immunospecific treatments such as molecular-targeted or specific T cell-targeted therapeutics.

## Disclosure statement

The authors have declared no conflicts of interest.

## Patient consent

The authors have declared in the published articles that the informed consent was obtained from the patients.

## Ethical approval

The authors have declared in the published articles that the protocols were approved by the institutional review board.

## Author details

Akira Takeda[1*] and Yoshiki Ishii[2]

*Address all correspondence to: akitake@iuhw.ac.jp

1 Division of Clinical Immunology & Rheumatology, International University of Health and Welfare Hospital, Nasu-Shiobara, Tochigi, Japan

2 Department of Pulmonary Medicine and Clinical Immunology, Dokkyo University School of Medicine, Mibu, Tochigi, Japan

## References

[1] American Thoracic Society. European Respiratory Society: American Thoracic Society/European Respiratory Society international multidisciplinary consensus classification of the idiopathic international pneumonias. American Journal of Respiratory and Critical Care Medicine. 2002;**165**:277-304

[2] Travis WD, Costabel U, Hansell DM, King TE Jr, Lynch DA, Nicholon AG, Ryerson CJ, Ryu JH, Selman M, Wells AU, Behr J, Bouros D, Brown KK, Colby TV, Collard HR, Cordeiro CR, Cottin V, Crestani B, Drent M, Dudden RF, Egan J, Flaherty K, Hogaboam C, Inoue Y, Johkoh T, Kim DS, Kitaichi M, Loyd J, Martinez FJ, Myers J, Myers J, Protzko S, Raghu G, Richeldi L, Sverzellati N, Swigris J, Valeyre D, on behalf of the ATS/ERS committee on idiopathic interstitial pneumonias. An official American Thoracic Society/European Respiratory Society statement: Update of the international multidisciplinary classification of the idiopathic international pneumonias. American Journal of Respiratory and Critical Care Medicine. 2013;**188**:733-748. DOI: 10.1164/rccm.201308-1483ST

[3] Margaritopoulos GA, Romagnoli M, Poletti V, Siafakas NM, Wells AU, Antoniou KM. Recent advances in the pathogenesis and clinical evaluation of pulmonary fibrosis. European Respiratory Review. 2012;**21**:48-56. DOI: 10.1183/09059180.00007611

[4] Antoniou KM, Margaritopoulos GA, Tomassetti S, Bonella F, Costabel U, Poletti V. Interstitial lung disease. European Respiratory Review. 2014;**23**:40-54. DOI: 10.1183/09059180.00009113

[5] Vij R, Strek ME. Diagnosis and treatment of connective tissue disease-associated interstitial lung disease. Chest. 2013;**143**:813-824. DOI: 10.1378/chest.12-0741

[6] Fukushima Y, Takeda A, Matsutani T, Fukushima F, Furihata T, Maezawa R, Miyoshi M, Hirata H, Sugiyama K, Okada M, Fukuda T. Involvement of antigen-driven mechanisms in interstitial pneumonia with polymyositis. Rheumatology. 2013;**52**:1537-1540. DOI: 10.1093/rheumatology/ket003

[7] Takeda A, Fukushima Y, Matsutani T, Rokutanda R, Suyama Y, Kishimoto M, Yamaguchi K-I, Okada M. Implication of antigen-driven mechanisms in the pathogenesis of interstitial pneumonia associated with polymyositis. Frontiers in Immunology. 2013; 15th International Congress of Immunology (ICI). DOI: 10.3389/conf.fimmu.2013.02.00414 (published online: Aug 22, 2013)

[8] Nakamura Y, Suda T. Idiopathic pulmonary fibrosis: Diagnosis and clinical manifestations. Circulatory Respiratory and Pulmonary Medicine. 2015;**9**(S1):163-171. DOI: 10.4137/CCRPM.S39897

[9] Raghu G, Collard HR, Egan JJ, et al. ATS/ERS/JRS/ALAT Committee on Idiopathic Pulmonary Fibrosis. An official ATS/ERS/JRS/ALAT statement: Idiopathic pulmonary fibrosis: Evidence-based guidelines for diagnosis and management. American Journal of Respiratory and Critical Care Medicine. 2011;**183**:788-824

[10] Raghu G, Rochwerg B, Zhang Y, et al. American Thoracic Society; European Respiratory society; Japanese Respiratory Society; Latin American Thoracic Association. An official ATS/ERS/JRS/ALAT clinical practice guideline: Treatment of idiopathic pulmonary fibrosis. An update of the 2011 clinical practice guideline. American Journal of Respiratory and Critical Care Medicine. 2015; **192**:e3-19. DOI: 10.1164/rccm.201506-1063ST

[11] de Lauretis A, Veeraraghavan S, Renzoni E. Aspects of interstitial lung disease: Connective tissue disease-associated interstitial lung disease: How does it differ from IPF? How should the clinical approach differ? Chronic Respiratory Disease. 2011;**8**:53-82. DOI: 10.1177/1479972310393758

[12] Castelino FV, Varga J. Interstitial lung diseases: Evolving concepts of pathogenesis and management. Arthritis Research & Therapy. 2010;**12**(4):213. DOI: 10.1186/ar3097

[13] Mathai SC, Danoff SK. Management of interstitial lung disease associated with connective tissue disease. BMJ. 2016;**352**:h6819. DOI: 10.1136/bmj.h6819

[14] Cottin V. Interstitial lung diseases: Are we missing formes frustes of connective tissue disease? The European Respiratory Journal. 2006;**28**:893-896

[15] Fischer A, West SG, Swigris JJ, et al. Connective tissue disease-associated interstitial lung disease: A call for clarification. Chest. 2010;**138**:251-256

[16] Bryson T, Sundaram B, Khanna D, Kazerooni E. Connective tissue disease-associated interstitial lung disease: Similarity and difference. Seminars in Ultrasound, CT and MRI. 2014;**35**:29-38

[17] Fischer A, du Bois R. Interstitial lung disease in connective tissue disorders. Lancer. 2012;**380**:689-698.

[18] Fischer A, Richeldi L. Cross-disciplinary collaboration in connective tissue disease-related lung disease. Seminars in Respiratory and Critical Care Medicine. 2014;**35**:159-165

[19] Tzelepis GE, Toya SP, Moutsopoulos HM. Occult connective tissue diseases mimicking idiopathic interstitial pneumonias. European Respiratory Review. 2008;**31**:11-20

[20] Bonella F, Costabel U. Biomarkers in connective tissue disease-associated interstitial lung disease. Seminars in Respiratory and Critical Care Medicine. 2014;**35**:181-220

[21] Prasse A, Muller-Quernheim J. Non-invasive biomarkers in pulmonary fibrosis. Respirology. 2009;**14**(6):788-795

[22] Pastva AM, Wright JR, Williams KL. Immunomodulatory roles of surfactant protein A and D: Implications in lung disease. Proceedings of the American Thoracic Society. 2007;**4**(3):252-257

[23] Takahashi H, Kuroki Y, Tanaka H, et al. Serum levels of surfactant proteins A and D are useful biomarkers for interstitial lung disease in patients with progressive systemic sclerosis. American Journal of Respiratory and Critical Care Medicine. 2000;**162**(1):258-263

[24] Ishikawa N, Hattori N, Yokoyama A, Kohno N. Utility of KL-6/MUC1 in the clinical management of interstitial lung diseases. Respiratory Investigation. 2012;**50**(1):3-13

[25] Ohshimo S, Yokoyama A, Hattori N, Ishikawa N, Hirasawa Y, Kohno N. KL-6, a human MUC1 mucin, promotes proliferation and survival of lung fibroblasts. Biochemical and Biophysical Research Communications. 2005;**338**(4):1845-1852

[26] Yamane K, Ihn H, Kubo M, et al. Serum levels of KL-6 as a useful marker for evaluating pulmonary fibrosis in patients with systemic sclerosis. The Journal of Rheumatology. 2000;**27**(4):930-934

[27] Papiris SA, Kagouridis K, Bouros D. Serologic evaluation in idiopathic interstitial pneumonias. Current Opinion in Pulmonary Medicine. 2012;**18**(5):433-440

[28] Lunardi F, Balestro E, Nordio B, et al. Undifferentiated connective tissue disease presenting with prevalent interstitial lung disease: Case report and review of literature. Diagnostic Pathology. 2011;**6**:50

[29] Olson AL, Brown KK, Fischer A. Connective tissue disease-associated lung disease. Immunology and Allergy Clinics of North America. 2012;**32**(4):513-536

[30] Mosca M, Tani C, Bombardieri S. Undifferentiated connective tissue diseases (UCTD): A new frontier for rheumatology. Best Practice & Research. Clinical Rheumatology. 2007;**21**(6):1011-1023

[31] Kinder BW, Collard HR, Koth L, et al. Idiopathic nonspecific interstitial pneumonia: Lung manifestation of undifferentiated connective tissue disease? American Journal of Respiratory and Critical Care Medicine. 2007;**176**:691-697

[32] Vij R, Noth I, Strek ME. Autoimmune-featured interstitial lung disease: A distinct entity. Chest. 2011;**140**:1292-1299

[33] Fischer A, Antoniou KM, Brown KK, et al. ERS/ATS Task Force on Undifferentiated Forms of CTD-ILD. An official European Respiratory Society/American Thoracic Society research statement: Interstitial pneumonia with autoimmune features. The European Respiratory Journal. 2015;**46**(4):976-987. DOI: 10.1183/13993003.00150-2015

[34] Collins BF, Spiekerman CF, Shaw MA, Ho LA, Hayes J, Spada CA, Stamato CM, Raghu G. Idiopathic interstitial pneumonia associated with autoantibodies a large case series followed over 1 year. Chest. 2017;**152**(1):103-112. DOI: org/10.1016/j.chest.2017.03.004

[35] Urisman A, Jones KD. Pulmonary pathology in connective tissue disease. Seminars in Respiratory and Critical Care Medicine. 2014;**35**:201-212

[36] Vivero M, Padera RF. Histopathology of lung disease in connective tissue diseases. Rheumatic Diseases Clinics of North America. 2015;**41**:197-211

[37] Kitaichi M. Pathologic features and the classification of interstitial pneumonia of unknown etiology. Bulletin of the Chest Disease Research Institute, Kyoto University. 1990;**23**:1-18

[38] Katzenstein A-LA, Fiorelli RF. Non-specific interstitial pneumonia/fibrosis. Histologic patterns and clinical significance. The American Journal of Surgical Pathology. 1994; **18**:136-147

[39] Nagai S, Kitaichi K, Itoh H, Nishimura K, Izumi T, Colby TV. Idiopathic nonspecific interstitial pneumonia/fibrosis: Comparison with idiopathic pulmonary fibrosis and BOOP. The European Respiratory Journal. 1998;**12**:1010-1019

[40] Travis WD, Matsui K, Moss J, Ferrans VJ. Idiopathic nonspecific nonspecific interstitial pneumonia: Prognostic significance of cellular and fibrosing pattrens: Survival comparison with usual interstitial pneumonia and desquamative interstitial pneumonia. The American Journal of Surgical Pathology. 2000;**24**:19-33

[41] Tanaka N, Kim JS, Newell JD, Brown KK, Cool CD, Meehan R, et al. Rheumatoid arthritis-related lung disease: CT findings. Radiology. 2004;**232**:81-91

[42] Lee HK, Kim DS, Yoo B, Seo JB, Rho JY, et al. Histopathologic pattern and clinical features of rheumatoid arthritis-associated interstitial lung disease. Chest. 2005;**127**:2019-2027

[43] Park LH, Kim DS, Park I, Jang SJ, Kitaichi M, Nicholson AG, et al. Prognosis of fibrotic interstitial pneumonia: Idiopathic versus collagen vascular disease-related subtypes. American Journal of Respiratory and Critical Care Medicine. 2007;**175**:705-711

[44] Song JW, Do K, Kim M, Jang SJ, Colby TV, Kim DS. Pathologic differences between idiopathic and collagen vascular disease-related usual interstitial pneumonia. Chest. 2009;**136**:23-30

[45] Hamman L, Rich AR. Fulminating diffuse interstitial fibrosis of the lungs. Transactions of the American Clinical and Climatological Association. 1935;**51**:154-163

[46] Katzenstein A-LA, Bloor CM, Leibow AA. Diffuse alveolar damage – the role of oxygen, shock, and related factors: A review. The American Journal of Pathology. 1976;**85**(1):209-228

[47] Katzenstein A-LA, Myers JL, Mazur MT. Acute interstitial pneumonia: A clinicopathologic, ultrastructural, and cell kinetic study. The American Journal of Surgical Pathology. 1986;**10**(4):256-267

[48] Mukhopadhyay S, Parambil JG. Acute interstitial pneumonia (AIP): Relationship to Hamman-Rich syndrome, diffuse alveolar damage, and acute respiratory distress syndrome (ARDS). Seminars in Respiratory and Critical Care Medicine. 2012;**33**:476-485

[49] Tomashefski JF Jr. Pulmonary pathology of acute respiratory distress syndrome. Clinics in Chest Medicine. 2000;**21**(3):435-466

[50] Brower RG, Matthay MA, Morris A, Schoenfeld D, Thompson BT, Wheeler A. Acute Respiratory Distress Syndrome Network. Ventilation with lower tidal volumes for acute lung injury and acute respiratory distress syndrome. The New England Journal of Medicine. 2000;**342**(18):1301-1308

[51] Parambil JG, Myers JI, Ryu JH. Diffuse alveolar damage: Uncommon manifestation of pulmonary involvement in patients with connective tissue diseases. Chest. 2006; **130**(2):553-558

[52] Zamora MR, Warner ML, Tuder R, Schwarz KI. Diffuse alveolar hemorrhage and systemic lupus erythematosus. Clinical presentation, histology, survival, and outcome. Medicine (Baltimore). 1997;**76**(3):192-202

[53] Tazelaar HD, Viggiano RW, Pickersgill J, Colvy TV. Interstitial lung disease in polymyositis/dermatomyositis. Clinical features and prognosis as correlated with histologic findings. The American Review of Respiratory Disease. 1990;**141**(3):727-733

[54] Douglas WW, Tazelaar HD, Hartman TE, et al. Polymyositis/dermatomyositis-associated interstitial lung disease. American Journal of Respiratory and Critical Care Medicine. 2001;**164**(7):1182-1185

[55] Fujisawa T, Suda T, Nakamura Y, et al. Differences in clinical features and prognosis of interstitial lung diseases between polymyositis and dermatomyositis. The Journal of Rheumatology. 2005;**32**(1):58-64

[56] Yousem SA, Colvy TV, Carrington CB. Lung biopsy in rheumatoid arthritis. The American Review of Respiratory Disease. 1985;**131**(5):770-777

[57] Katzenstein A-LA, Myers JL. Nonspecific interstitial pneumonia and the other idiopathic interstitial pneumonias: Classification and diagnostic criteria. The American Journal of Surgical Pathology. 2000;**24**(1):1-3

[58] Henriet AC, Diot E, Marchand-Adam S, et al. Organizing pneumonia can be the inaugural manifestation in connective tissue diseases, including Sjögren's syndrome. European Respiratory Review. 2010;**19**(116):161-163

[59] Tansey D, Wells AU, Colby TV, et al. Variations in histological patterns of interstitial pneumonia between connective tissue disorders and their relationship to prognosis. Histopathology. 2004;**44**(6):585-596

[60] Bouros D, Wells AU, Nicholson AG, et al. Histopathologic subsets of fibrosing alveolitis in patients with systemic sclerosis and their relationshio to outcome. American Journal of Respiratory and Critical Care Medicine. 2002;**165**(12):1581-1586

[61] Nicholson AG. Lymphocytic interstitial pneumonia and other lymphoproliferative disorders in the lung. Seminars in Respiratory and Critical Care Medicine. 2001;**22**(4):409-422

[62] Deheinzelin D, Cpelozzi VL, Kairalla RA, BarbasFilho JV, Saldiva PH, de Carvalho CR. Interstitial lung disease in primary Sjögren's syndrome. Clinical-pathological evaluation and response to treatment. American Journal of Respiratory and Critical Care Medicine. 1996;**154**:794-799.

[63] Steen VD. Clinical manifestations of systemic sclerosis. Seminars in Cutaneous Medicine and Surgery. 1998;**17**:48-54 A comprehensive review of the general clinical features of systemic sclerosis

[64] D'Angelo WA, Fries JF, Masi AT, et al. Pathologic observations in systemic sclerosis (scleroderma). A study of fifty-eight autopsy cases and fifty-eight matched controls. The American Journal of Medicine. 1969;**46**:428-440

[65] Gabrielli A, Avvedimento EV, Krieg T. Scleroderma. The New England Journal of Medicine. 2009;**360**(19):1989-2003

[66] Cutolo M, Sulli A, Smith V. Assessing microvascular changes in systemic sclerosis diagnosis and management. Nature Reviews Rheumatology. 2010;**6**(10):578-587

[67] Huguhes M, Herrick AL. Raynaud's phenomenon. Best Practice & Research. Clinical Rheumatology. 2016;**30**(1):112-132

[68] van den Hoogen F, Khanna D, Fransen J, et al. 2013 classification criteria for systemic sclerosis: An American College of Rheumatology/European League against Rheumatism collaborative initiative. Arthritis and Rheumatism 2013;**65**(11):2737-2747

[69] Reveille JD, Solomon DH. Evidence-based guidelines for the use of immunologic tests: Anticentromere, Scl-70, and nucleolar antibodies. Arthritis and Rheumatism. 2003;**49**:399-412

[70] Shah AA, Hummers LK, Casciola-Rosen L, et al. Examination of autoantibody status and clinical features associated with cancer risk and cancer-associated scleroderma. Arthritis and Rheumatism. 2015;**67**(4):1053-1061

[71] Parra ER, Otani LH, de Carvalho EF, et al. Systemic sclerosis and idiopathic interstitial pneumonia: Histomorphometric differences in lung biopsies. Jornal Brasileiro de Pneumologia 2009;**35**:529-540

[72] Fujita J, Yoshinouchi T, Ohtsuki Y, et al. Non-specific interstitial pneumonia as pulmonary involvement of systemic sclerosis. Annals of the Rheumatic Diseases. 2001;**60**:281-283

[73] Tashkin DP, Elashoff R, Clements PJ, Goldin J, Roth MD, Furst DE, et al. Cyclophosphamide versus placebo in scleroderma lung disease. The New England Journal of Medicine. 2006;**354**:2655-2666

[74] Hoyles RK, Ellis RW, Wellsbury J, Lees B, Newlands P, Goh NS, et al. A multicenter, prospective, randomized, double-blind, placebo-controlled trial of and intravenous cyclophosphamide followed by oral azathioprine for the treatment of pulmonary fibrosis in scleroderma. Arthritis and Rheumatism. 2006;**54**:3962-3970

[75] Kelly C, Hamilton J. What kills patients with rheumatoid arthritis? Rheumatology (Oxford). 2007;**46**(2):183-184

[76] Bongartz T, Nannini C, et al. Incidence and mortality of interstitial lung disease in rheumatoid arthritis: A population-based study. Arthritis and Rheumatism. 2010;**62**(6):1583-1591

[77] Turesson C. Extra-articular rheumatoid arthritis. Current Opinion in Rheumatology. 2013;**25**(3):360-366

[78] Hyland RH, Gordon DA, Broder I, Davies GM, Russell ML, Hutcheon MA, et al. A systematic controlled study of pulmonary abnormalities in rheumatoid arthritis. The Journal of Rheumatology. 1983;**10**:395-405

[79] Jurik AG, Davidsen D, Graudal H. Prevalence of pulmonary involvement in rheumatoid arthritis and its relationship to some characteristics of the patients. A radiological and clinical study. Scandinavian Journal of Rheumatology. 1982;**11**:217-224

[80] Gabbay E, Tarala R, Will R, Carroll G, Adler B, Cameron D, Lake FR. Interstitial lung disease in recent onset rheumatoid arthritis. American Journal of Respiratory and Critical Care Medicine. 1997;**156**:528-535

[81] Youssef AA, Machaly SA, El-Dosoky ME, El-Maghraby NM. Respiratory symptoms in rheumatoid arthritis: Relation to pulmonary abnormalities detected by high-resolution CT and pulmonary functional testing. Rheumatology International. 2012;**32**(7):1985-1995

[82] Saag KG, Cerhan JR, Kolluri S, Ohashi K, Hunninghake GW, Schwartz DA. Cigarette smoking and rheumatoid arthritis severity. Annals of the Rheumatic Diseases. 1997; **56**:463-469

[83] Cipriani NA, Strek M, Noth I, et al. Pathologic quantification of connective tissue disease-associated versus idiopathic usual interstitial pneumonia. Archives of Pathology & Laboratory Medicine. 2012;**136**:1253-1258

[84] Yoshinouchi T, Ohtsuki Y, Fujita J, et al. Nonspecific interstitial pneumonia pattern as pulmonary involvement of rheumatoid arthritis. Rheumatology International. 2005; **26**:121-125

[85] Nakamura Y, Suda T, Kaida Y, et al. Rheumatoid lung disease: Prognostic analysis of 54 biopsy-proven cases. Respiratory Medicine. 2012;**106**:1164-1169

[86] Cherin P, Herson S, Crevon MC, et al. Mechanisms of lysis by activated cytotoxic cells expressing perforin and granzyme-B genes and the protein TIA-1 in muscle biopsies of myositis. The Journal of Rheumatology. 1996;**23**:1135-1142

[87] Dalakas MC. Molecular immunology and genetics of inflammatory muscle diseases. Archives of Neurology. 1998;**55**:1509-1512

[88] Chevrel G, Page G, Miossec P. Novel aspects on the contribution of T cells and dendritic cells in the pathogenesis of myositis. Autoimmunity. 2006;**39**(3):171-176

[89] Medsger TA Jr, Dawson WN Jr, Masi AT. The epidemiology of polymyositis. The American Journal of Medicine. 1970;**48**:715-723

[90] Bohan A, Peter JB. Polymyositis and dermatomyositis (first part). The New England Journal of Medicine. 1975;**292**:344-347

[91] Bohan A, Peter JB. Polymyositis and dermatomyositis (second part). The New England Journal of Medicine. 1975;**292**:403-407

[92] Dalakas MC, Hohlfeld R. Polymyositis and dermatomyositis. Lancet. 2003;**362**:971-982

[93] Briani C, Doria A, Sarzi-Puttini P, Dalakas MC. Update on idiopathic inflammatory myopathies. Autoimmunity. 2006;**39**(3):161-170

[94] Nirmalananthan N, Holton JL, Hanna MG. Is it really myositis? A consideration of the differential diagnosis. Current Opinion in Rheumatology. 2004;**16**:684-691

[95] Dickey BF, Myers AR. Pulmonary disease in polymyositis/dermatomyositis. Seminars in Arthritis and Rheumatism. 1984;**14**:60-76

[96] Lakhanpal S, Lie JT, Conn DL, WJ M. Pulmonary disease in polymyositis/dermatomyositis: A clinicopathological analysis of 65 autopsy cases. Annals of the Rheumatic Diseases. 1987;**46**:23-29

[97] Marie I, Hatron PY, Hachulla E, Wallaert B, Michon-Pasturel U, Devulder B. Pulmonary involvement in polymyositis and in dermatomyositis. The Journal of Rheumatology. 1998;**25**:1336-1343

[98] Marie I, Hachulla E, Hatron PY, Hellot MF, Levesque H, Devulder B, Courtois H. Polymyositis and dermatomyositis: Short term and longterm outcome, and predictive factors of prognosis. The Journal of Rheumatology. 2001;**28**:2230-2237

[99] Marie I, Hachulla E, Chèrin P, Dominique S, Hatron P, Hellot MF, et al. Interstitial lung disease in polymyositis and dermatomyositis. Arthritis and Rheumatism. 2002;**47**:614-622

[100] Fathi M, Lundberg IE, Tornling G. Pulmonary complications of polymyositis and dermatomyositis. Seminars in Respiratory and Critical Care Medicine. 2007;**28**:451-458

[101] Connors GR, Christopher-Stine L, Oddis CV, et al. Interstitial lung disease associated with the idiopathic inflammatory myopathies: what progress has been made in the past 35 years? Chest. 2010;**138**:1464-1474

[102] Lega J-C, Reynaud Q, Belot A, Fabien N, Durieu I, Cottin V. Idiopathic inflammatory myopathies and the lung. European Respiratory Review. 2015;**24**:216-238. DOI: 10.1183/16000617.00002015

[103] Cottin V, Thivolet-Bèjui F, Reynaud-Gaubert M, Cadranel J, Delaval P, Ternamian PJ, et al. Groupe d'Etudes et de Recherche sur les Maladies "Orphelines" Pulmonaires. Interstitial lung disease in amyopathic dermatomyositis, dermatomyositis and polymyositis. The European Respiratory Journal. 2003;**22**:245-250

[104] Devaraj A, Wells AU, Hansell DM. Computed tomographic imaging in connective tissue diseases. Seminars in Respiratory and Critical Care Medicine. 2007;**28**:389-397

[105] Ikezoe J, Johkoh T, Kohno N, Takeuchi N, Ichikado K, Nakamura H. High-resolution CT findings of lung disease in patients with polymyositis and dermatomyositis. Journal of Thoracic Imaging. 1996;**11**:250-259

[106] Mino M, Noma S, Taguchi Y, Tomii K, Kohri Y, Oida K. Pulmonary involvement in polymyositis and dermatomyositis: Sequential evaluation with CT. American Journal of Roentgenology. 1997;**169**:83-87

[107] Akira M, Hara H, Sakatani M. Interstitial lung disease in association with polymyositis/dermatomyositis: Long-term follow-up CT evaluation in seven patients. Radiology. 1999;**210**:333-338

[108] Arakawa H, Yamada H, Kurihara Y, Nakajima Y, Takeda A, Fukushima Y, Fujioka M. Nonspecific interstitial pneumonia associated with polymyositis and dermatomyositis: Serial high-resolution CT findings and functional correlation. Chest. 2003;**123**(4):1096-1103. DOI: 10.1378/chest.123.4.1096

[109] Euwer RL, Sontheimer RD. Amyopathic dermatomyositis: A review. The Journal of Investigative Dermatology. 1993;**100**(1):124S-127S

[110] Sontheimer RD. Would a new name hasten the acceptance of amyopathic dermatomyositis (dermatomyositis sine myositis) as a distinctive subset within the idiopathic inflammatory dermatomyopathies spectrum of clinical illness? Journal of the American Academy of Dermatology. 2002;**46**:626-636

[111] Suda T, Fujisawa T, Enomoto N, et al. Interstitial lung diseases associated withamyopathic dermatomyositis. The European Respiratory Journal. 2006;**28**(5):1005-1012

[112] Ye S, Chen XX, Lu XY, et al. Adult clinically amyopathic dermatomyositis with rapid progressive interstitial lung disease: A retrospective cohort study. Clinical Rheumatology. 2007;**26**(10):1647-1654

[113] Sato S, Hirakata M, Kuwana M, et al. Autoantibodies to a 140-kd polypeptide, CADM-140, in Japanese patients with clinically amyopathic dermatomyositis. Arthritis and Rheumatism. 2005;**52**(5):1571-1576

[114] Targoff IN. Immune manifestations of inflammatory muscle disease. Rheumatic Diseases Clinics of North America. 1994;**20**(4):857-880

[115] Yoshifuji H, Fujii T, Kobayashi S, Imura Y, Fujita Y, Kawabata D, Usui T, Tanaka M, Nagai S, Umehara H, Mimori T. Anti-aminoacyl-tRNA synthetase antibodies in clinical course prediction of interstitial lung disease complicated with idiopathic inflammatory myopathies. Autoimmunity. 2006;**39**(3):233-241

[116] Nishikai M, Reichlin M. Heterogeneity of precipitating antibodies in polymyositis and dermatomyositis. Characterization of the Jo-1 antibody system. Arthritis and Rheumatism. 1980;**23**(8):881-888

[117] Yoshida S, Akizuki M, Mimori T, et al. The precipitating antibody to an acidic nuclear protein antigen, the Jo-1, in connective tissue diseases. A marker for a subset of polymyositis with interstitial pulmonary fibrosis. Arthritis and Rheumatism. 1983;**26**:604-611

[118] Reeves WH, Nigam SK, Blobel G. Human autoantibodies reactive with the signal-recognition particle. Proceedings of the National Academy of Sciences of the United States of America. 1986;**83**(24):9507-9511

[119] Okada N, Mimori T, Mukai R, Kashiwagi H, Hardin JA. Characterization of humanautoantibodies that selectively precipitate the 7SL RNA component of the signal recognition particle. Journal of Immunology. 1987;**138**(10):3219-3223

[120] Targoff IN, Reichlin M. The association between Mi-2 antibodies and dermatomyositis. Arthritis and Rheumatism. 1985;**28**(7):796-803

[121] Nakashima R, Imura Y, Kobayashi S, et al. The RIG-I-like receptor IFIH1/MDA5 is a dermatomyositis-specific autoantigen identified by the anti-CADM-140 antibody. Rheumatology (Oxford). 2010;**49**(3):433-440

[122] Sato S, Hoshino K, Satoh T, Fujita T, Kawakami Y, Kuwana M. RNA helicase encoded by melanoma differentiation associated gene 5 is a major autoantigen in patients with clinically amyopathic dermatomyositis: Association with rapidly progressive interstitial lung disease. Arthritis and Rheumatism. 2009;**60**(7):2193-2200

[123] Targoff IN, Mamyrova G, Trieu EP, et al. Childhood Myositis Heterogeneity Study Group; International Myositis Collaborative Study Group. A novel autoantibody to a 155-kd protein is associated with dermatomyositis. Arthritis and Rheumatism. 2006;**54**(11):3682-3689

[124] Kaji K, Fujimoto M, Hasegawa M, et al. Identification of a novel autoantibody reactive with 155 and 140 kDa nuclear proteins in patients with dermatomyositis: An association with malignancy. Rheumatology (Oxford). 2007;**46**(1):25-28

[125] Genth E, Mierau R, Genetzky P, et al. Immunogenetic associations of scleroderma related antinuclear antibodies. Arthritis and Rheumatism. 1990;**33**(5):657-665

[126] Kuwana M, Okano Y, Kaburaki J, Tojo T, Medsger TA Jr. Racial differences in the distribution of systemic sclerosis-related serum antinuclear antibodies. Arthritis and Rheumatism 1994;**37**(6): 902-906.

[127] Betteridge ZE, Gunawardena H, Chinoy H, et al. UK Adult Onset Myositis Immunogenetic Collaboration. Clinical and human leucocyte antigen class II haplotype associations of autoantibodies to small ubiquitin-like modifier enzyme, a dermatomyositis-specific autoantigen target, in UK Caucasian adult-onset myositis. Annals of the Rheumatic Diseases. 2009;**68**(10):1621-1625

[128] Nakashima R, Mimori T. Clinical and pathophysiological significance of myositis-specific and myositis-associated autoantibodies. International Journal of Clinical Rheumatology. 2010;**5**(5):523-536

[129] Sato S, Kuwana M. Utility of dermatomyositis-specific autoantibodies for diagnosis and clinical subsetting. International Journal of Clinical Rheumatology. 2015;**10**:257-271. DOI: 10.2217/ijr.15.27

[130] Hozumi H, Fujisawa T, Nakashima R, Johkoh T, Sumikawa H, Murakami A, Enomoto N, Inui N, Nakamura Y, Hosono Y, Imura Y, Mimori T, Suda T. Comprehensive assessment of myositis-specific interstitial lung disease. Respiratory Medicine. 2016;**121**:91-99

[131] Satoh M, Tanaka S, Ceribelli A, Calise SJ, Chan EK. A comprehensive overview on myositis-specific antibodies: New and old biomarkers in idiopathic inflammatory myopathy. Clinical Reviews in Allergy & Immunology. 2017;**52**:1-19

[132] Abraham DJ, Krieg T, Distler J, Distler O. Overview of pathogenesis of systemic sclerosis. Rheumatology (Oxford). 2009;**48**(Suppl. 3):iii3-iii7. DOI: 10.1093/rheumatology/ken481 (published online: May 28, 2009)

[133] Wells AU, Denton CP. Interstitial lung disease in connective tissue disease – mechanisms and management. Nature Reviews Rheumatology. 2014;**10**:728-739. DOI: 10.1038/nrrheum.2014.149

[134] Denton CP. Therapeutic targets in systemic sclerosis. Arthritis Research & Therapy. 2007;**9**(Suppl. 2):S6. DOI: 10.1186/ar2190

[135] Kim KK, Kugler MC, Wolters PJ, et al. Alveolar epithelial cell mesenchymal transition develops in vivo during pulmonary fibrosis and is regulated by the extracellular matrix. Proceedings of the National Academy of Sciences of the United States of America. 2006;**103**:13180-13185

[136] Jain R, Shaul PW, Borok Z, Willis BC. Endothelin-1 induces alveolar epithelial mesenchymal transition through endothelin type A receptor-mediated production of TGF-beta 1. American Journal of Respiratory Cell and Molecular Biology. 2007;**37**:38-47

[137] Mauviel A. Transforming growth factor-beta: A key mediator of fibrosis. Methods in Molecular Medicine. 2005;**117**:69-80

[138] Varga J, Abraham D. Systemic sclerosis: A prototypic multisystem fibrotic disorder. The Journal of Clinical Investigation. 2007;**117**:557-567

[139] Clozel M, Salloukh H. Role of endothelin in fibrosis and anti-fibrotic potential of bosentan. Annals of Medicine. 2005;**37**:2-12

[140] Abraham DJ, Vancheeswaran R, Dashwood MR, et al. Increased levels of endothelin-1 and differential endothelin type A and B receptor expression in scleroderma-associated fibrotic lung disease. The American Journal of Pathology. 1997;**151**:831-841

[141] Tager AM, LaCamera P, Shea BS, Campanella GS, Selman M, Zhao Z, Polosukhin V, Wain J, Karimi-Shah BA, Kim ND, Hart WK, Pardo A, Blackwell TS, Xu Y, Chun J, Luster AD. The lysophosphatidic acid receptor LPA1 links pulmonary fibrosis to lung injury by mediating fibroblast recruitment and vascular leak. Nature Medicine. 2008;**14**:45-54

[142] Hamaguchi Y, Fujimoto M, Matsushita T, Hasegawa M, Takehara K, Sato S. Elevated serum insulin-like growth factor (IGF-1) and IGF binding protein-3 levels in patients with systemic sclerosis: Possible role in development of fibrosis. The Journal of Rheumatology. 2008;**35**:2363-2371

[143] Perbal B. CCN proteins: Multifunctional signaling regulators. Lancet. 2004;**363**:62-64

[144] Ponticos M, Holmes AM, Shi-wen X, Leoni P, Khan K, Rajkumar VS, Hoyles RK, Bou-Gharios G, Black CM, Denton CP, Abraham DJ, Leask A, Lindahl GE. Pivotal role of connective tissue growth factor in lung fibrosis: MAPK dependent transcriptional activation of type I collagen. Arthritis and Rheumatism. 2009;**60**:2142-2155

[145] Hoyles RK, et al. Fibroblast-specific perturbation of transforming growth factor β signaling provides insight into potential pathogenic mechanisms of scleroderma-associated lung fibrosis: Exaggerated response to alveolar epithelial injury in a novel mouse model. Arthritis and Rheumatism. 2008;**58**:1175-1188

[146] Christmann RB, Wells AU, Capelozzi VL, Silver RM. Gastroesophageal reflux incites interstitial lung disease in systemic sclerosis: Clinical, radiologic, histopathologic, and treatment evidence. Seminars in Arthritis and Rheumatism. 2010;**40**:241-249

[147] Walker N, et al. Resident tissue-specific mesenchymal progenitor cells contribute to fibrogenesis in human lung allografts. The American Journal of Pathology. 2011; **178**:2461-2469

[148] Hoyles RK, et al. An essential role for resident fibroblasts in experimental lung fibrosis is defined by lineage-specific deletion of high-affinity type II transforming growth factor β receptor. American Journal of Respiratory and Critical Care Medicine. 2011;**183**:249-261

[149] Borie R, et al. Detection of alveolar fibrocytes in idiopathic pulmonary fibrosis and systemic sclerosis. PLoS One. 2013;**8**:e53736. DOI: 10.1371/journal.pone.0053736 (published online: Jan 16, 2013)

[150] Nihtyanova SI, et al. Prediction of pulmonary complications and long-term survival in systemic sclerosis. Arthritis & Rhematology. 2014;**66**:1625-1635

[151] Wynn TA. Fibrotic disease and the TH1/TH2 paradigm. Nature Reviews. Immunology. 2004;**4**:583-594

[152] Wells AU, Lorimer S, Majumdar S, Harrison NK, Corrin B, Black CM, et al. Fibrosing alveolitis in systemic sclerosis: Increase in memory T-cells in lung interstitium. The European Respiratory Journal. 1995;**8**:266-271

[153] Yurovsky VY, Wigley FM, Wise RA, White B. Skewing of the CD8-T cell repertoire in the lungs of systemic sclerosis patients. Human Immunology. 1996;**48**:84-97

[154] Atamas SP, Yurovsky VV, Wise R, Wigley FM, Goter Robinson CJ, Henry P, et al. Production of type 2 cytokines by CD8+ lung cells is associated with greater decline in pulmonary function in patients with systemic sclerosis. Arthritis and Rheumatism. 1999;**42**:1168-1178

[155] Yamadori I, Fujita J, Kajitani H, Bandoh S, Tokuda M, Yang Y, et al. Lymphocyte subsets in lung tissues of non-specific interstitial pneumonia and pulmonary fibrosis associated with collagen vascular disorders: Correlation with CD4/CD8 ratio in bronchoalveolar lavage. Lung. 2000;**178**:361-370

[156] Luzina IG, Atamas SP, Wise R, Wigley FM, et al. Occurrence of an activated, profibrotic pattern of gene expression in lung CD8+ T cells from scleroderma patients. Arthritis and Rheumatism. 2003;**48**:2262-2274

[157] Radstake TR, van Bon L, Broen J, et al. Increased frequency and compromised function of T regulatory cells in systemic sclerosis (SSc) is related to a diminished CD69 and TGFbeta expression. PLoS One 2009; **4**(6): e5981–e5992. DOI: 10.1371/journal.pone.0005981

[158] Kolahian S, Fernandez IE, Eickelberg O, Hartl D. Immune mechanisms in pulmonary fibrosis. American Journal of Respiratory Cell and Molecular Biology. 2016;**55**:309-322

[159] Matsutani T, Yoshioka T, Tsuruta Y, et al. Analysis of TCRAV and TCRBV repertoires in healthy individuals by microplate hybridization assay. Human Immunology. 1997;**56**:57-69

[160] Hirokawa M, Matsutani T, Saitoh H, et al. Distinct TCRAV and TCRBV repertoire and CDR3 sequence of T lymphocytes clonally expanded in blood and GVHD lesions after human allogeneic bone marrow transplantation. Bone Marrow Transplantation. 2002;**30**:915-923

[161] Matsutani T, Ohashi Y, Yoshioka T, et al. Skew in T-cell receptor usage and clonal T-cell expansion in patients with chronic rejection of transplanted kidneys. Transplantation. 2003;**75**:398-407

[162] Lehmann PV, Sercarz EE, Forsthuber T, et al. Determinant spreading and the dynamics of the autoimmune T-cell repertoire. Immunology Today. 1993;**14**:203-208

[163] Englund P, Wahlstrom J, Fathi M, et al. Restricted T cell receptor BV gene usage in the lungs and muscles of patients with idiopathic inflammatory myopathies. Arthritis and Rheumatism. 2007;**56**:372-383

[164] Wucherpfennig KW, Ota K, Endo N, et al. Shared human T cell receptor Vβ usage to immunodominant regions of myelin basic protein. Science. 1990;**248**:1016-1019

[165] Kaushansky N, Kerlero de Rosbo N, Zilkha-Falb R, et al. Multi-epitope-targeted immune-specific therapy for a multiple sclerosis-like disease via engineered multi-epitope protein is superior to peptides. PLoS One. 2011;**6**:e27860. DOI: 10.1371/journal.pone.0027860 (published online: Nov 29, 2011)

[166] Rosas IO, Kaminski N. Update in diffuse parenchymal lung disease 2013. American Journal of Respiratory and Critical Care Medicine. 2015;**191**:270-274. DOI: 10.1164/rccm.201405-0856UP

[167] Haubitz M, Schellong S, Gobel U, Schurek HJ, Schaumann D, Koch KM, et al. Intravenous pulse administration of cyclophosphamide versus daily oral treatment in patients with antineutrophil cytoplasmic antibody-associated vasculitis and renal involvement: A prospective, randomized study. Arthritis and Rheumatism. 1998;**41**:1835-1844

[168] Tashkin DP, Elashoff R, Clements PJ, Roth MD, Furst DE, Silver RM, et al. Scleroderma Lung Study Research Group. Effects of 1-year treatment with cyclophosphamide on outcomes at 2 years in scleroderma lung disease. American Journal of Respiratory and Critical Care Medicine. 2007;**176**:1026-1034

[169] Poormoghim H, Moradi Lakeh M, et al. Cyclophosphamide for scleroderma lung disease: A systematic review and meta-analysis. Rheumatology International. 2012; **32**:2431-2444

[170] Giacomelli R, Liakouli V, Berardicurti O, Ruscitti P, Di Benedetto P, Carubbi F, Guggino G, Di Bartolomeo S, Ciccia F, Triolo G, Cipriani P. Interstitial lung disease in systemic sclerosis: Current and future treatment. Rheumatology International. 2017;**37**:853-863. DOI: 10.1007/s00296-016-3636-7

[171] Sem M, Molberg O, Lund MB, Gran JT. Rituximab treatment of the anti-synthetase syndrome: A retrospective case series. Rheumatology (Oxford). 2009;**48**:968-971

[172] Oddis CV, Reed AM, Aggarwal R, et al. RIM Study Group. Rituximab in the treatment of refractory adult and juvenile dermatomyositis and adult polymyositis: A randomized, placebo-phase trial. Arthritis and Rheumatism. 2013;**65**:314-324. DOI: 10.1002/art.37754

[173] Gruhn WB, Diaz-Buxo JA. Cyclosporine treatment of steroid resistant interstitial pneumonitis associated with dermatomyositis/polymyositis. The Journal of Rheumatology. 1987;**14**:1045-1047

[174] Maeda K, Kimura R, Komuta K, Igarashi T. Cyclosporine treatment for polymyositis/dermatomyositis: Is it possible to rescue the deteriorating cases with interstitial pneumonitis? Scandinavian Journal of Rheumatology. 1997;**26**(1):24-29

[175] Nawata Y, Kurasawa K, Takabayashi K, Miike S, Watanabe N, Hiraguri M, Kita Y, Kawai M, Saito Y, Iwamoto I. Corticosteroid resistant interstitial pneumonitis in dermatomyositis/polymyositis: Prediction and treatment with cyclosporine. The Journal of Rheumatology. 1999;**26**(7):1527-1533

[176] Harigai M, Hara M, Kamatani N, Kashiwazaki S. Nation-wide survey for the treatment with cyclosporin A of interstitial pneumonia associated with collagen diseases. Ryūmachi. 1999;**39**:819-828

[177] Nagasaka K, Harigai M, Tateishi M, Hara M, Yoshizawa Y, Koike T, Miyasaka N. Efficacy of combination treatment with cyclosporin A and corticosteroids for acute interstitial pneumonitis associated with dermatomyositis. Modern Rheumatology. 2003;**13**:231-238

[178] Takada K, Nagasaka K, Miyasaka N. Polymyositis/dermatomyositis and interstitial lung disease: A new therapeutic approach with T-cell-specific immunosuppressants. Autoimmunity. 2005;**38**(5):383-392

[179] Koreeda Y, Higashimoto I, Yamamoto M, Takahashi M, Kaji K, Fujimoto M, Kuwana M, Fukuda Y. Clinical and pathological findings of interstitial lung disease patients with anti-aminoacyl-t RNA synthetase autoantibodies. Internal Medicine. 2010;**49**(5):361-369

[180] Cavagna L, Caporali R, Abdi-Ali L, Dore R, Meloni F, Montecucco C. Cyclosporine in anti-Jo1-positive patients with corticosteroid-refractory interstitial lung disease. The Journal of Rheumatology. 2013;**40**:484-492

[181] Nagai K, Takeuchi T, Kotani T, Hata K, Yoshida S, Isoda K, Fujiki Y, Shiba H, Makino S, Hanafusa T. Therapeutic drug monitoring of cyclosporine microemulsion in interstitial pneumonia with dermatomyositis. Modern Rheumatology. 2011;**21**(1):32-36

[182] Oddis CV, Sciurba FC, Elmagd KA, Starzl TE. Tacrolimus in refractory polymyositis with interstitial lung disease. Lancet. 1999;**353**(9166):1762-1763

[183] Ochi S, Nanki T, Takada K, Suzuki F, Komano Y, Kubota T, Miyasaka N. Favorable outcomes with tacrolimus in two patients with refractory interstitial lung disease associated with polymyositis/dermatomyositis. Clinical and Experimental Rheumatology. 2005;**23**:707-710

[184] Wilkes MR, Sereika SM, Fertig N, Lucas MR, Oddis CV. Treatment of antisynthetase-associated interstitial lung disease with tacrolimus. Arthritis and Rheumatism. 2005; **52**(8):2439-2446

[185] Kurita T, Yasuda S, Oba K, Odani T, Kono M, Otomo K, Fujieda Y, Oku K, Bohgaki T, Amengual O, Horita T, Atsumi T. The efficacy of tacrolimus in patients with interstitial lung diseases complicated with polymyositis or dermatomyositis. Rheumatology (Oxford). 2015;**54**(1):39-44. DOI: 10.1093/rheumatology/keu166

[186] Kurita T, Yasuda S, Amengual O, Atsumi T. The efficacy of calcineurin inhibitors for the treatment of interstitial lung disease associated with polymyositis/dermatomyositis. Lupus. 2015;**24**:3-9. DOI: 10.1177/0961203314554849

[187] Suda M, Kataoka Y, Tomishima Y, Jinta T, Rokutanda R, Kishimoto M, Okada M. Effectiveness of multi-target therapy in anti-melanoma differentiation-associated gene 5 antibody-positive dermatomyositis with early-stage interstitial lung disease. Scandinavian Journal of Rheumatology. Jun 26, 2017:1-2. DOI: 10.1080/03009742.2017.1314004 (published online: Jun 26, 2017)

[188] Ishikawa H. Mizoribine and mycophenolate mofetil. Current Medicinal Chemistry. 1999;**6**:575-597

[189] Rokutanda R, Kishimoto M, Ohde S, Shimizu H, Nomura A, Suyama Y, Ohara Y, Yamaguchi K, Okada M. Safety and efficacy of mizoribine in patients with connective tissue diseases other than rheumatoid arthritis. Rheumatology International. 2014; **34**:59-62

[190] Nomura A, Shimizu H, Kishimoto M, Suyama Y, Rokutanda R, Ohara Y, Yamaguchi K, Okada M. Efficacy and safety of multitarget therapy with mizoribine and tacrolimus for systemic lupus erythematosus with or without active nephritis. Lupus. 2012; **21**:1444-1449

# Chapter 8

# Pneumonia of Viral Etiologies

Al Johani Sameera and Akhter Javed

Additional information is available at the end of the chapter

http://dx.doi.org/10.5772/intechopen.71608

**Abstract**

Pneumonia is a common illness that continues to cause significant morbidity and mortality in both adults and children. Bacteria such as *Streptococcus pneumonia, Staphylococcus aureus* and *Haemophilus influenzae* are generally considered as the main pathogens in community-acquired pneumonia and Legionella species, *Chlamydia pneumoniae* and *Mycoplasma pneumonia* in atypical pneumonias. In contrast the proportion of pneumonias due to viruses has been both difficult to detect and quantify with any precision. However, with the advent of powerful molecular techniques and rapidly developing technologies a greater number of viruses are being implicated as pathogens and co-pathogens in pneumonia. In the case of adults, the most commonly detected viruses are influenza virus, RSV and parainfluenza. Other viruses that have recently received considerable attention, are H5N1 influenza virus and coronaviruses. Infectious causes of pneumonia in immunocompromised patients include measles, HSV, CMV, HHV-6 and Influenza viruses. Pneumonias caused by other viruses are more rarely reported and include outbreaks of rhinovirus, adenovirus (particularly serotype 14 in military institutions), coronavirus, and metapneumovirus. A range of promising therapeutic targets have been identified and numerous innovative therapeutic treatments demonstrated to improve lung injury due to viral infections.

**Keywords:** pneumonia, etiology, viruses, diagnosis, treatment

## 1. Introduction

Pneumonia was once known as Winter Fever and is an acute infection and inflammation of the lung parenchyma. It was first described by Hippocrates around 460 BC [1] . However, it wasn't until the 19th century that pneumonia was established as a true infection, and not just a symptom of other diseases. Edwin Klebs a German pathologist in 1875 observed bacteria under a microscope in cases of pneumonia [2]. Then, Carl Friedlander and Albert Frankel in

INTECH
open science | open minds

© 2017 The Author(s). Licensee InTech. This chapter is distributed under the terms of the Creative Commons Attribution License (http://creativecommons.org/licenses/by/3.0), which permits unrestricted use, distribution, and reproduction in any medium, provided the original work is properly cited.

1884 and 1884 respectively identified two of the most common bacterial causes of pneumonia, *Streptococcus pneumoniae* and *Klebsiella pneumonia* [3]. By the 1930s, treatment for pneumonia had been developed with the introduction of penicillin playing a key role.

Pneumonia remains the leading cause of childhood mortality under the age of 5 and the most common reason for adult hospitalisation in low and middle income countries, despite advances in preventative and management strategies [4]. Pneumonia usually causes symptoms for 3–4 weeks, and daily activities may be impaired for a further 3 weeks on average. Community-acquired pneumonia (CAP) refers to pneumonia acquired outside of hospitals or extended-care facilities. Nosocomial pneumonia and hospital-acquired pneumonia describe infections acquired in the hospital setting. These are usually defined as pneumonia that occurs 48 h or more after hospital admission, and which was not incubating at the time of admission. Community-acquired pneumonia continues to be a significant health issue [5]. Annually in the United States there are around 4 million cases of which 20% of cases may require hospitalization. As a result there are more than 65 million days of reduced activity overall. Mortality rates can range from 1 to 30% making it the sixth leading cause of death [6]. In developing countries pneumonia is either the first or second leading cause of death. In Europe, around 14.4 per 10,000 children aged over 5 years and 33.8 per 10,000 under 5 years are diagnosed with CAP. CAP is more common in the developing world, estimated at 0.28 episodes per child per year and accounting for 95% of all cases [7].

## 2. Pathophysiology

Pneumonia is an inflammatory process in lung parenchyma most commonly caused by bacteria and viruses. Less common etiologies include mycoplasma, fungi and parasites. Organisms spread to the lungs through aerosolization, aspiration, or hematogenous spread due to inhalation of droplet or by aspiration of fluids in the oropharynx [8] Pneumonia results if host defense mechanisms are unable to keep the respiratory network infection free. The pathophysiology varies depending on etiology. In the case of bacterial pneumonia there is an intra-alveolar suppurative exudate with consolidation [9].

In the case of viral pneumonia there is an inflammatory interstitial inflammation with infiltrate in the alveolar, causing damage to ciliated epithelium surfaces. The lungs become congested, hemorrhagic and Intracellular viral inclusions may form. Local host defenses, such as mucociliary clearance, or secretion of specific secretory IgA antibodies can remove some of the virus particles. However, if mucociliary clearance is impaired or secretory anti-influenza IgA antibodies are absent, infection continues to spread. Respiratory epithelial cells are invaded, and viral replication occurs. Newer viruses then infect larger numbers of epithelial cells, shut off the synthesis of critical proteins, and ultimately lead to host cell death [10].

There can be numerous types of immune response depending on how cytokine is produced. For example, cell-mediated immunity is initiated in type 1, while type 2 cytokines are responsible for allergic responses. Children infected with respiratory syncytial virus (RSV) with more serious acute bronchiolitis often have impaired type 1 immunity or augmented type 2 immunity [11].

Respiratory viruses such as RSV or rhinovirus that damage the respiratory tract cause release of multiple humoral factors, including leukotriene C4, and histamine. In the case of RSV virus-specific immunoglobulin E is released. Rhinovirus infections can cause release of bradykinin, interleukin 1, interleukin 6, and interleukin 8. A further complication of RSV infections is that they can increase bacterial adherence to respiratory epithelium, impair mucociliary clearance, and cause changes in bacterial phagocytosis by host cells [12].

In co infections, secondary bacterial superinfection makes for a poor prognosis of the original viral infection [13]. Interleukin-10, is purported to attract large numbers of macrophages and neutrophils to the lung. The presence of these cytokines increases the immune response, causing inflammatory damage and preventing the proper removal of bacteria.

## 3. Epidemiology

Numerous studies by the WHO have estimated there are over 450 million cases of pneumonia globally with approximately 3 million deaths particularly prone are the elderly and children [14]. The annual rate of CAP increases from 6/1000 in the 18–39 age group to 34/1000 in 75 years and over age group. Incident rates tend to be higher in colder climates of the North and hospitalization is required in 20–40% cases. In severe cases mortality can vary from 5 to 10% of cases [15] .

Viral pneumonias are common in the Mideast. In an Iranian study viruses causing pneumonia were Influenza A (7.4%), influenza B (3.5%), RSV (12.9%), and adenovirus (5.9%). Parainfluenza-1,2 and 3 were 6.4, 6.4 and 15.8% respectively [16]. More recently, avian influenza has become endemic in some parts of the Middle East, especially Egypt and Turkey [17].

WHO data published in May 2014 Influenza and Pneumonia Deaths in Saudi Arabia reached 5689 or 7.08% of total deaths. The age adjusted death rate is 44.89 per 100,000 of population [18]. Middle East respiratory syndrome is caused by a novel coronavirus (MERS-CoV) first isolated in the Kingdom of Saudi Arabia in 2012 from the respiratory tract secretions of a Saudi businessman who died from viral pneumonia [19]. Subsequently, cases were identified in patients living outside the Arabian Peninsula and the Middle East, who were infected either during a stay in the Middle East or by close contact with an individual from an endemic country. Most affected patients were previously healthy men with a median age of 50 years [20]. In 2016, the World Health Organization (WHO) published a report on 1698 laboratory-confirmed cases of MERS-CoV infection. The mortality rate was 36%. All cases were directly or indirectly linked through residence or travel to Saudi Arabia, the UAE, Jordan, Qatar, Oman, Lebanon, Kuwait, Yemen, Egypt, and Iran. There were also reports of sporadic reports in other countries including the United Kingdom, France, Malaysia, Tunisia, Italy, Austria, Greece, Turkey, the United States of America, Germany, Philippines, and Thailand [21]. The largest outbreak of the virus outside its endemic region was recorded in 2015, in South Korea. One-hundred and eighty-six additional cases were confirmed, including the first in China, with a total of 36 deaths. MERS-CoV is a zoonotic virus that can lead to secondary human infections. Dromedary camels are considered as the intermediate host, with closely related virus sequences in bats. Human-to-human transmission has been noted in households and health care setting. But community-wide transmission has not been observed [22].

### 3.1. Pneumonia in children

The World Health Organization (WHO) established the Child Health Epidemiology Reference Group (CHERG) to monitor the incidence of childhood [23]. In 2000, CHERG compiled pneumonia statistics in children under age 5. It was found that there were 150 million new cases of pneumonia in children under 5. Of these, approximately 4 million occurred in developed countries, while the majority occurred in developing nations [24]. Hospitalization rates for pneumonia were approximately 9%. More than half of all worldwide cases of childhood pneumonia occurred in just five countries: India, China, Pakistan, Indonesia, Nigeria and Bangladesh. Europe had the lowest rate (0.06 episodes per child-year), while Southeast Asia and Africa had the highest overall incidence rates (0.36 and 0.33 episodes per child-year, respectively). Factors that increased the risk of developing childhood pneumonia included low birth weight, malnutrition, crowded living quarters, indoor air pollution, insufficient breast feeding, and lack of vaccinations. Other possible contributing factors included pre-existing medical conditions such as asthma, and annual rainfall levels. Also, parents who smoked and lack of parent education [25].

### 3.2. Pneumonia in adults

Pneumonia is a serious concern in adults and viruses cause 15–30% of cases in immunocompetent adults hospitalized with pneumonia [26]. Increased rates of pneumonia-associated hospitalizations have been reported in the United States, Denmark, United Kingdom, and the Netherlands. In 2010, approximately 1.1 million patients in the USA were hospitalized for pneumonia with an average length of hospital stay 5.2 days [27]. In the UK, the number of hospitalizations due to pneumonia increased by 34% during the period from 1997 to 2005. This was particularly notable in older adults. Approximately 26,000 people died from pneumonia and influenza in England and Wales in 2013 according to national statistics. Contributing factors may be due to other chronic diseases such as heart disease, diabetes, and immunocompromised patients [28].

## 4. Atypical pneumonia

Atypical pneumonia refers to pneumonia caused by atypical bacteria, including *Legionella* species, *Chlamydia pneumoniae* and *Mycoplasma pneumoniae* [29]. It is called "atypical" because the symptoms and signs differ from those of pneumonia due to other common organisms. It is generally regarded that *M. pneumoniae, Legionella* spp., *C. pneumoniae, Chlamydophila psittaci and Coxiella burnetii* are the key CAP pathogens not readily identified by standard culture methods [30]. Other atypical pathogens include viruses, atypical mycobacteria, *Francisella tularensis* and an extensive list of agents of bioterrorism.

### 4.1. Organisms that cause atypical pneumonias include

*Mycoplasman pneumoniae,* the most common atypical pneumonia organism spreads when someone carrying the infection comes in close contact with others. The condition, also known as "walking pneumonia," is generally mild and seen in the outpatient setting. It appears to occur mostly in school-aged children and young adults. Less common is *Chlamydia pneumoniae* which causes 10% of all CAP cases and is usually mild but usually more severe in the elderly [31]. *Legionella pneumophila* causes Legionnaires' disease commonly found in hotels, cruise ships, hospitals and commercial buildings, where people come into contact with contaminated droplets from cooling towers and evaporative condensers. Other reports of infection have been noted near whirlpools and saunas [32]. It is believed the organism causes up to 4% of all pneumonia cases. Known viral causes of atypical pneumonia include respiratory syncytial virus (RSV), influenza A and B, parainfluenza, adenovirus, severe acute respiratory syndrome (SARS) and measles [33].

## 5. Viral pneumonia

The advent of molecular diagnostics has greatly improved the identification of viruses in patients with CAP. Over the last decade, several studies have used PCR to establish the importance of viruses in the etiology of CAP. Globally, it is estimated that 200 million cases of viral pneumonia occur annually. Most commonly are influenza viruses (A and B), parainfluenza viruses 1, 2 and 3, rhinoviruses, and coronaviruses [34].

Viral pneumonia prevails mostly in young children and older adults. Etiologies include influenza, adenovirus, parainfluenza, H1N1 and respiratory syncytial virus (RSV). Influenza A and B occurs in the winter and spring. Symptoms include, headache, fever, and muscle aches. Respiratory syncytial virus (RSV) is most common in the spring and infects young children. Adenovirus and parainfluenza viral pneumonias exhibit cold symptoms (runny nose and conjunctivitis). Post-influenza pneumonia is often accompanied by secondary bacterial infection due to *Staphylococcus pneumoniae* and *Staphylococcus aureus.* Pneumonia in immunocompromised patients is attributed to measles, HSV, CMV, HHV-6 and Influenza viruses. There is also an increased risk of secondary bacterial lower respiratory tract infection (LRTI). The known complication following influenza infection is *Staphylococcus aureus* pneumonia [35].

Respiratory syncytial virus (RSV) has been identified as an important cause of pneumonia in adults, especially in the elderly. The rate of RSV, overall is between 2 and 5% throughout the year and between 5 and 14% during winter. Adults with severe immunodeficiency are at particular risk of severe RSV infection [36].

Viral pneumonia infections include both DNA and RNA viruses. Some are well-known lung pathogens that produce common clinical and radiologic manifestations. Others are rarely involved as lung pathogens. Many viruses can cause pneumonia, either directly or indirectly. They include:

### 5.1. Adenoviruses

Adenoviruses are enveloped DNA viruses and a diverse group that cause a wide spectrum of clinical illnesses. At least 52 serotypes exist, classified into 7 subgroups or species (A-G). Adenovirus pneumonia typically is limited to newborns, immunocompromised hosts, and school or military camp populations. Severe adenovirus pneumonia has been more commonly described in immunocompromised patients. Respiratory infection in immunocompetent patients is usually self-limited and mild [37]. However, with advances in molecular techniques, adenovirus has been increasingly discovered to be involved in sporadic cases and in severe CAP in healthy adults. Pulmonary disease is predominantly caused by serotypes 1, 2, 3, 4, 5, 7, 14, and 21. Adenovirus infection accounts for up to 20% of childhood pneumonias, primarily in those children younger than 5 years of age, but such pneumonias occur infrequently in the non-military adult population. Types 4 and 7 viruses can cause outbreaks of respiratory disease in military recruits, whereas Type 7 viruses can cause bronchiolitis and pneumonia in infants. A virulent strain of Adenovirus, serotype 14 (subgroup B) has been reported to cause greater symptoms of respiratory illness and pneumonia. It was first observed in 2005 among civilian and military populations. Outbreaks occurred subsequently at military academies throughout the United States and in the Pacific Northwest [38].

### 5.2. Coronavirus

Coronaviruses are from the family Coronaviridae and are single-stranded RNA viruses. As the name indicates the surface is covered by crown like projections. This virus is spread via droplet and fomite exposure. Coronaviruses were not thought to significantly cause pneumonia until recently. However, the severe acute respiratory syndrome (SARS) pandemic in 2003 brought the ability of this virus to cause life-threatening pneumonia to worldwide attention.

There are six human coronaviruses (HCoVs) that are established human pathogens with world-wide distribution, causing upper and lower respiratory tract infections: HCoV-229E, OC43, HKU1, NL63, MERS-COV (Middle East respiratory syndrome) and SARS-COV (severe acute respiratory syndrome) [39].

MERS-COV was first identified in Saudi Arabia in September 2012, approximately 2000 MERS-CoV cases have been detected in over 20 countries. The newly reported cases lift Saudi Arabia's MERS-CoV total since the virus was first detected in humans in 2012 to 1598 cases, 661 of them fatal and the majority of MERS-CoV cases continue to be reported from the Middle East. The source of the virus has remained a mystery but transmission and virological studies point toward dromedary camels in the Middle East by which humans may become infected through zoonotic transmission. Human-to-human transmission is then exacerbated through close household contacts and in healthcare settings [40].

### 5.3. Cytomegalovirus

Cytomegalovirus (CMV) is a herpesvirus that is a common cause of infections. In hosts who are immunocompetent, acute CMV infection causes a mononucleosis-like syndrome. CMV pneumonia may occur and is often fatal in immunocompromised individuals, primarily hematopoietic stem cell transplant (HSCT) and solid organ transplant (SOT) recipients. The severity of pneumonia is related to the extent of immunosuppression [41]. CMV pneumonia has a prevalence of 15% and a mortality rate of approximately 85% in cancer patients receiving allogeneic bone marrow transplants. The major risk factor for CMV pneumonia in these patients is acute graft-versus-host disease.

Pneumonia is the most common presentation of CMV disease following lung transplantation CMV infection in lung transplant recipients is approximately 50%. Lung is a CMV latency site and viral reactivation has been associated with direct systemic infection and indirect effects such as acute rejection. The risk of CMV infections in these cases is dependent on the immunosuppressive therapy and serologic status of the donor and recipient.

Moreover CMV pneumonia is identified to be a predictive factor for the later development of chronic rejection in lung transplant. Several studies have been carried to find the optimal preventive strategy to avoid CMV infection after lung transplantation. An effective treatment strategy has been valganciclovir prophylaxis for at least 180 days following combined prophylaxis together with ganciclovir and CMV-immune globulin (CMV-IG) [42].

### 5.4. Epstein-Barr virus

Epstein-Barr virus (EBV) is well-known to be transmitted through infected saliva. The virus can cause pneumonia without mononucleosis. Lung involvement secondary to EBV infections usually only occurs in immunocompromised people. However, in 25% of pediatric patients with HIV infection, the virus can cause lesions due to lymphocytic interstitial pneumonia or pulmonary lymphoid hyperplasia.

Infectious mononucleosis occurs in young adults aged 15–30 years and usually resolves without *sequelae*. This disorder may cause chronic tiredness and fevers but can also be complicated by life-threatening problems. Pulmonary involvement associated with Epstein-Barr virus infection is uncommon but can occur as a complication of infectious mononucleosis. Pathologically, mononuclear inflammatory cells are evident along interlobular septa in interstitial pulmonary infiltrates [43].

### 5.5. Herpes simplex virus

Herpes simplex virus (HSV) is primarily implicated in severely immunocompromised patients primarily, e.g., solid organ transplant recipients, patients who are undergoing chemotherapy or are neutropenic, or those who have congenital immunodeficiency. Herpes simplex virus is spread by viral shedding from asymptomatic excreters or from active lesions. It is a rare cause of lower respiratory tract infections. HSV pneumonia can occur as a secondary infection to upper airway infection or following viremia due to genital or oral lesions [44]. Herpes simplex virus can also cause pneumonia in compromised hosts, with a mortality rate of 80%.

Herpes simplex virus type 1 pneumonia is relatively uncommon that generally affects patients who are immunocompromised. It often occurs as a polymicrobial infection and is frequently associated with coexisting bacterial pneumonia. Pneumonia is usually characterized by a proteinaceous exudate and alveolar necrosis. There is a variable polymorphonuclear inflammatory response [45].

### 5.6. Human metapneumovirus

Human metapneumovirus (hMPV) is in the Paramyxoviridae family and was initially described in the Netherlands in 2001 [46]. It is a pleomorphic-shaped virus with protein projections from the surface. hMPV is a ubiquitous organism and almost all children have been exposed to it by age 5 years, Morbidity in lower respiratory tract infections in children and infants was reported to bronchiolitis (59%), croup (18%), asthma (14%), and pneumonia (8%) [47]. Reinfection continues to occur throughout life. The virus is spread via droplet and fomite exposure.

The severity of infection increases with older age and with complications such as immunosuppressive conditions or cardiopulmonary disease. Adult hospitalizations with hMPV infection are associated with chronic obstructive pulmonary disease (COPD) exacerbations, pneumonia and bronchitis. Severe pneumonitis requiring intensive care is required in immunocompromised hosts (e.g., hematologic malignancies).

### 5.7. Influenza virus

The influenza viruses are RNA viruses in the family Orthomyxoviridae, they are enveloped, single-stranded, and are the most common viral cause of pneumonia. Influenza has three serotypes A, B, and C. Influenza type A can infect livestock allowing a reservoir for infection and opportunity for epidemics in humans. For this reason it is usually the most virulent pathogen. The structure of influenza virus includes two envelope glycoproteins, known as hemagglutinin (H) and neuraminidase (N).The hemagglutinin enables infectivity of the virus by attaching to cellular sialic acid residues, whereas the N protein allows spread of the virus to other cells through cleavage of the new virus. Severe pneumonia complications can occur in high-risk individuals [48]. Two influenza types have emerged of particular importance: H5N1 avian influenza strain and the novel H1N1 swine influenza strain. In the influenza A (H1N1) pandemic of 2009–2010, the World Health Organization estimated approximately 16,000 deaths. The majority of these deaths corresponded to patients with underlying risk factors contributing to worse outcomes Influenza type B causes illness seems to occur more in closed populations, e.g., boarding schools. Influenza type C is less common and occurs as sporadic cases [49].

### 5.8. Measles virus

Measles is a respiratory tract virus that causes a febrile illness with rash in children and a mild pneumonia in healthy adults. It is a single-stranded RNA virus in the Paramyxoviridae family and the genus *Morbillivirus*. It comprises a nucleocapsid surrounded by an envelope. Measles is a highly contagious disease that results from infection with measles virus and is still responsible for more than 100,000 deaths every year [50]. Measles virus is transmitted by the respiratory route and illness begins with fever, cough, coryza. Complications of measles affect most organ systems, with pneumonia accounting for most measles-associated morbidity and mortality.

Pulmonary disease from measles virus infection can occur as a primary measles virus pneumonia with secondary bacterial pneumonia or as an atypical measles virus pneumonia. Measles virus can cause pneumonia in 3–4% of infected patients mostly with secondary bacterial infection such as Haemophilus influenzae and Neisseria meningitides. The prevalence of measles virus pneumonia is higher in immunocompromised patients and pregnant women. Measles virus pneumonia without a secondary bacterial infection appears with diffuse alveolar damage and epithelial hyperplasia. Epithelial hyperplasia is seen in bronchioles and peribronchial alveoli as well as in the tracheobronchial epithelium with cystic dilatation of mucous glands. Histologically, measles virus pneumonia displays multinucleated giant cells containing up to 50 nuclei within the bronchiolar and tracheobronchial epithelium [51].

### 5.9. Parainfluenza virus

Parainfluenza virus (PIV) consists of nucleocapsids, which propagate in the cytoplasm of infected cells, with hemagglutinin present in the virion envelope. PIV is a common virus infection of childhood. PIV is second in importance to only RSV in causing children pneumonia and bronchiolitis in infants younger than 6 months and lower respiratory tract disease. Transmission is through direct contact or large-droplet spread.

Although there are four subtypes of PIV, PIV types 1 and 2 tend to peak during the fall season where as type 3 is endemic year-round. Recurrent upper or lower respiratory tract infections occur throughout life because Immunity is short term. The infections vary from a self-limiting illness to life-threatening pneumonia especially in immunocompromised hosts leading to lung injury and respiratory failure [52]. In one study, hematopoietic stem cell transplant (HSCT) patients with PIV progressed to develop pneumonia. Of 44% of these patients with pneumonia there was a mortality rate of 37% [53].

### 5.10. Respiratory syncytial virus

Respiratory syncytial virus (RSV) consists of only one serotype and is in the Paramyxoviridae family. Structurally, it consists of 10 viral polypeptides, 4 of which are associated with virus envelope, and 2 of these (F and G) are important for infectivity and pathogenicity. RSV is highly contagious, spreading via droplet and fomite exposure. RSV is the most frequent cause of lower respiratory tract infections among infants and children and the second most common viral cause of pneumonia in adults [54]. The majority of children are infected by the age of 5 years in settings such as daycare centers but the resulting immunity is incomplete. Reinfection when it occurs in older children and young adults is mild. But, with advancing age there is a greater likelihood severe disease and pneumonia. Diagnosed adult RSV hospitalizations have increased significantly in the United States. Respiratory syncytial virus hospitalizations appear to be greater in severity than influenza hospitalizations, especially immunocompromised and in older adults [55].

### 5.11. Rhinovirus

Many reports from the literature report that rhinovirus accounts for approximately 30% of cases of all virus-related pneumonia. Rhinovirus is considered the second most frequently recognized agent associated with pneumonia and bronchiolitis in the young. The virus is associated with asthma hospitalizations in both old and young patients [56].

Rhinovirus is genetically diverse with more than 100 serotypes identified. In addition to common colds, reports have suggested that rhinovirus is associated with bronchiolitis, bronchitis, pneumonia and acute asthma exacerbation. Rhinovirus has been detected by molecular methods in 10–30% of hospitalized children with lower respiratory tract infections. Rhinovirus is also considered to be the second most common cause of bronchiolitis after respiratory syncytial virus (RSV) [57]. Rhinoviruses have long been known to cause common colds and exacerbations of Chronic obstructive pulmonary disease (COPD), but because rhinoviruses grow poorly at 37°C lower respiratory tract infections were thought to be rare. However, it has been demonstrated that rhinoviruses can replicate at body temperature and infect cells of the lower respiratory tract. Molecular studies have consistently identified rhinoviruses in nasopharyngeal or pharyngeal specimens from children and adults with lower respiratory tract infections. Rhinovirus has also been detected in 2–17% of adults and 4–45% of children with CAP [58].

### 5.12. Varicella-zoster virus

Varicella-zoster virus (VZV) is a highly contagious herpes virus and primary infection manifests as chickenpox. The reactivation in later life results in zoster (shingles). It is spread by the respiratory route or direct contact with skin lesions. This pneumonia is rare in otherwise healthy children but does occur in immunocompromised children causing life-threatening complications [59]. VZV-related community-acquired pneumonia (VZV-CAP) has become increasingly recognized as a very serious and life-threatening complication invasive mechanical ventilation in more than half of the cases. Complications include secondary bacterial infections, encephalitis, hepatitis, and, with concomitant aspirin use, Reye syndrome. VZV pneumonia also tends be more severe in individuals who smoke. In fatal cases of pneumonia, laboratory findings include extensive alveolar hemorrhage, pulmonary edema and mononuclear cell infiltration with histological evidence of intranuclear inclusion bodies.

Varicella-zoster virus pneumonia is a serious complication of disseminated varicella-zoster virus infection with mortality rates of 9–50%. In adults prevalence of varicella-zoster virus pneumonia has varied from 5 to 50% of all varicella infections. Varicella-zoster virus is a self-limited benign disease in children known as chickenpox. But in adults it causes significant complications such as varicella-zoster virus pneumonia and over 90% of cases occur in patients with lymphoma and immunocompromised patients. Patients exhibit diffuse alveolar damage, spherical nodules are seen throughout the lung parenchyma. The nodules are composed of an outer fibrous capsule enclosing areas of necrotic tissue [60].

### 5.13. Zoonotic viral pneumonias

Zoonotic viral pneumonias include those caused by avian influenza, hantavirus, severe acute respiratory syndrome (SARS), and H1N1 (swine) influenza. In 1997, an influenza virus (H5N1 virus) which normally only infects only birds was found to infect humans In Hong Kong. Manifestations included pneumonia, which in some cases led to fatal acute respiratory distress syndrome (ARDS) or multisystem organ failure. The rising incidence and widespread reporting of disease from H5N1 influenza viruses can probably be attributed to the increasing spread of the virus from existing reservoirs in domestic waterfowl and live bird markets, leading to greater environmental contamination [61]. Recombinations of viruses in animals are a global concern. The H5N1 outbreak in Southeast Asia, H3N2 variant in the USA in 2012, and H7N9 avian cases in China 2013 are examples of such new threats. Effective surveillance is required to monitor such developments [62].

There is a growing danger that in the future avian influenza, a subtype of influenza A, may result in a worldwide pandemic. A/H5N1 exhibits several serious characteristics, such as increased virulence and human-to-human transmission in some cases, rather than bird-to-human transmission. The disease causes high morbidity and mortality due to pneumonia and respiratory failure [63].

H1N1 was first reported in Mexico and spread to the United States. The infection from a novel swine-origin influenza A (H1N1) virus rapidly spread to become a worldwide pandemic in 2009. Virus-associated hemophagocytic syndrome may play an important role in development of multiorgan failure and ensuing death in H1N1 infection [64].

SARS is a respiratory infection caused by a coronavirus, which appears to have jumped from animals to humans. The disease was first reported in China in 2003 and rapidly spread from to the rest of the world in a 1 year period. It resulted in more than 8000 patients in 29 countries causing 774 deaths [65].

### 5.14. Co-infections

Co-infection Infections involving both respiratory bacteria and viruses or are common. Viral infection usually occurs first, followed by a secondary bacterial infection, as observed in the influenza pandemics of 1918, 1957, and 1968 where most deaths occurred due to secondary bacterial infection. In some infections however, especially H5N1 avian influenza, the associated pneumonia appears to be caused by direct viral action.

Co-infections are particularly common in 45% of children with CAP, and mainly involve pneumococcus [66], Mycoplasma pneumoniae and several species of *Chlamydophila*. CAP of mixed etiology has been characterized less in adults than in children, and prevalence is estimated at less than 5%. The most common combinations reported are pneumococcus with rhinovirus or influenza A virus [67].

## 6. Laboratory testing

Laboratory diagnosis of viral pneumonia has relied on detection of virus or viral antigen in upper-respiratory specimens (e.g., nasopharyngeal aspirates) and lower respiratory samples (e.g., induced sputum) by culture or immunofluorescence microscopy.

Traditional microbiological methods for detection of respiratory tract pathogens are relatively slow, often are not sensitive and are influenced by previous antibiotic therapy. Molecular diagnostics on the other hand hold much potential for detection of both common and atypical pathogens causing CAP. Analysis can be completed in hours, rather than days, for detection of typical pathogens and weeks for detection of atypical pathogens [68].

There are >200 known respiratory viruses, but accurate data on how many are etiological agents in CAP are lacking. The discovery of 6 new respiratory viruses since 2000—including metapneumovirus (hMPV), the severe acute respiratory syndrome coronavirus, influenza virus strain H5N1, coronavirus strains NL63 and Hku1, and human bocavirus—has presented new challenges for comprehensive viral diagnostics [69]. The significance of respiratory viral infections in patients with sepsis is underestimated. During the winter season, viral such as coronavirus, influenza A virus, human metapneumovirus, and respiratory syncytial virus are clinically underdiagnosed in 70% of patients detected by the multiplex PCR assay [70].

Quantitative multiplex PCR testing of respiratory secretions is recognized as a highly sensitive method for the diagnosis with the ability to detect viral pathogens and atypical bacterial pathogens. An acute viral infection can be confirmed with detection of influenza virus, parainfluenza virus, RSV, or hMPV. The presence of nucleic acid from adenoviruses, bocaviruses, coronaviruses or rhinoviruses is often found in asymptomatic persons. In the future the study of the virus concentration over time will contribute to distinguishing acute infections from protracted nucleic acid excretion [71].

## 7. Treatment

Antiviral drugs have been developed targeting viral proteins that can be inhibited by small molecular receptors or larger biotherapeutics. Consequently, most approved antiviral drugs are highly specific for a particular virus or family of viruses (e.g., neuraminidase inhibitors and adamantanes for influenza). The benefits of this approach are that there is greater selectivity and may lower the risk of adverse host effects. The disadvantages are that there is a limited antiviral spectrum, and greater risk of antiviral resistance [72].

Treatment of Influenza Virus Neuraminidase, is essential interrupting intercellular viral propagation. Selective inhibitors, e.g., oseltamivir, peramivir, and zanamivir have been used to prevent infection during the first 24–72 hours, improving clinical symptoms and reducing morbidity and mortality. Reductions in the incidence of pneumonia in patients has been observed in numerous studies who received treatment in the early stages of infection [73].

http://dx.doi.org/10.5772/intechopen.71608

| Virus family | Virus | Morphology | Treatment | Prevention | Seasonality |
|---|---|---|---|---|---|
| Adenoviridae | Adenoviruses | 90–100 nm, non-envelope, icosahedral nucleocapsid, double-stranded DNA | Cidofovir and brincidofovir | Hand hygiene, oral vaccine for military recruits | All year |
| Coronaviridae | (Coronaviruses)—SARS, MERS | 75–160 nm, envelope, helical, nucleocapsid, ssRNA (positive sense) | Supportive therapy | Preventive measures, e.g., hand hygiene | Winter |
| Bunyaviridae | (Arboviruses)—Hantavirus | 90–100 nm, envelope spherical virions. RNA- single stranded | Supportive therapy | Preventive measures, e.g., limit vector breeding | Widespread, all year |
| Herpesviridae | Herpes simplex virus 1 (HSV-1) herpes simplex virus 2 (HSV-2), herpesvirus 6, herpesvirus 7, and herpesvirus 8 Varicella-zoster virus (VZV), Cytomegalovirus (CMV), Epstein-Barr virus (EBV) | 130-300 nm, enveloped, double-stranded DNA | Acyclovir, ganciclovir, and foscarnet | V-Z immunoglobulin<br>Intravenous immunoglobulin<br>Vaccine | All year |
| Orthomyxoviridae | (Orthomyxoviruses)—Influenza A,B virus, H1N1 | 200–300 nm enveloped pleomorphic RNA single stranded | Oseltamivir, peramivir, zanamivir, amantadine, and rimantadine | Influenza vaccine chemoprophylaxis | End of autumn and winter |
| Papovaviridae | (Polyomavirus)—JC virus, BK virus | 18–28 nm non-envelope Icosahedral DNA single strand | Limited treatments, surgical removal | Vaccines, e.g., Gardasil, Cervarix | All year |
| Paramyxoviridae | (Paramyxoviruses)—parainfluenza virus, respiratory syncytial virus (RSV), human metapneumovirus (hMPV), measles virus | 150–200 nm, enveloped helical symmetry RNA-negative strand | Ribavirin protease inhibitors (e.g., lopinavir/ritonavir)<br>Ribavirin | Preventive measures, measles vaccination for immune serum immunoglobulin | End of autumn, beginning of winter |
| Picornaviridae | (Picornaviruses)—enteroviruses, coxsackievirus, echovirus, enterovirus 71, rhinovirus | 20–30 nm non-envelope cubic symmetry RNA-positive strand | Pleconaril | Alfa interferon (intranasal) | All year |

| Virus family | Virus | Morphology | Treatment | Prevention | Seasonality |
|---|---|---|---|---|---|
| Retroviridae | (Retroviruses)—human immunodeficiency virus (HIV), human lymphotropic virus type 1 (HTLV-1) | 80–100 nm envelope helical RNA-single strand | Nucleoside reverse transcriptase inhibitors (NRTIs), protease inhibitor (PI), non-nucleoside reverse transcriptase inhibitor (NNRTI) | Education, preventive measures | All year |

**Table 1.** Characteristic features of viral pathogens causing pneumonia.

Laninamivir octanoate, a new neuraminidase inhibitor administered by inhalation, can be effective in the treatment of IV infection, including oseltamivir-resistant strains. They are exclusively specific to influenza virus type A. However, side effects and rapid development of resistances, has meant that they have fallen into disuse. Immunomodulators are also being studied for reducing viral-mediated inflammation and its effect on the host [74].

Ribavirin has shown effectiveness in the management of acute episodes of pneumonia or for improving respiratory parameters during recovery. Meta-analysis studies performed in children, indicated that inhaled ribavirin can reduce hospital stay and time on ventilator times during pneumonia, however, the overall mortality rates are not affected. Ribavirin has also been used in severely immunocompromised patients, e.g., lung transplant recipients with positive outcomes. General use of bronchodilators, antibiotics, or corticosteroids are not recommended in the American pediatric guidelines for SRV bronchiolitis [75].

Acyclovir (Zovirax), inhibits viral DNA synthesis by competitively binding to viral DNA polymerase. Due to poor absorption, intravenous acyclovir at a dosage of 250 $mg/m^2$ every 8 hours is currently the treatment of choice for HSV pneumonia. The dosage of acyclovir should be decreased in patients with underlying renal insufficiency. Adverse reactions are infrequent, but renal impairment secondary to precipitation of acyclovir in the tubules can occur in 5–10% of patients if not properly rehydrated. Having a proven HSV pneumonia appears to be associated with high morbidity in solid tumor patients. This group of patients have been shown to benefit from acyclovir therapy [76]. There is little doubt that intravenous acyclovir is beneficial in the rare cases of varicella-zoster pneumonia in immunocompromised patients.

Supportive treatment was only available for other respiratory viruses until recently, However, some antiviral drugs are currently under investigation. Cidofovir is an acyclic nucleoside phosphonate analog of cytidine monophosphate. Upon conversion to its diphosphate form it leads to viral DNA chain termination. Limitations of cidofovir include poor cellular uptake and nephrotoxicity. Brincidofovir, a derivative of cidofovir which is active against double-stranded DNA viruses, is a major improvement in anti-adenovirus therapy [77]. Lung transplant recipients with metapneumovirus infections have been treated with success using intravenous ribavirin. Rhinovirus and Enterovirus, have been successfully used in limited studies using Pleconaril, which is incorporated into the virus capsid (**Table 1**) [78].

## 8. Prevention

Measures in infectious infection control, particularly of the respiratory tract, involve using barrier methods preventing infection. Use of gloves, masks and hand-washing have been shown to be effective in reducing transmission rates in the health care centers. Isolation of patients during the clinical phase of the disease is also strongly recommended and reduces overall incidence. Immunization plays a very important role in prevention, but is only available for a few viruses. As the population ages and rates of pneumonia increase. Hospitalizations for pneumonia will continue to show an upward trend unless effective intervention strategies are devised and implemented. This includes recommending immunization with PPV and annual influenza vaccinations. Although the effectiveness of these vaccines decreases with age and comorbid conditions [79].

## 9. Future strategies

Vaccines are still considered the great hope in disease prevention and control strategies. However, among respiratory viruses there has been little progress, only influenza has vaccines. A different approach is needed in developing new vaccines with longer term efficacy and broader response. Current vaccines are prone to changing antigenicity and need to be administered annually. Vaccine development has been in progress for decades but faces numerous technical challenges. Respiratory viruses such as RSV, PIV and hMPV initiate incomplete immune responses and so reinfections tend to occur. The pace of progress is slow both for Both live-attenuated and subunit vaccines. It may be years before such vaccines are available in the market place. However, once available then adult immunization may offer protection to young infants as is the case with influenza vaccines [80].

### 9.1. Stem cell

Stem cells are unique in that they possess the capacity to self-renew and capable of differentiation into many cell types hence leading to the regeneration of injured organs. In lung injury, stem cells have been shown to promote endothelial and epithelial repair by engrafting into tissue and interacting with neighboring cells. Furthermore, stem cells beneficially influence the host's immune response by reducing harmful inflammatory reactions. Paracrine mediators and mitochondria-containing micro-vesicles released by stem cells appear responsible for the beneficial effects on immune responses and cellular functions [81].

### 9.2. Gene expression

Gene expression profiles of peripheral blood leukocytes can differentiate viral from bacterial infections with 95% accuracy. They can also identify unique profiles in patients with bacterial and viral respiratory tract infections. Application of gene expression profile analysis in children with CAP can significantly enhance the ability to classify patients according to the class of pathogen causing the infection and disease severity. Molecular distance to health (MDTH) is a novel metric that in a single score can provide a global assessment of the perturbation of the patient immune profile compared to healthy controls. It has been shown to accurately classify the severity of the disease in for example cases of bacterial sepsis, staphylococcal infections, as well as in children with respiratory viral infections [82].

## Author details

Al Johani Sameera* and Akhter Javed

*Address all correspondence to: johanis@ngha.med.sa

King Abdulaziz Medical City, Riyadh, Saudi Arabia

## References

[1] Prioreschi P. A history of medicine. In: vol II: Greek Medicine, chapter five, "Hippocrates". 2nd ed. NE: Horatius Press; 1996. p. 201-205

[2] Centers for Disease Control and Prevention. *Klebsiella pneuminae* in Healthcare Settings. Available at: http://www.cdc.gov/HAI/organisms/klebsiella/klebsiella.htm

[3] Austrian R. The Gram stain and the etiology of lobar pneumonia, an historical note. Bacteriological Reviews. 1960;**24**(3):261-265

[4] Rudan I, Tomaskovic L, Boschi-Pinto C, Campbell H, WHO Child Health Epidemiology Reference Group. Global estimate of the incidence of clinical pneumonia among children under five years of age. Bulletin of the World Health Organization. 2004;**356**:895-903

[5] Musher D, Anna R, Thorner AR. Community-acquired pneumonia. The New England Journal of Medicine. 2014;**371**:1619-1628

[6] File TM, Marrie TJA. Burden of community-acquired pneumonia in North American adults. Postgraduate Medicine. 2010;**122**(2):130-141

[7] Haq IJ, Battersby AC, Eastham K, McKean M. Community acquired pneumonia in children. BMJ. 2017;**356**:j686

[8] Alcón A, Fàbregas N, Torres A. Pathophysiology of pneumonia. Clinics in Chest Medicine. 2005;**26**(1):39-46

[9] Lee KH, Gordon A, Foxman B. The role of respiratory viruses in the etiology of bacterial pneumonia: An ecological perspective. Evolution, Medicine and Public Health. 2016; **2016**(1):95-109

[10] Mogensen TH. Pathogen recognition and inflammatory signaling in innate immune defenses. Clinical Microbiological Reviews. 2009;**22**(2):240-273

[11] Legg JP, Hussain IR, Warner JA, Johnston SL, Warner JO. Type 1 and type 2 cytokine imbalance in acute respiratory syncytial virus bronchiolitis. American Journal of Respiratory and Critical Care Medicine. 2003;**168**(6):633-639

[12] Wack A, Openshaw P, Ogarra A. Contribution of cytokines to pathology and protection in virus infection. Current Opinion in Virology. 2011;**1**(3):84-195

[13] Cauley LS, Vella AT. Why is coinfection with influenza virus and bacteria so difficult to control? Discovery Medicine. 2015;**19**(102):33-40

[14] Rudan I, Boschi-Pinto C, Biloglav Z, Mulholland K, Campbell H. Epidemiology and etiology of childhood pneumonia. Bulletin of the World Health Organization. 2008;**86**:408-16.3

[15] Blasi F, Aliberti S, Pappalettera M, Tarsia P. 100 years of respiratory medicine: pneumonia. Respiratory Medicine. 2007;**101**(5):875-881

[16] Farshad N, Saffar MJ, Khalilian AR, et al. Respiratory viruses in hospitalized children with acute lower respiratory tract infections, Mazandaran Province, Iran. Indian Pediatrics. 2008;**45**:590-592

[17] Ozbay B, Sertoğullarindan B, Tekin M, et al. Influenza-associated pneumonia in a Turkish area with endemic avian influenza. Respirology. 2008;**13**:444-446

[18] Saudi Arabia: Influenza and Pneumonia. LeDuc Media, USA: WHO; May 2014. http://www.worldlifeexpectancy.com/saudi-arabia-influenza-pneumonia

[19] Saeed AA, Abedi GR, Alzahrani AG, Salameh I, Abdirizak F, Alhakeem R, Algarni H, El Nil OA, Mohammed M, Assiri AM, Alabdely HM, Watson JT, Gerber SI. Surveillance and testing for Middle East respiratory syndrome coronavirus, Saudi Arabia, April 2015-February 2016. Emerging Infectious Diseases. 2017 Apr;**23**(4):682-685

[20] Shapiro M, London B, Nigri D, Shoss A, Zilber E, Fogel I. Middle East respiratory syndrome coronavirus: Review of the current situation in the world. Disaster and Military Medicine. 2016; May 4;**2**:9

[21] Middle East Respiratory Syndrome cCronavirus (MERS-CoV)—Saudi Arabia. World Health Organization; Feb 29, 2016 http://www.who.int/csr/don/29-february-2016-mers-saudi-arabia/en/

[22] Chen X, Chughtai AA, Dyda A, MacIntyre CR. Comparative epidemiology of Middle East respiratory syndrome coronavirus (MERS-CoV) in Saudi Arabia and South Korea. Emerging Microbes and Infection. 2017;**6**(6):e51

[23] Rudan I, Tomaskovic L, Boschi-Pinto C, Campbell H. Global estimate of the incidence of clinical pneumonia among children under five years of age. Bulletin of the World Health Organization. 2004;**82**:895-903

[24] Williams BG, Gouws E, Boschi-Pinto C, Bryce J, Dye C. Estimates of world-wide distribution of child deaths from acute respiratory infections. The Lancet Infectious Diseases. 2002;**2**:25-32

[25] Chang AB, Brown N, Toombs M, Marsh RL, Redding GJ. Lung disease in indigenous children. Paediatric Respiratory Reviews. 2014;**15**(4):325-332

[26] Jain S, Self WH, Wunderink RG, Fakhran S, Balk R, Bramley AM, et al. Community-acquired pneumonia requiring hospitalization among U.S. adults. The New England Journal of Medicine. 2015;**373**(5):415-427

[27] Rozenbaum MH, Marie-Josee J, Mangen MJJ, Huijts SM, Van Der Werf TS, Postma MJ. Incidence, direct costs and duration of hospitalization of patients hospitalized with community acquired pneumonia: A nationwide retrospective claims database analysis. Vaccine. 2015;**33**(28):3193-3199

[28] Trotter CL, Stuart JM, George R, Miller E. Increasing Hospital Admissions for Pneumonia, England. Emerging Infectious Diseases. 2008;**14**(5):727-733. DOI: 10.3201/eid1405.071011

[29] Waterer GW. Diagnosing viral and atypical pathogens in the setting of community-acquired pneumonia. Clinics in Chest Medicine. 2017;**38**(1):21-28

[30] Sharma L, Losier A, Tolbert T, Dela Cruz CS, Marion CR. Atypical pneumonia: Updates on Legionella, Chlamydophila, and Mycoplasma Pneumonia. Clinics in Chest Medicine. 2017; **38**(1):45-58

[31] Parrott GL, Kinjo T, Fujita J. A compendium for Mycoplasma pneumoniae. Frontiers in Microbiology. 2016;**7**:513. DOI: 10.3389/fmicb.2016.00513

[32] Cunha BA, Burillo A, Bouza E. Legionnaires' disease. Lancet. 2016;**387**(10016):376-385

[33] Smyth A. Pneumonia due to viral and atypical organisms and their sequelae: Childhood respiratory infections. British Medical Bulletin. 2002;**61**(1):247-262

[34] Walter JM, Wunderink RG. Severe Respiratory Viral Infections: New Evidence and Changing Paradigms. Infectious Disease Clinics of North America. 2017;Jul 5. pii:S0891-5520(17)30034-X. DOI: 10.1016/j.idc.2017.05.004 [Epub ahead of print]

[35] Burk M, El-Kersh K, Saad M, Wiemken T, Ramirez J, Cavallazzi RA. Viral infection in community-acquired pneumonia: A systematic review and meta-analysis. European Respiratory Review. 2016;**25**(140):178-188

[36] Falsey AR, Walsh EE. Respiratory syncytial virus infection in adults. Clinical Microbiology Reviews. 2000;**13**(3):371-384

[37] Ison MG, Hayden RT. Adenovirus. Microbiology Spectrum. 2016 Aug;**4**(4):217-232. DOI: 10.1128/microbiolspec.DMIH2-0020-2015.

[38] Lamson DM, Kajon A, Shudt M, Girouard G, St. George K. Detection and genetic characterization of adenovirus type 14 strain in students with influenza-like illness, New York, USA, 2014-2015. Emerging Infectious Diseases. 2017;**23**(7):1194-1197. DOI: 10.3201/eid2307.161730.

[39] Zahradnik JM. Adenovirus pneumonia. Seminars in Respiratory Infections. 1987;**2**(2): 104-111

[40] Dingyu Tan, Huadong Zhu, Yangyang Fu, Fei Tong, Dongqi Yao, Joseph Walline, Jun Xu, Xuezhong Yu. Severe Community-Acquired Pneumonia Caused by Human Adenovirus in Immunocompetent Adults: A Multicenter Case Series. Published: March 11, 2016. https://doi.org/10.1371/journal.pone.0151199

[41] Boeckh M, Ljungman P. How we treat cytomegalovirus in hematopoietic cell transplant recipients. Blood. 2009;**113**(23):5711-5719. DOI: 10.1182/blood-2008-10-143560

[42] Corona-Nakamura AL, Arias-Merino MJ. In: Price P, editor. Management of CMV-Associated Diseases in Immunocompromised Patients, Manifestations of Cytomegalovirus Infection. InTech; 2013. DOI: 10.5772/56141 Available from: https://www.intechopen.com/books/manifestations-of-cytomegalovirus-infection/management-of-cmv-associated-diseases-in-immunocompromised-patients

[43] Perk M, Marrie TJ. Epstein-Barr virus pneumonia. In: Marrie TJ, editor. Community-Acquired Pneumonia. Boston, MA: Springer; 2002

[44] Jain M, Duggal S, Chugh TD. Cytomegalovirus infection in non-immumosuppressed critically ill patients. Journal of Infection in Developing Countries. 2011;**5**(8):571-579

[45] C1 C, Sidoti F, Saldan A, Sinesi F, Balloco C, Simeone S, Lorusso M, Mantovani S, Merlino C, Solidoro P, Cavallo R. Clinical impact of HSV-1 detection in the lower respiratory tract from hospitalized adult patients. Clinical Microbiology and Infection. 2012;**18**(8):E305-E307

[46] Van den Hoogen BG, de Jong JC, Groen J, et al. A newly discovered human pneumovirus isolated from young children with respiratory tract disease. Nature Medicine 2001; **7**:719.

[47] Bénet T, Picot VS, Awasthi S, Pandey N, Bavdekar A, Kawade A, Robinson A, Rakoto-Andrianarivelo M, Sylla M, Diallo S, Russomando G, Basualdo W, Komurian-Pradel F, Endtz H, Vanhems P, Paranhos-Baccalà G, For The Gabriel Network. Severity of pneumonia in under 5-year-old children from developing countries: A multicenter, prospective, observational study. The American Journal of Tropical Medicine and Hygiene. 2017;**97**(1):68-76

[48] Joseph C, Togawa Y, Shindo N. Bacterial and viral infections associated with influenza. Influenza and Other Respiratory Viruses. 2013;**7**(2):105-113

[49] Mauskopf J, Klesse M, Lee S, Herrera-Taracena G. The burden of influenza complications in different high-risk groups: A targeted literature review. Journal of Medical Economics. 2013;**16**(2):264-277

[50] Moss WJ. Measles. Lancet. 2017 Jun 30. pii: S0140-6736(17)31463-0. DOI: 10.1016/S0140-6736(17)31463-0

[51] Rota PA, Moss WJ, Takeda M, de Swart RL, Thompson KM, Goodson JL. Measles. Nature Reviews Disease Primers. 2016;**2**:16049

[52] Pawełczyk M, Kowalski ML. The role of human parainfluenza virus infections in the immunopathology of the respiratory tract. Current Allergy and Asthma Reports. 2017 Mar;**17**(3):16. DOI: 10.1007/s11882-017-0685-2.A

[53] Branche AR, Falsey AR. Parainfluenza virus infection. Seminars in Respiratory and Critical Care Medicine. 2016;**37**(4):538-554

[54] Hall CB. Respiratory syncytial virus and parainfluenza virus. The New England Journal of Medicine. 2001;**344**:1917-1928

[55] Pastula ST, Hackett J, Coalson J, Jiang X, Villafana T, Ambrose C, Fryzek J. Hospitalizations for Respiratory Syncytial Virus Among Adults in the United States, 1997-2012. Open Forum Infectious Diseases. 2017 Jan 9;**4**(1):1-7. DOI: 10.1093/ofid/ofw270 eCollection 2017 Winter

[56] Drysdale SB, Mejias A, Ramilo O. Rhinovirus—Not just the common cold. The Journal of Infection. 2017;**74**(1):S41-S46

[57] Xiao Q, Zheng S, Zhou L, Ren L, Xie X, Deng Y, Tian D, Zhao Y, Fu Z, Li T, Huang A, Liu E. Impact of human rhinovirus types and viral load on the severity of illness in hospitalized children with lower respiratory tract infections. The Pediatric Infectious Disease Journal. 2015;**34**(11):1187-1192

[58] Pavia AT. What is the role of respiratory viruses in community acquired pneumonia; What is the best therapy for influenza and other viral causes of CAP? Infectious Disease Clinics of North America. 2013;**27**(1):157-175. DOI: 10.1016/j.idc.2012.11.007.

[59] Heininger U, Seward JF. Varicella. Lancet. 2006;**368**(9544):1365-1376

[60] Mirouse A, Vignon P, Piron P, Robert R, Papazian L, Géri G, Blanc P, Guitton C, Guérin C, Bigé N, Rabbat A, Lefebvre A, Razazi K, Fartoukh M, Mariotte E, Bouadma L, Ricard JD, Seguin A, Souweine B, Moreau AS, Faguer S, Mari A, Mayaux J, Schneider F, Stoclin A, Perez P, Maizel J, Lafon C, Ganster F, Argaud L, Girault C, Barbier F, Lecuyer L, Lambert J, Canet E. Severe varicella-zoster virus pneumonia: A multicenter cohort study. Critical Care. 2017;**21**(1):137. DOI: 10.1186/s13054-017-1731-.0

[61] Gao R, Cao B, Hu Y, Feng Z, Wang D. Human infection with a novel avian-origin influenza A (H7N9) virus. The New England Journal of Medicine. 2013;**368**:1888-1897

[62] Medina RA, Garcia-Sastre A. Influenza A viruses: New research developments. Nature Reviews. Microbiology. 2011;**9**:590-603

[63] Cunha BA. Swine influenza (H1N1) pneumonia: Clinical considerations. Infectious Disease Clinics of North America. 2010;**24**:203-228

[64] Mena I, Nelson MI, Quezada-Monroy F, Dutta J, Cortes-Fernández R, Lara-Puente JH, Castro-Peralta F, Cunha LF, Trovão NS, Lozano-Dubernard B, Rambaut A, Van Bakel H, García-Sastre A. Origins of the 2009 H1N1 influenza pandemic in swine in Mexico. eLife. 2016;**5**:1-21. DOI: 10.7554/eLife.16777

[65] Morens DM, Taubenberger JK, Fauci AS. Predominant role of bacterial pneumonia as a cause of death in pandemic influenza: Implications for pandemic influenza preparedness. The Journal of Infectious Diseases. 2008;**198**:962-970

[66] Johnstone J, Majdumar SR, Fox JD, Marrie TJ. Viral infections in adults hospitalized with community-acquired pneumonia: Prevalence, pathogens, and presentation. Chest. 2008;**134**:1141-1148

[67] Gadsby NJ, Russell CD, McHugh MP, Mark H, Conway Morris A, Laurenson IF, et al. Comprehensive molecular testing for respiratory pathogens in community-acquired pneumonia. Clinical Infectious Diseases. 2016;**62**(7):817-823

[68] Murdoch DR. How recent advances in molecular tests could impact the diagnosis of pneumonia. Expert Review of Molecular Diagnostics. 2016;**16**(5):533-540

[69] Berry M, Gamieldien J, Fielding BC. Identification of new respiratory viruses in the new millennium. Viruses. 2015;**7**(3):996-1019

[70] Ljungström LR, Jacobsson G, Claesson BEB, Andersson R, Enroth H. Respiratory viral infections are underdiagnosed in patients with suspected sepsis. European Journal of Clinical Microbiology & Infectious Diseases. 17-05-2017. DOI: 10.1007/s10096-017-2990-z [Epub ahead of print]

[71] Krause JC, Panning M, Hengel H, Henneke P. The role of multiplex PCR in respiratory tract infections in children. Deutsches Ärzteblatt International. 2014;**111**(38):639-645

[72] Hermann T. Small molecules targeting viral RNA. WIREs RNA. 2016. DOI: 10.1002/wrna.1373

[73] Kamali A, Holodniy M. Influenza treatment and prophylaxis with neuraminidase inhibitors: A review. Infection and Drug Resistance. 2013;**6**:187-198

[74] Watanabe SC, Chang MJ, Kim DW, Chu YO, MARVEL Study Group. Long-acting neuraminidase inhibitor laninamivir octanoate versus oseltamivir for treatment of influenza: a double-blind, randomized, noninferiority clinical trial. Clinical Infectious Diseases. 2010;**51**:1167-1175

[75] Galván JM, Rajas O, Aspa J. Review of non-bacterial infections in respiratory medicine: Viral pneumonia. Archivos de Bronconeumología. 2015;**51**(11):590-597

[76] GM1 A, Torres HA, Tarrand J, Safdar A, Bodey G, Chemaly RF. Herpes simplex virus lower respiratory tract infection in patients with solid tumors. Cancer. 2009;**115**(1):199-206. DOI: 10.1002/cncr.24011

[77] Wold WSM, Toth K. New drug on the horizon for treating adenovirus. Expert Opinion on Pharmacotherapy. 2015;**16**(14):2095-2099

[78] Smee DF, Evans WJ, Nicolaou KC, Tarbet EB, Day CW. Susceptibilities of enterovirus D68, enterovirus 71, and rhinovirus 87 strains to various antiviral compounds. Antiviral Research. 2016;**131**:61-65

[79] Assaad U, El-Masri I, Porhomayon J, El-Solh AA. Pneumonia immunization in older adults: Review of vaccine effectiveness and strategies. Clinical Interventions in Aging. 2012;**7**:453-461. DOI: 10.2147/CIA.S29675

[80] Rey-Jurado E, Kalergis AM. Immunological features of respiratory syncytial virus-caused pneumonia—Implications for vaccine design. International Journal of Molecular Sciences. 2017;**18**(3):556. DOI: 10.3390/ijms18030556.

[81] Hogan BLM, Barkauskas CE, Chapman HA, Epstein JA, Jain R, Hsia CCW, Niklason L, Calle E, Le A, Randell SH, Rock J, Snitow M, Krummel M, Stripp BR, Vu T, White ES, Whitsett JA, Morrisey EE. Repair and regeneration of the respiratory system: Complexity, plasticity, and mechanisms of lung stem cell function. Cell Stem Cell. 2014;**15**(2):123-138

[82] Xu X, Yuan B, Liang Q, et al. Gene expression profile analysis of ventilator-associated pneumonia. Molecular Medicine Reports. 2015;**12**(5):7455-7462. DOI: 10.3892/mmr.2015.4389